NUTRITIONAL ASPECTS OF HUMAN PHYSICAL AND ATHLETIC PERFORMANCE

Nutritional Aspects of Human Physical and Athletic Performance

By

MELVIN H. WILLIAMS, Ph.D., F.A.C.S.M.

Director, Human Performance Laboratory
Old Dominion University, Norfolk, Virginia

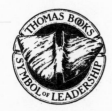
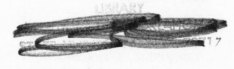

CHARLES C THOMAS • PUBLISHER
Springfield • Illinois • U.S.A.

Published and Distributed Throughout the World by
CHARLES C THOMAS ● PUBLISHER
Bannerstone House
301-327 East Lawrence Avenue, Springfield, Illinois, U.S.A.

© *1976, by* CHARLES C THOMAS ● PUBLISHER

ISBN 0-398-03548-2

Library of Congress Catalog Card Number: 75-44115

Printed in the United States of America
R-1

Library of Congress Cataloging in Publication Data

Williams, Melvin H
   Nutritional aspects of human physical and
athletic performance.

   Bibliography: p.
   Includes Indexes.
   1. Athletes--Nutrition. 2. Nutrition.
I. Title. [DNLM: 1. Sport medicine. 2. Nu-
trition. 3. Exertion. 4. Energy metabolism.
QU145 W725n]
QP141.W515   613.7'1   75-44115
ISBN 0-398-03548-2

Dedicated with Love to Five Beautiful Young Girls

Serena Michele Williams
Shirley Anne Barnard
Barbara Suzanne Barnard
Nancy Leigh Barnard
Doreen Frances Barnard

PREFACE

THROUGHOUT the years, athletes have constantly been searching for a diet or dietary ingredient which would increase their physical performance capacity. Since the various nutrients in foods provide energy and regulate various physiological processes associated with exercise, there is some theoretical basis linking dietary modification to improvement in athletic performance. Thus, nutritionists, biochemists, exercise physiologists and others involved in sports medicine have investigated the influence of selected nutrients as they may affect the physical performance parameters related to athletic ability.

Many of these experimental studies have been published, and hence, some notable reviews of the literature relative to nutrition and athletic performance have been presented previously. There are several books in the foreign literature dealing directly and totally with the topic of nutrition for the athlete; however, no English translations were uncovered. There are also many books which contain a chapter or two on nutrition for the athlete; however, they are usually limited in scope due to space restrictions, as are reviews in leading periodicals in the area of sports medicine. Thus, it was deemed important to compile, in one volume, materials in the area of nutrition and physical performance which may be of interest to athletes, physical educators, coaches, trainers and other allied personnel in sports medicine.

As the reader is probably aware, the literature relative to nutritional effects upon health is voluminous. Needless to say, any dietary deficiency that adversely affects the health of the individual is likely to impair his or her physical performance capacity. Most athletes in industrialized countries, however, are on a balanced diet, and if they utilize nutritional substances as ergogenic aids, they take them in excess of recommended daily dietary allowances. Thus, when studying the role of a particular nutrient and its effect upon physical performance, both deficiency effects and supplementation effects may be important considerations. Although the effects of certain deficiency states are discussed throughout this monograph, the main thrust centers around dietary modifications in the athlete who is adequately nourished.

As an overview, the first chapter discusses the historical aspects of nutrition and athletic performance, leading into the nutritional faddism current in athletics today. The second chapter concerns energy and metabolic concepts, while the next six chapters elaborate upon the role of the major nutrients, i.e. carbohydrate, fat, protein, vitamins, minerals and water, in the diet of athletes. Chapter Nine represents a review of the literature relative to the efficacy of certain purported ergogenic foods. Chapter Ten discusses the concepts underlying weight control, and the last chapter deals with the practical aspects of feeding the athlete.

This monograph is not intended to be a nutrition book per se. It is not designed to review the literature relative to the effects of nutrition upon disease processes, intellectual performance, animal performance, or other such parameters. It is primarily concerned with the effects of nutrition on human physical performance related to athletic abilities.

Within this context, the intent of this monograph is to incorporate, as much as possible, the literature that is critical to the effect of nutrition on human physical performance, i.e. those investigations which have directly studied the problem. However, allied literature is utilized when necessary to explain underlying mechanisms.

I would like to thank the staff of the National Library of Medicine and the Old Dominion University Library for their assistance during the literature search. Special thanks are due also to Guenther Dietz for his help in translating numerous foreign reports, and to Miss Betty Williams and Miss Janis McDonald for their expertise in typing the final manuscript.

M.H.W.

CONTENTS

                                                              Page

Preface v

Chapter

One. INTRODUCTION 3
  Historical Aspects 7
  Diets of Athletes................................. 10
  Nutritional Faddism and Athletics 13
  Reasons for Quackery in Sports 15
  Research and Educational Needs 20
Two. ENERGY AND METABOLIC CONCEPTS 24
  Measures of Energy 27
  Energy Expenditure 30
  Basal Metabolic Rate 30
  Energy Sources During Physical Activity........... 32
  Energy Expenditure During Physical Activity 35
Three. THE ROLE OF CARBOHYDRATES IN PHYSICAL ACTIVITY .. 43
  Carbohydrates — Types, Source, Digestion 43
  Storage and Metabolism of Carbohydrates........... 45
  Blood Glucose, Hypoglycemia and Physical
   Performance 48
  Carbohydrate Intake Prior to Performance 50
  Carbohydrate Intake and Blood Glucose
   Utilization During Exercise.................... 51
  Practical Application of Oral Glucose Ingestion ... 57
  Glycogen Storage Techniques 58
  Liver Glycogen................................ 60
  Selective Depletion of Muscle Glycogen........... 61
  Time Phases for Depletion and Repletion

Chapter   *Page*

　　　　of Muscle Glycogen............................ 62

　　　　Diet Modification to Increase Muscle
　　　　　　Glycogen Levels.............................. 63

　　　　Fuel for Energy During Exercise: Carbohydrates
　　　　　　and Fat...................................... 69

Four. THE ROLE OF FAT IN PHYSICAL ACTIVITY 76

　　Source, Type and Digestion 76

　　Storage and Metabolism.......................... 78

　　　　Fat as an Energy Source During Exercise 82

　　Dietary Fat, Exercise and Coronary Heart Disease 83

　　　　Role of Diet in Coronary Heart Disease........... 85

　　　　Dietary Modifications to Reduce Blood Lipids..... 88

　　　　Exercise Effects Upon Blood Lipids 91

Five. THE ROLE OF PROTEIN IN PHYSICAL ACTIVITY 96

　　Source, Type and Digestion 97

　　Storage and Metabolism.......................... 100

　　Athletic Training and Protein Needs 102

Six. THE ROLE OF VITAMINS IN PHYSICAL ACTIVITY 113

　　Use of Vitamins by Athletes 115

　　Vitamin A (Retinol) 118

　　The B Vitamins 119

　　　　Vitamin B$_1$ (Thiamine) 120

　　　　Vitamin B$_2$ (Riboflavin) 124

　　　　Vitamin B$_3$ (Niacin) 124

　　　　Vitamin B$_6$ (Pyridoxine) 127

　　　　Vitamin B$_{12}$ (Cyanocobalamin) 128

　　　　Pantothenic Acid 129

　　　　Folic Acid (Folacin) 130

　　　　Other B Complex Vitamins or Factors 130

　　　　Vitamin B Complex Supplementation 131

　　　　B Complex and Other Vitamins.................. 134

　　Vitamin C (Ascorbic Acid)........................ 136

　　Vitamin D 145

　　Vitamin E 147

　　Summary 152

Seven. THE ROLE OF MINERALS IN PHYSICAL ACTIVITY 153

　　Calcium, Phosphorus, Magnesium and the Trace

Chapter	Page
Elements	154
Sodium, Potassium and Chloride	156
Iron	159
Iron Requirements and Metabolism	160
Anemia and Physical Performance	161
Iron Supplementation for Athletes	165
Eight. THE ROLE OF WATER AND MAJOR ELECTROLYTES IN PHYSICAL ACTIVITY	169
Functions of Water in the Body	170
Temperature Regulation in Man	173
Dehydration and Physical Performance	177
Effect of Dehydration on Strength	178
Effect of Dehydration Upon Submaximal Work Performance	179
Effect of Dehydration Upon Maximal Work Performance	180
Rehydration and Hyperhydration	181
Electrolyte Replacement	186
Salt Tablets	187
Potassium Depletion	190
Electrolyte Solutions	192
Ergogenic Aspects of Glucose-Electrolyte Solutions	195
Heat Illnesses	199
Prevention of Heat Illness	202
Nine. ERGOGENIC FOODS	208
Glucose and Dextrose	209
Honey	210
Gelatin	212
Lecithin	215
Phosphates	216
Multiple Supplements	217
Wheat Germ Oil	218
Alkaline Salts	225
Aspartates	229
Alcohol	232
Caffeine	239

Chapter   *Page*
   Ten. WEIGHT CONTROL AND PHYSICAL ACTIVITY 244
         The Calorie Concept in Weight Control Programs ... 245
         Body Composition................................. 247
         Weight Gaining 251
         Obesity 254
            Disadvantages of Obesity 255
            Etiology of Obesity 257
            Prevention and Treatment of Obesity 259
         Weight Loss for Sports Competition................ 272
            Starvation Techniques 274
            Theoretical Health Hazards of Making Weight 278
Eleven. FEEDING THE ATHLETE 282
         Basic Nutrition.................................. 284
            Essential Nutrients and the Recommended
              Daily Allowances (RDA) 284
            Adequate Diet Based Upon the Basic Four Food
              Groups 288
            Daily Food Intake 292
            Low Calorie Diets 295
         Special Considerations for the Athlete 297
            Energy Requirement 297
            Endurance Athletes 299
            The Female Athlete............................. 300
            Vegetarian Athletes 301
            Pregame Meals 303
            Breakfast and Physical Performance 311
            Myths, Misconceptions and Education 313

         Bibliography 315
         Appendices 351
         Glossary.. 413
         Author Index 423
         Subject Index 431

NUTRITIONAL ASPECTS OF HUMAN PHYSICAL AND ATHLETIC PERFORMANCE

CHAPTER **ONE** ⸺

INTRODUCTION

ATHLETES IN TRAINING for competition are always searching for the ultimate ingredient which may give them that extra winning edge over their opponents. Thus, over the years a number of theoretical ergogenic, or work producing, aids have been utilized in attempts to increase athlete performance capability. Due to the diverse nature of these substances or treatments, there are varied hypotheses which account for the beneficial effects they are alleged to produce. The rationale for their use may be reduced to two categories: (a) the substances may directly influence the physiological capacity of a particular body system which contributes to success in the athletic performance, or (b) the substance may remove psychological restraints which may limit physiological capacity. Excellent coverage of the theory and research relative to a number of ergogenic aids may be found in a book edited by Morgan (1972).

There are four different classifications of ergogenic aids, grouped according to the general nature of their application. The mechanical ergogenic aids, such as heat, cold, ultraviolet rays and massage, are used primarily for their theoretical beneficial effects on local or general circulation. Thus, application of heat to the legs may serve as a passive form of warm-up, and has been theorized to increase performance due to increased speed of contraction and relaxation of the muscles, and greater efficiency due to decreased muscular viscosity. A second categorization, the psychological ergogenic aids, is best represented by hypnosis. With the proper application of hypnotic or posthypnotic suggestion, it has been suggested that the athlete may remove certain psychic limitations and possibly perform at a higher level. The pharmacological aids, characterized primarily by the amphetamines and anabolic steroids although a number of diverse pharmaceutical agents have been used, have become increasingly more prominent in the athletic scene during the past decade and have prompted

3

athletic governing bodies such as the International Olympic Committee (IOC), International Amateur Athletic Federation (IAAF), National Collegiate Athletic Association (NCAA) and others to proscribe their use in conjunction with athletic events. The term doping has been applied to the use of drugs to increase athletic performance, and a number of theories have been advanced relative to their mode of action, dependent, of course, upon the nature of the drug and the type of athletic performance. The fourth general classification, the nutritional ergogenic aids, is replete with foods, vitamins, minerals or dietary regimens which are hypothesized to increase performance, either by renewing energy stores in the body, facilitating the biochemical reactions that yield the energy, modifying the biochemical changes contributing to fatigue, or maintaining optimal body weight. Thus, glycogen storage techniques, vitamin supplementation, ingestion of alkaline salts, and protein supplementation may be nutritional techniques which are associated, respectively, with the four physiological rationale advanced in the preceding sentence.

Although the theoretical rationale exists for the beneficial application of numerous substances within these four categories of ergogenic aids to athletics, the experimental literature is generally controversial relative to their effectiveness in increasing performance. For example, in some well-designed studies, application of cold packs, passive warm-up, hypnosis, amphetamines, anabolic steroids and vitamin supplementation have all been shown to facilitate physical performance of one type or another; on the other hand, equally well-designed studies have evidenced no significant effect of the same substances. Controlled research is necessary to document the efficacy of the varied substances or treatments within each category.

Although it is important for coaches, trainers and others associated with the conduct of athletics to understand the theoretical basis and experimental evidence relative to the usefulness of ergogenic aids within each of the four general categories, special consideration should be directed towards the pharmacological and nutritive agents. It is incumbent upon athletic personnel to comprehend the legal, ethical and medical aspects of doping, as the utilization of drugs to increase performance has been judged to be unethical and consequently banned, and has also been implicated as causing the death of a number of athletes over the years. In the nutritional area, the international authority J. V. Durnin (1967) has stated that there is still no sphere of nutrition in which faddism and ignorance are more obvious than in athletics. Many athletes still believe there is a special diet or special nutritional ingredient essential to their success. To cite a few examples, Dave Meggysey, although talking about drug abuse in athletics, noted that in professional football many players receive shots of vitamin B_{12}. As Meggysey noted, "One of the ballplayers . . . had some experience with shooting cows and he would regularly give the shots to the players." (United States Senate, 1973). Harold Connolly, an Olympic Champion, noted that when he began his athletic career, athletes consumed a number of compounds such as vitamin B, protein supplements and wheat germ oil, rather than amphetamines and anabolic steroids. Phil Shinnick, another Olympic contender, stated that prior to the 1964 Olympics in Tokyo, a certain individual was disbursing free vitamins, minerals, protein tablets and similar items to the American athletes. Dr. John Boyer, in a report to a Senate subcommittee investigating the use of drugs in sports, reported that inorganic phosphates, massive amounts of vitamin C, and other compounds are often passed out by coaches and trainers without the knowledge of the chemistry and pharmacology of these substances (United States Senate, 1973).

In a general context, there appears to be a fundamental relationship between pharmacological and nutritional ergogenic aids. Both are usually ingested or injected in one form or another in order to enhance physical performance. Indeed, as early as 1939 Boje (1939) contended that apart from actual drugs such as Benzedrine®, cocaine and others, agents used for doping purposes also include dietetic preparations such as glucose, vitamins, and nontoxic salts such as the phosphates. However, there appears to be an essential difference between the two general classes, at least as related to the present discussion about athletics. The IOC specifies that pharmacological agents are prohibited in conjunction with athletic performance, whereas nutritional agents are not.

There are some gray areas in distinguishing between the use of certain substances as either drugs or nutrients. For example, both alcohol and caffeine are classified as drugs, but they are essential ingredients of many commonly consumed beverages. Alcohol is found in varying quantities in wine and beer, while caffeine is also present in coffee, tea and certain cola drinks. In the 1968 Olympic Games, the utilization of alcohol and caffeine was grounds for disqualification. However, they were removed from the proscribed drug list of the IOC prior to the 1972 games in Munich, mainly because beverages with alcohol and caffeine may be a part of the normal dietary habits of athletes. Moreover, vitamins are considered to be nutrients, but if they are prescribed by a physician, they may legally be considered a drug. However, in most cases there appears to be a clear distinction between a drug and a nutrient.

An analysis of drug use in athletics has been presented previously (Williams, 1974). In the area of nutrition and physical performance, the most prominent book in English is *Nutrition and Physical Fitness* (Bogart, and others, 1973). Overall it is an excellent book on nutrition in general as it relates nutritional knowledge to physical health. There is a small chapter concerning nutrition and physical work performance, and although the coverage is not detailed, the main points are stressed. A good bibliography of reviews of various aspects of nutrition and health has recently been developed by Rechcigl (1973). A number of excellent books published in German, Polish, French, Italian, and Russian are available, but very few have been translated into English. Some excellent foreign books include those authored by:

Creff (1964)
Creff and Berard (1966)
Bideau and Pagliuchi (1955)
Debigne (1970)
Grafe (1964)
Jannot (1968)
LaCava (1963)
Lodispoto (1968)
Nocker and Glatzel (1963)
Sidorowicz and Zawistowska (1962)

Yakovlev (1967)

A French periodical, *Sport Jeunesse et Alimentation*, is an official publication of a sport institute in France devoted specifically to athletic nutrition. In the United States, a number of excellent reviews of nutrition and athletic performance have appeared in leading periodicals and as chapters in major textbooks; however, the space limitations imposed by these methods of presenting the broad topic of nutrition and physical performance generally restrict the authors' scope. With these thoughts in mind, it was deemed worthwhile to consolidate and update, in one volume, a wide variety of information relative to the nutritional aspects of human physical performance.

HISTORICAL ASPECTS

In *A History of Nutrition,* McCollum (1957) noted that primitive man endowed objects of nature, both animate and inanimate, with various characteristics such as courage, power, weakness and fear. These characteristics were also attributed to animals and the foods they generated. Eating the heart or meat of various animals which were strong or aggressive would confer courage or strength, whereas those organs or meats of more timid animals would convey those characteristics. These thoughts persist to a limited degree even today, as Moore (1957) indicated that foods such as meat are considered masculine while vegetables are associated with femininity. She noted that steaks are the most masculine food in our society, raw steaks being the extreme. The strength and power of animals is also used to promote certain products. Consider the animal names given to automobiles, i.e. Cougar, Mustang, Barracuda, Impala, Skyhawk, etc. It is highly unlikely that GM or Ford will label one of their products Chicken. Thus, psychological factors which may have influenced the diet of athletes in preChristian times may still be operational with modern day athletes. Whereas powdered lions teeth may have been the popular ergogenic aid in ancient Rome, rare meat may serve the same psychological purpose in the 1970's. Indeed, from the time a child can comprehend words, he is admonished to eat, for it will make him big and strong.

The history of nutritional modification for increased physical performance is filled with tales indicating the success of a particular dietary program. One of the earliest recordings of nutritional advice was by Daniel, who requested his soldiers in training with Nebuchadnezzar not to eat the king's delicacies, but rather subsist on vegetables and water. The apparent result was a better appearance than those youths who did partake of the delicacies.

Probably the oldest application of nutrition to athletic performance was in the early Greek civilization. Harris (1966) cited the early relationship of the medical profession to athletics, noting that the emphasis which Greek doctors placed on the diet of the average citizen was probably an outgrowth of their interest in the diet of athletes. Tatkon (1968) noted that training for the Olympic games inspired the first preplanned system of dietetics, and the concept of a certain dietary regimen to maintain good health was soon prescribed by Greek physicians for nonathletes. However, Gardiner (1930), in talking about athletes in the early Grecian times, noted that they were not particular about their food, living primarily on porridge, unleavened bread and available meat. Thompson (1971) noted that the normal diet of the Greek athletes during these early centuries was composed of barley bread and unleavened wheat bread, vegetables, cheese, figs and a limited amount of meat.

According to Harris (1966) the earliest Greek athlete who supposedly trained on a special diet was Charmis of Sparta, who reportedly trained on dried figs as a major staple in his daily food intake. However, most reports of this time period center upon the emergence of the meat diet. As the rise of professionalism occurred in Grecian athletics, athletes began to specialize in particular events rather than be generalists. Although the diet of the old athletes was similar to that of the average Greek citizen, a change occurred shortly after the Persian wars when a meat diet was introduced. Dromeus of Stymphalus, a distance runner around 480 B.C., was reported by Pausanias in the second century A.D. to be the first athlete to train on meat. Harris (1966) feels it is more likely that Eurymenes of Samos, a heavyweight around 580 B.C., was probably the first to utilize meat as a training diet. However, even earlier in time is the story of Milo of Croton, an outstanding

Greek athlete who was a wrestling champion at seven successive Olympiads. His daily diet was supposedly twenty pounds of bread, twenty pounds of meat and eighteen pints of wine (a type of high carbohydrate, high protein drinking man's diet). Legend has it that he carried a four-year-old bull around an athletic stadium, killed it with a single blow, and ate it in one day. According to Pliny (Unsigned 1948), the athletes of this era were given much meat and little water, a practice observed down to the present century. However, the diets of athletes were not without criticism, as the philosopher and playwright Euripedes noted that the athlete was a slave to his jaw and belly.

There exists a general lack of information relative to nutrition and athletic performance throughout the dark and middle ages. In the late eighteenth and during the nineteenth centuries, several dietary practices were noted among athletes. Writing at the end of the eighteenth century, Sir John Sinclair recorded that the common practice for the athlete was to take an emetic, followed by purgatives, and then eat meat and drink a little fluid (Unsigned, 1948). Van Itallie and others (1956), citing Drummond and Wilbraham, noted that the Oxford crew in the sixties trained on a diet of underdone beef or mutton, bread, tea and beer, with a little jelly or water cress as a treat at the evening meal. Instructions were given that no vegetables were to be eaten. Cambridge, on the other hand, suffered no restrictions regarding potatoes, greens or even fruit. From 1861 to 1869 there was an unbroken succession of Oxford victories, the inference being that their diet played a role in the victory string. In the nineteenth century the myth of meat superiority was again revived, as Liebig incorrectly indicated that during exercise the muscle substance was used up.

Up until this period of time little scientific experimental evidence, at least as compared to modern research techniques, was utilized to justify these nutritional practices with athletes. Nutrition is a relatively young science, and Mayer (1968) classified the history of nutritional science into four eras: (1) the prescientific period up to the year 1750, when Lavoisier introduced heat measuring concepts; (2) the nineteenth century with investigations into caloric and nitrogen balance; (3) the period between 1900 and 1940, involving the study of trace elements, vitamins and amino acids; and (4) post-1945 involving the relation of nutrition to disease.

Thus, from the beginning of the twentieth century, scientists have been able to more effectively discern the general physiological roles of many of the essential nutrients, and a tremendous increase in nutritional knowledge occurred. A large percentage of research, dealing with optimal nutrition for men engaged in hard physical labor, was generated by World War II. Much of the literature during the 1938-46 time period involves the implications of nutritive aspects as they relate to military situations, namely the interaction of prolonged hard physical activity with caloric and water restriction. During this time frame, a number of studies also were conducted relative to the effects of variant nutrient supplementation upon different feats of athletic performance. Vitamin supplementation, alkaline salts, gelatin and other nutritive substances were studied, with the general intent of finding a useful ergogenic aid or disproving the alleged usefulness of such compounds. This general type of research was continued following World War II, and topics studied within recent years include iron supplementation, vitamin B complex, vitamin E, wheat germ oil, electrolyte solutions, glycogen storage techniques and other nutritional practices designed to maximize athletic potential. The efficacy of these nutritional practices, at least as determined by the available experimental evidence, is discussed in the following chapters.

DIETS OF ATHLETES

A quasi-logical approach to the determination of the optimal diet for athletes would be to study the diet of highly successful athletes. Consequently, a number of studies have been undertaken to ascertain the caloric intake and nutrient composition of Olympic athletes. Examination of the diets of American collegiate athletes have also been reported.

In one of the earlier studies, Cureton (1969b) indicated that the Japanese Olympic swimming team of 1932 could partly attribute their victory over the Americans to careful medical regulation of the diet, which consisted of B_1 supplementation, baked and raw fish, shell fish, bamboo shoots, moochi beans, kali and rice. No milk, cream, butter or foods fried in animal grease were included in the diet. The Japanese also ate citrus fruits in abundance. Cureton noted that replication of this diet was effective in improving the swimming performance of a Springfield College team. Bohm (1938) after questioning many athletes, coaches and trainers following the 1936 Berlin Olympics, noted a wide variety of diets in use by athletes from various nations. However, he concluded that the common tendency was to eat a balanced diet. However, Schenk (1936), studying a total of 4700 competitors from forty-two nations in the 1936 Olympics, noted that the average consumption was 7300 cal/day. He reported an average consumption of 320 g protein, 270 g fat and 800 g carbohydrate. However, Abrahams (1948) indicated that in his experience with Olympians, although the caloric intake was dependent upon the event, the average daily intake was approximately 3600 calories, about one-half the value reported by Schenk. Berry and his colleagues (1949) also studied the diets of the Olympic athletes in London during the 1948 games and reported a mean daily caloric intake of 3350 cal, with a range of 2113-4739 cal. The mean protein consumption was 139 g/day, due largely to huge intakes of meat, milk and eggs. Fat intake was 137 g/day and carbohydrate was 390 g/day. The apparent differences between the report by Schenk and those of Abrahams and Berry is probably due to the nature of analyzing food intake. Schenk did not actually measure food eaten, while the other investigations were meticulous in determining actual food intake. Berry and his associates reported no consistent differences in diets between the types of athletes. They did note that in those athletes studied, the majority stressed the value of milk, meat and eggs, while several regarded sugar as an aid. Some athletes also took vitamin supplements.

Jokl (1964) studied the dietary intake of athletes participating in the Helsinki Olympics in 1952. He reported a caloric intake of 4500 cal/day, composed of 40 percent carbohydrate, 21 percent protein and 39 percent fat. He noted the comparison of this value to the average American diet of 3000 cal/day and the Keys' ideal diet of 2300 cal/day. The caloric values reported in Jokl's study are similar to those found by Mays and Scoular (1961) in an evaluation of American college athletes. They studied the diet of sixty athletes throughout the preseason prior to competition, during the competitive season, and throughout the postseason period. The total caloric means were similar for the three different time periods, averaging respectively 4400, 4400 and 4535 calories. The general composition of the meals was 13 to 16 percent protein, 42 to 46 percent fat and 38 to 44 percent carbohydrate. The authors noted these rather high caloric diets contributed minerals and vitamins in excess of the adjusted Recommended Dietary Allowances (RDA), with the possible exception of thiamine and ascorbic acid.

At the 1968 Olympic games in Mexico City, Steel (1970) studied the diets and nutritional practices of the Australian team consisting of sixty-six male and fourteen female athletes. He noted that the nutrient intake varied tremendously, some taking less than the RDA for average Australians. Although the average percentage of protein in the diet was only approximately 15 percent of the total caloric intake, Steel noted that the belief still persists that the consumption of large quantities of meat is necessary for athletes participating in competition requiring strength and stamina. Sixty-two of the eighty athletes received no dietary advice whatsoever from coaches or trainers. However, twenty-five of these athletes ingested vitamin or mineral supplements, one took phosphate compounds, and two were utilizing lecithin, all probably in the hope of improving performance.

There still exists a wide variety of nutritional practices among world class athletes. According to Bogart and her associates (1973), some dietary modifications are based upon sound scientific knowledge, and diets based on the principle of improving the fuel for muscular work have been developed and enthusiastically adopted in Europe. However, they note that it is difficult to ascertain whether or not this technique, often called glycogen storage, has any significant effect upon the outcome of athletic competition. It has also been documented that international class athletes are still utilizing various food supplements. A world record holder in the 440 yard run reportedly uses a multivitamin/mineral supplement and protein supplementation daily (Unsigned, 1973), while some Olympic athletes still favor wheat germ oil and other such theoretical aids (Darden, 1974).

This brief historical review does not purport to have covered all the studies evaluating food consumption practices by athletes, but it is representative of the major surveys conducted and provides some data relative to caloric consumption, general diet composition, and other nutritional practices of international class athletes. As the informed reader notes, however, the review offers no insight into the optimal diet, if any such diet exists, for maximal physical performance.

NUTRITIONAL FADDISM AND ATHLETICS

If the reader has been a casual observer of major nutritional news over the past decade or so, he has seen nationwide publicity directed toward such topics as the possible dangers of cyclamates, coffee, monosodium glutamate, saturated fats, refined sugar and cholesterol, the nutrient wasteland of most dry cereals, the controversy over vitamins, the organic food cult and a host of other food related issues. Since eating subserves one of man's primary physiological drives, it should be a basic assumption that the individual will be deeply interested in the composition and quality of his diet. However, such is not the case, and the task of determining what is an adequate diet is left to the nutritional scientist, who attempts to have his research findings implemented through appropriate governmental agencies. Thus, in general, the public is fairly well assured that the composition of foods purchased in the local supermarket is free of ingredients which may be hazardous to their health.

Although hunger is an innate physiological drive, appetite is responsive to environmental factors or the general culture within which the individual develops. Thus, dog meat and octopus may be delicacies to some but are not generally appealing to the American palate. Even in the United States there are diverse regional preferences for specific foods, e.g. grits are popular in the South. A recent article also noted that the general color and texture of hot dogs are tailored to specific tastes of a given region in the United States. Thus, physiological needs and psychological preferences usually determine the appetite of a given individual, and Campbell and his associates (1971) have noted that it is difficult to dichotomize the physiological from the nonphysiological factors that influence human eating behavior. Since eating is a major part of life and is controlled partly by psychological processes, and because of the percentage of the family budget that is directed towards food purchases, it is no wonder that there is a high prevalance of food cultism and nutritional quackery. Blix (1970) noted that nutritional quackery and food cultism, in general, are major problems in industrialized as well as emerging countries.

Although the purpose of this book is not to discuss food faddism in general, there is a high degree of commonality between food cultism in the general public, for example, the organic food movement, and food cultism in athletics. Olson (1958) indicated that the problem exists because food has emotional rather than intellectual value to the average person; thus, food faddists appeal to the emotional drives of the average individual. George P. Larrick, a former United States Commissioner of the Food and Drug Administration, noted that the most widespread and expensive type of quackery in the United States was the promotion of vitamin products, special dietary foods and food supplements. It is a known fact that there is a great deal of quackery in the food industry, for the average consumer is not getting the most nutritious value for his money, as the current high cost and trend towards convenience foods dilutes his food purchasing power. However, with current labeling practices on food containers, the individual with a good background in nutrition should be able to ascertain the nutritional quality of the product he purchases. For the interested reader, an excellent book on the food industry, and how you can get more for your money, is *The Great American Food Hoax* by Sidney Margolius (1971). As Engel (1959) has noted, the food faddists are not likely to be legislated out of existence; thus, the more appropriate approach is to disseminate the truth through vigorous youth and adult education programs. Jalso and others (1965) advocated a supplementation of the direct educational approach with a mass media program (newspapers, magazines, television) designed to present valid nutritional information to the public. As will be noted below, similar approaches should be applied to nutritional quackery in sports.

There exists a variety of reasons why nutritional quackery in sports should be attacked by those individuals responsible for the education of the athlete. First, from a health standpoint, certain complications may arise from the indiscriminate consumption of various nutrients. In one report (United States Senate, 1973), a team doctor for the United States Olympic team in 1968 noticed some athletes consuming as many as 10,000 mg vitamin C in one day. Some Olympic athletes have experienced tremendous allergic reactions to vitamins, as noted by Phil Shinnick, an Olympic contestant in Tokyo in 1964. In the same report, Dr. John Boyer indicated that the combination of large amounts of vitamin D, plus prolonged exposure to ultraviolet light, increases the hazard of vitamin D intoxication. The liberal consumption of salt tablets by athletes exercising in hot environments may predispose them to gastrointestinal disturbances and possible electrolyte imbalance in the body fluids. In addition, the development of a belief that a particular nutritional substance may help improve performance may lead the athlete to experiment with stronger agents, such as drugs, at a later time. Secondly, the athlete may rely on one particular compound to the exclusion of others necessary for a balanced diet, and consequently may suffer nutritionally. Thirdly, on an intellectual basis, the particular ingredient the athlete is consuming may have no scientific basis for increasing his performance capacity. In addition, the athlete may credit part of his success if he does win, to an extraneous substance, thus depriving his ego of the fact that his success was due to the natural development of his innate resources. Finally, the nutritional ergogenic aids may impose a financial burden on the athlete, as some of the compounds are relatively expensive.

REASONS FOR QUACKERY IN SPORTS

As indicated previously by Durnin (1967), there is still no area of nutrition where faddism, misconceptions and ignorance are more obvious than in athletics. Why? Durnin himself has noted that there are no ordinary foods which man eats which are of any special value or, for that matter, contraindicated in athletic training. He has also emphasized the point that the nutritional requirements for the athlete in training depend upon the same fundamental principles which govern human beings in general. Durnin's viewpoint is buttressed by a number of other nutritionists, exercise physiologists and others involved in sports medicine. Ernst Simonson (1951), an international expert in work physiology, concluded that in general, no type of diet supplementation will improve any type of performance in a normal person on a normal diet. J. Williams (1962), the renowned British authority in sports medicine, stated that no specific diet will change a moderately endowed athlete into a champion, but a sound dietary regimen is necessary to produce maximal fitness. Roger Banister (1974), a prominent physician and the first human to break the four-minute mile, indicated that there is no proof that special foods or extra vitamin supplements are necessary as long as athletes eat a well-balanced diet. The National Research Council (1974) noted that even though athletic activity increased energy expenditure, the increased needs for any essential nutrients should be met by the larger quantities of foods consumed, provided they are well-selected. Jean Mayer (1972b), an international authority on nutrition and exercise, and a host of other investigators, have supported the general concept of these statements.

The general consensus of these authorities is that the athlete, aside from possible increases in caloric intake due to increased energy expenditure, does not need additional nutrients beyond those found in a balanced diet. To amplify this point, Sheehan (1972), talking about nutrition and success in athletics, noted that a prominent swimming coach prescribed the following dietary regimen for his athletes:

- Breakfast of Champions — Long workouts for stamina
- Lunch of Champions — Gruelling sessions for strength
- Supper of Champions — Exhausting practice for speed

Even though these eminent authorities contend that diet manipulation will not enhance athletic performance, some coaches, trainers and athletes continue to search for the super diet. There are various reasons for their pursuit, ranging from collective food faddism to rather reputable research. The plight of the coach and athlete is to separate fact from fancy, to discern what is quackery and what may possibly be a useful dietary technique to apply to their sport. The sports world is replete with nutritional faddism and misinformation which appears to be propagated by coaches, athletes themselves and some forms of media, thus enticing the gullible athlete to reach for that ultimate ingredient. This is not to say that there are not any important dietary concerns for the athlete beyond the normal diet, for there may be some useful application of selected nutritional techniques to some athletic activities. Nevertheless, nutritional quackery does exist in athletics, and the following paragraphs will attempt to delineate the major reasons why.

Olson (1958) has described the phenomenon of collective food faddism, whereby the general public may pattern their food habits after a particular individual. This phenomenon is readily apparent in the sporting world, whereby dietary practices of successful athletes or teams become the *sine qua non* of the aspiring athlete. If a freshman wrestler observes the senior star consume tea laced with honey an hour before his match, there is a strong possibility he will do the same. Hanley (1968) reported the story of the New York Giants who ate meatball sandwiches prior to one of their games and did so well that it became the popular food for the pregame meal. Some current professional athletes are devoted to organic foods or are vegetarians, and it is assumed that young athletes who emulate these stars may experiment with their diets. Thus, the phenomenon of collective food faddism may be one of the main reasons for unscientific nutritional behavior in sports.

Another reason for food faddism in sports may be due to the directives of those individuals administering the program. Mayer and Bullen (1960a) reported that through perusal of the daily newspaper, inquiries into university athletic training table practices and study of the diets of professional and Olympic athletes lend testimony to the fact that a number of team physicians, coaches and trainers are convinced that there are some very special nutritional factors involved in the preparation of athletes. Krause and Hunscher (1972) indicated that coaches have contributed to the belief that certain foods will enable the athlete to do more and better work, win more medals or gain greater victories. To document this point, Phil Shinnick (United States Senate, 1973), an Olympic contender, testified before a Senate subcommittee that he was given a list of substances, including vitamins B_{12} and C, that would make him great if he took them. He also noted that just prior to the 1964 Tokyo games, vitamins, minerals, proteins and other supplements were distributed in his hotel, although he did not indicate the official position of the individual dispensing them.

These sports administration personnel may have obtained their nutritional information from respected journals, which have in some cases published research indicative of an ergogenic effect of some particular ingredient, or a review by some authorities recommending some specific diet modifications for athletes. Simonson (1971b) has severely criticized some of the research done in this area, noting that in one rather uncontrolled study the authors indicated that one of the properties of orange juice provided resistance to fatigue. Simonson noted that such uncritical claims are unfortunately abundant in the literature dealing with nutrition and performance. Nevertheless, in a relatively recent issue of a prominent sports medicine journal, Bobb (1969) recommended that the athletic department may wish to give orange juice or vitamin-mineral supplements to their athletes. Recent Russian research (Ranson, 1973) has claimed that athletes need special food supplements. The translation of their research has indicated that enrichment of the diet may regulate and activate biochemical reactions in a desired direction and therefore increase the efficiency of the athlete. Due to the high stress on their bodies, especially in endurance events, athletes require additional vitamin B complex and vitamin C, probably a two-fold increase. They also indicated that vitamin E, wheat germ, wheat germ oil and citric acid may be essential in the athletes' diet, the citric acid actively stimulating the oxygen-using processes in the blood and contributing to athletic efficiency. They note that a tennis player or trackman who sucks on a lemon or orange may help his performance more than he thinks. Cureton (1969a; 1969b) also noted it would appear to be wise for people involved in hard stressful work to be committed to the use of extra B complex and C vitamins as well as the extra use of fresh, natural, unheated oils such as wheat germ oil. Moreover, Horstman (1972), after a review of the literature, concluded that optimal nutritional status for physical performance may be dependent upon more than just a well-balanced diet. With statements such as these, presented in popular coaching magazines such as *Swimming Technique* and *Athletic Journal*, a coach or athlete might assume that vitamin supplementation and wheat germ oil are essential.

In addition to the periodical articles noted above, a book entitled *Super Food for Super Athletes* (Fleming, 1968) has been on the market for nearly eight years, advising athletes and coaches about such topics as competition meals, quick-energy competition snacks, high protein super energy drinks, meals to build stamina and a miscellany of other nutritional concerns for athletes. Fleming states that the purpose of the book is to show athletes how to use the diet to extract every ounce of energy and muscle-building material out of the efficient food they put in their bodies. The secret magic pill is high protein natural food and specially prepared dishes like banana dynamite.

Aside from these previous reasons for the development of nutritional quackery in athletics, the athlete and coach are subjected to direct advertisements extolling the virtues of a given product relative to increased performance capacity. For example, a product called "world champion protein" has been marketed in Europe, and the box of 250 tablets included a total of 34 g protein at a cost ten times that of an equivalent amount of milk protein — and no better (Blix, 1970). Similar compounds are advertised in the United States. One advertisement suggests that most coaches know the deciding factor in a winning team is often the training diet, and that its super high protein mixture and germ oil concentrate have energizing properties. The Carnation Company advertised one of their products, Carnation Instant Breakfast® in a leading athletic journal. Bold faced type read "High-powered liquid meal increases speed of swimmers," and the remaining content of the advertisement reported that according to their research, the Instant Breakfast produced an "energy edge" and allowed swimmers to beat their own best times. Another company, the General Health and Fitness Corporation, advertised four different products, indicating they could be applied for conditioning your athletes to top performance. The four products, Protein Weight Gainer, Protein Powerizer, Protein Energizer, and Protein Slimmer, were designed for specific athletic purposes, as the names imply. Their report indicated that all products had been university tested, and implied that they would be effective in improving athletic records. Both the Carnation Company and the General Health and Fitness Corporation indicated that reports of their research were available upon request. Upon receiving and analyzing these reports, the general conclusion is that they would not appear to meet acceptable standards for reporting research dealing with dietary supplements and their role in human athletic performance. These reports will be discussed in further detail in later chapters.

According to Clarke (1968), numerous companies have been profiting on the sale of nutritional supplements to athletes. In several instances, the Food and Drug Administration (FDA) has seized food supplements to athletes because of false or misleading advertising. However, although the FDA has taken some action in this area, a number of products still exist on the market.

In summary, although many authorities indicate that there are no magic nutritional ingredients available which will improve performance of an athlete on a well-balanced diet, reports from other authoritative sources, advice from coaches, the nutritional practices of star athletes, and well-designed product advertisements in major athletic journals, all give the impression that certain substances may increase athletic potential.

RESEARCH AND EDUCATIONAL NEEDS

In the search for knowledge concerning general nutrition, White, Handler and Smith (1973) have noted that one of the major research areas in biochemistry today is the determination of the substances that are required to satisfy the nutritional requirements of man and the physiological roles of these compounds. They indicated that the knowledge relative to the number of substances needed in man is perhaps complete. In other words, the knowledge is adequate to manage the nutritional affairs of mankind. The apparent problem, it would seem, is the proper implementation of this knowledge to the general public.

Williams (1962) has noted that diet and nutrition in relation to athletic performance is the subject of much debate and controversy, and there has been little practical research and accumulated knowledge. Cureton (1969b) also noted a dearth of research in this area, especially in controlled parallel group studies which also should be of a double-blind, placebo experimental design. On the other hand, Horstman (1972) noted there has been considerable research in this area. If one includes the pre-1940 studies, which suffered from improper experimental methodology at least in comparison to contemporary experimental design, his statement is correct. Nevertheless, Horstman still concludes there is no definitive statement as to the role that various foodstuffs play in aiding performance. Van Itallie (1968) supported this viewpoint with his statement that in the present state of physiologic science, we are not able to sufficiently separate truth from fancy in order to really know whether or not we can change physical performance through diet.

Although it may be difficult to assess the effect of one particular food or nutritional ingredient on athletic performance due to the confounding effect of other variables, controlled research is absolutely essential if we are to separate fact from fancy. Harper (1974), an expert in nutrition, has indicated there is no evidence that intakes of specific nutrients, greater than those that support satisfactory growth and prevent body stores from falling below accepted norms, increase vigor, promote better health or prolong life. However, he did note that the possibility that large amounts of certain nutrients may have some beneficial pharmaceutical or pharmacological effect in special circumstances deserves exploration. Thus, the possibility exists that large quantities of certain nutritional ingredients, based upon their physiological role in the body, *may* facilitate performance in selected athletic endeavors.

However, as Simonson (1971b) has declared, general recommendations concerning the best composition of the athlete's diet are difficult to make, but any suggestions we do make would have to be based on what one considers to be the best supported evidence. One of the basic purposes of this text is to present, in the following chapters, the available evidence so that coach and athlete may be able to discern the role of selected nutritional ingredients in sports performance.

As noted earlier by Engel (1959), educational programs are needed to eliminate food faddism in general. In the case of nutritional quackery in athletics, the coaches should be the main target for nutritional education programs, so they may disseminate the knowledge to their athletes. According to a recent report (American Alliance for Health, Physical Education and Recreation, 1971), the majority of coaches throughout the country base their nutritional advice to youngsters upon their own nutritional experiences. Some of their experiences may not be based upon sound scientific evidence, as Nelson (1961), in a survey of high school coaches in Utah, reported that 50 percent of the respondents recommended some type of food supplement, including a number of so-called "quick energy" foods such as dextrose tablets, honey, chocolate, sugar and coke. The coaches believed their athletes would benefit immediately after the ingestion of these foods. Furthermore, in a recent nutritional knowledge survey of physical education majors, reported by Cho and Fryer (1974a), the male students indicated that a significant source of their knowledge about nutrition was obtained from both their high school and college coaches. It should also be noted that the mean nutritional knowledge of the physical education majors, who were juniors, seniors and graduate students, was rather low, averaging about 40 percent correct responses concerning such basic nutritional concepts as digestion, metabolism, energy expenditure, weight control, protein, lipids, vitamins and minerals. In a subsequent report, Cho and Fryer (1974b) found that although the physical education majors did utilize some basic nutritional principles in their recommendations for athletes, they did make a number of recommendations that have no scientific basis. They emphasized the value of such supplements as protein, iron and multivitamins, along with honey, wheat germ, gelatin and Gatorade®. The implication is that these coaches of tomorrow have not acquired substantial knowledge regarding basic nutritional concepts, giving some credence to the notation by Mayer (1968; 1975) that nutrition is poorly taught, not only to the public but also to the health professions.

The education of the modern coach and physical educator should include a broad range of knowledge on a number of subjects, including nutrition, that are of interest to athletes and students involved in physical education. Based on this knowledge, sound educational programs may be directed towards the students to help eliminate quackery in sports and promote sound health practices. Hein (1967) indicated that physical education and athletics in the public school can make an important impact upon the health behavior of both participants and nonparticipants, especially in the area of food selection. Other studies, documented later in the chapter concerning weight control and obesity, demonstrate the effectiveness of educational programs coordinated between nutritionists and physical educators.

The time is rapidly passing when the roles of the health educator and physical educator should be combined. Many states are currently offering separate certification in health and physical education, although some still maintain dual certification. Due to the expanding amount of information in the health sciences, and the increasing diversity of physical activities being offered by public school systems, specialization in teacher preparation becomes increasingly important. However, the historical background indicates a close liaison between nutrition and sports, and it is to be hoped that physical educators and coaches, due to their influential role in the development of young men and women, will attempt to keep well-informed concerning basic nutritional principles as they apply to everyday health and athletic performance.

CHAPTER TWO

ENERGY AND METABOLIC CONCEPTS

ENERGY EXISTS IN a variety of forms in life, and there exists a varity of different classifications, including such forms as chemical, thermal, mechanical, electrical, light and nuclear energy. The basic purpose of living cells is to transform chemical energy into other forms for bodily functions, namely electrical, thermal, mechanical, other chemical forms, and in some organisms, light. The sum total of these energy transformations and utilization in the living organism represents metabolism.

In the human organism, the major energy sources are provided by coupling the oxidation of carbohydrate and fats to the synthesis of adenosine triphosphate (ATP), the organic high-energy phosphate used for virtually all endergonic cellular processes. With the oxidation of the food in the cell, some energy is trapped and harnessed before it is degraded and lost as heat. The classical formula $(1) C_6H_{12}O_6 + 6O_2 \rightarrow 6CO_2 + 6H_2O + \Delta F$ $(2) \Delta F + ADP + P \rightarrow ATP$, represents the conversion of energy in glucose $(C_6H_{12}O_6)$ by oxidation to free energy (ΔF), some of the free energy being harnessed as ATP and the reminder being released as heat, helping to maintain normal body temperture at 98.6°F (37°C). The energy stored in ATP is made available when the ATP is hydrolyzed and can be utilized for diverse physiological processes in the body, including muscular contraction, synthesis of proteins and other compounds and conduction of the nerve impulse, among others. During a resting situation, the majority of the energy resulting from the oxidation processes in the body is released as heat; however, during muscular work an increasing percentage of the energy is utilized to produce mechanical work, although 75 to 80 percent is still released as heat due to the relative inefficiency of man doing work.

To review a little basic biology, Figure 2-1 represents the essential processes involved in the conversion of the chemical energy in carbohydrate (glucose), fats and proteins into a physiologically

24

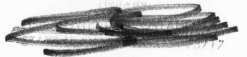

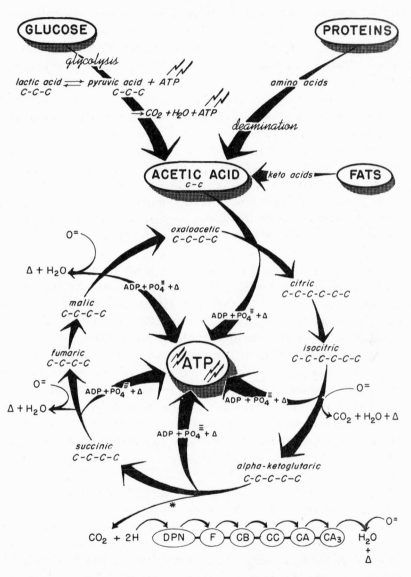

Figure 2-1 A summary of the major events in the production of ATP. The arrow with an asterisk (*) beside it indicates the mechanism by which hydrogen is passed along the various coenzymes and finally reacts with oxygen to yield water and energy. DPN (diphosphopyridine nucleotide), F (flavoprotein), CB (cytochrome B), CC (cytochrome C), CA (cytochrome A), and CA_3 (CYTOCHROME A_3) are the coenzymes. From Brooks, S., *Integrated Basic Science*, 1966. Courtesy of the C. V. Mosby Company, St. Louis, Missouri.

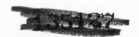

useful form of energy, ATP. The major reactions occur within the cell mitochondria, within which are contained the enzymes of the citric acid cycle, also known as the Krebs and tricarboxylic cycle. Also within the mitochondria are the various coenzymes such as DPN (also known as NAD), the flavoproteins (F) and the cytochromes (CB, CC, CA, CA_3). These coenzymes serve as electron carrier systems and facilitate the transfer of numerous hydrogen ions from the substrate in the cycle to eventually combine with oxygen for the formation of water. During this electron flow, an oxidation occurs when hydrogen is removed from a particular substrate and energy is released. Some of this energy is stored as ATP. This overall process is called oxidative phosphorylation. The essential factor of this process is that a continual supply of oxygen is necessary for its operation. Hence, this is an aerobic process.

To backtrack a little, it is known that the ultimate source of energy on earth is the sun. The energy radiated by the sun is harnessed by plants and stored as either carbohydrate, fats or protein. In the human body, although all three compounds may be utilized for energy, only carbohydrate and fats are normally used, protein being spared for tissue maintenance and growth. These compounds are transformed in the digestive process and eventually formed into acetyl CoA, represented in Figure 2-1 as acetic acid. In the conversion of glucose to acetyl CoA, some ATP may be produced without the necessity for oxygen. The process of glycolysis is thus anaerobic in nature and allows man to produce energy rapidly without a readily available supply of oxygen. A more detailed discussion of the metabolism of carbohydrate, fat and protein, and their respective roles during exercise, is presented in the respective chapters.

Other sources of energy in the form of organic phosphates are present in human muscle in limited amounts and may be utilized to form ATP. In summary, Bergstrom (1967), using needle biopsy techniques to sample muscle tissue, reported that ATP in the muscle is resynthesized primarily from three processes:

1. oxidative phosphorylation via the citric acid cycle
2. anaerobic glycolysis
3. transphosphorylation of phosphocreatine, an organic phosphate.

The first process is aerobic; the second process is anaerobic and may result in the accumulation of lactic acid; and the third process is also anaerobic but produces no lactic acid. The percentual participation of each source of ATP for muscular contraction is presented in the section of this book dealing with energy demands of physical activities.

As is obvious from this discussion, dietary carbohydrates and fats play a central role in the energy supply of the body. What may not be so obvious is the role of several vitamins and minerals in the energy transformations. For example, thiamine (vitamin B_1) is essential for the conversion of pyruvic acid to acetyl CoA; pantothenic acid is bound in an ester linkage to acetyl CoA; riboflavin and niacin are components, respectively of flavoproteins (FAD) and DPN (NAD); and iron is a major constituent of the cytochrome system. Their roles will be delineated later in the text.

Although energy is utilized for diverse processes in the body, the main concern here is its relationship to muscular performance. Before discussing energy expenditure during physical activity, some methods of expressing energy will be covered.

MEASURES OF ENERGY

Although there are a variety of ways to express energy, the basic unit in the area of nutrition is a calorie. One small calorie represents the amount of heat needed to heat one gram of water one degree Centigrade (at 15°C). One large calorie, or kilocalorie, equals 1000 small calories, and it is the general measure used when one speaks of the caloric cost of exercise or the caloric content of foods. Unless noted otherwise, the term *calorie* in this text will refer to the kilocalorie (kc).

According to the principles underlying the first law of thermodynamics, energy can be equated from one form to another. Thus, the calorie, which represents thermal energy, can be equated to mechanical, chemical and other forms of energy. Relative to our discussion concerning physical work and nutrition, it is important to equate the calorie with mechanical work and chemical energy released with oxidative processes in the body. Thus, Table 2-I represents some equivalent energy values in common measures used today.

TABLE 2-I

EQUIVALENT ENERGY VALUES FOR THE CALORIE,

MECHANICAL WORK AND OXYGEN

---

1 Calorie Equals:

3086 Foot Pounds
426.4 Kilogram Meters (KGM)
198 ml Oxygen when metabolizing carbohydrate
213 ml Oxygen when metabolizing fat

1 Liter of Oxygen Equals:

15,575 Foot Pounds
2,153 Kilogram Meters (KGM)
5.047 Calories when metabolizing carbohydrate
4.863 Calories when metabolizing a mixed diet
4.686 Calories when metabolizing fat
4.600 Calories when metabolizing protein

Another aspect of energy which will permeate the discussions in several chapters is the energy equivalent of the three basic foodstuffs. The caloric values of one gram of carbohydrate, fat and protein have been determined by use of a bomb calorimeter, whereby the heat content was measured when the food was completely oxidized. Depending upon the structure of the carbohydrate, fat or protein, different caloric values have been reported, but in general one gram of each of the compounds yields the following calories: Carbohydrate = 4.30; Fat = 9.45; and Protein = 5.65. However, man does not get all the energy that is contained in food, for the body is not as efficient as the bomb calorimeter. Thus, in man food is not completely absorbed and the nitrogen in protein is not completely changed to nitrous oxide. According to Wyndham (1974), about 97 percent of the dietary carbohydrate is absorbed, 95 percent of the fat, and 92 percent of the protein; in addition, the protein is not completely oxidized in the body and some of the nitrogen is excreted in the urine. According to White,

Handler and Smith (1973), the caloric values of carbohydrate, fat and protein in the body may be rounded to 4, 9, 4, respectively, if the above absorption and digestion factors are considered. Mayer and Bullen (1959) noted that this is not entirely accurate but may serve as a good practical guide for caloric determination of foods. When great precision is necessary, only a chemical determination will suffice. Thus, for the practical considerations throughout this text, the caloric value system of 4-9-4 for carbohydrate, fat and protein respectively, will be utilized.

As noted in Table 2-I, one liter of oxygen will yield more calories when metabolizing glycogen (carbohydrate) than when metabolizing either fat or protein. The determination of which food is being metabolized is accomplished by measuring oxygen consumption and carbon dioxide production in the individual. The respiratory quotient (RQ), a relative measure of the food being metabolized, is represented by the formula $RQ = CO_2/O_2$. The RQ for carbohydrate is 1.0, for fat 0.70, and for protein 0.80. The caloric values for different RQ levels are presented in Table 2-II.

TABLE 2-II

CALORIC VALUES FOR NONPROTEIN

RESPIRATORY QUOTIENTS

R. Q.	Calories per Liter O_2
0.707	4.686
0.75	4.739
0.80	4.801
0.85	4.862
0.90	4.924
0.95	4.985
1.00	5.047

As may be discerned, carbohydrate yields more calories per liter of oxygen, and hence should be the most efficient fuel. This concept will be explored in Chapter Three.

ENERGY EXPENDITURE

Since man consumes a prodigious amount of food, approximately a ton per year in the average adult American male, with a substantial amount of energy content, he must expend that energy or suffer the consequences of creeping obesity. If an individual consumes more calories than he expends, he is in a state of positive caloric balance, and the excess calories are converted to fat and stored as reserve depots of energy. On the other hand, if caloric expenditure exceeds caloric intake, a negative caloric balance is achieved, and the body will mobilize energy from the adipose tissue. When caloric intake and output are equal, the individual is in a state of caloric balance. During the developmental years of the child, when the anabolic aspect of metabolism dominates, positive caloric balance occurs and the child accumulates body mass. As he enters adulthood, hopefully caloric balance occurs; a slight negative caloric balance is advised during middle age and the advanced years.

The living human body expends energy at all times, ranging from a low value during sleep to over a fifty-fold increase during maximal anaerobic exercise. During a resting state the energy is utilized to operate the basic bodily functions that help maintain normal internal homeostasis, but during exercise, large amounts of energy are necessary for muscular contraction.

Basal Metabolic Rate

One of the most important factors governing caloric expenditure is the basal metabolic rate (BMR). This represents the energy requirements of the various cellular and tissue processes that are necessary and continuing activities in a resting, postabsorptive state. The determination of BMR is usually done following an overnight fast, with the subject resting in a lying position. The oxygen consumption and carbon dioxide production of the subject is measured, the respiratory quotient is determined, and the appropriate caloric equivalent for one liter oxygen consumption is calculated. From this value, the BMR is expressed either as cal/kg body weight/hour, or cal/square meter body surface/hour; minute or day may be substituted for day or hour. It should be noted that this is not the minimal value to sustain life as the value is lower during sleep. In total, the BMR is approximately 50 percent of the daily energy expenditure.

The BMR decreases with age and is approximately 10 percent lower in females than in males (Mayer and Bullen, 1959). A good rule of thumb to apply over a twenty-four hour period is 1 cal/hr/kg body weight. Thus, a 110 pound woman, who would weight 50 kg (1 kg = 2.2 pounds), would have an estimated BMR of 1200 cal/day (50 x 24). A 70 kg man would have a BMR of 1680 cal/day. If more accurate measurements are necessary, especially for medical or research purposes, laboratory methods would have to be applied.

Ofttimes the BMR is expressed in the literature as cal/sq. m/hr. In the case of our 70 kg man, an average value of his body surface area would be 1.85 square meters. Therefore, since his BMR is 70 cal/hour, the resultant value for cal/sq. m/hr would be 37.8 cal (70 ÷ 1.85).

A number of factors may affect the BMR. The specific dynamic action of food, first noted by Max Rubner in 1902, is an important point to consider since some contend there is a useful application to dieting practices. Following a meal, in the postprandial state, heat production normally increases. White, Handler and Smith (1973) reported the following values for the three major foodstuffs: protein, 30 percent; carbohydrate, 6 percent; and fat, 4 percent of the energy value of the food ingested. Thus, the ingestion of 50 g protein, equivalent to 200 calories, would result in 60 calories of heat loss due to the specific dynamic action. An equivalent intake of carbohydrate would create a loss of only 12 calories as heat. Bray and his associates (1974) have hypothesized that the specific dynamic action of food is due to the work of intestinal absorption and the metabolic effects of hepatic metabolism directed mainly at the disposition of amino acids from the ingested protein. The normal value for a mixed meal is a specific dynamic action approximating 8 to 10 percent. Although some contend that the high effect of protein makes it the preferential source of food during a dieting program, Wilson and others (1967) noted that in order to be effective, the diet would have to contain a considerable amount of protein above the percentage found in the normal diet, which is approximately 15 percent. They noted that in one experiment, in diets with equal caloric value, the specific dynamic action in a high protein diet with 122 g protein/day was 8 percent, while it was 6 percent in a low protein diet with 34 g protein/day. It appears the difference is not too appreciable.

Energy Sources During Physical Activity

According to a recent review (Unsigned, 1970b), the problem of defining energy sources for metabolic requirements during exercise is difficult. The effects of fat, carbohydrates (blood glucose, liver glycogen and muscle glycogen), diet, insulin, previous training, level of muscular work, oxygen supply and other factors all interrelate and must be identified. However, in many instances the level of work fixes certain sources of energy for exercise.

For the purpose of this discussion, energy sources will be classified as either, (1) aerobic sources reflecting the oxidation of carbohydrates or fats, (2) lactacid sources, reflecting the breakdown of glycogen to lactic acid or (3) alactacid anaerobic sources, reflected by the breakdown of stored phosphagens, mainly ATP and phosphocreatine (PC). These classifications are patterned after the work of Cerretelli (1974), who evaluated common physical activities on an energetic basis. Corresponding to the three classes above, respectively, his schema included: (1) exercise lasting from ten minutes to several hours, (2) exercise producing exhaustion in one to ten minutes, and (3) exercises producing exhaustion in a very short time, less than twenty seconds. It should be noted that man does not usually derive energy from just one of the three sources; most athletic activities involve all three sources. However, one source may predominate, dependent primarily upon the intensity of the activity. For example, a sprinter will utilize primarily the anaerobic alactacid mechanism, while a marathoner will function almost totally aerobically. These general statements have been documented by painstaking research. Bergstrom (1967) noted that PC concentration in the muscle is inversely related to work intensity. The heavier the work load, the lower the PC. At very high work loads, the PC concentration drops to near zero, and contractile activity of the muscle ceases. Margaria (1968) noted that the energy for an event such as the 100 meter dash is derived almost exclusively from the phosphagen breakdown (ATP-PC). Some calories are derived from the breakdown of glycogen to lactic acid, and a very small percentage comes from oxidative processes. Karlsson and Saltin (1970), studying the effect of exhaustive exercise on blood lactate, ATP and PC, noted that when exhaustion was elicited in tests of five to seven minutes duration and fifteen to twenty minutes duration, lactate accumulation progressively increased throughout the test, and they suggested it could be a causative factor of fatigue.

Margaria and his colleagues (1964b) have calculated the approximate capacity and power of the energetic processes in the muscle. They rated the maximal power, in cal/kg body weight/hour as follows: alactacid oxygen debt, 45.0; lactacid oxygen debt, 21.5; and, aerobic sources, 15.0. Thus, if one desired maximal power, alactacid mechanisms predominate as the energy source. However, one can only utilize these sources for a very limited amount of time. If one desires to perform for a longer period of time, he must decrease the intensity of his work output. Thus, the speed of a given individual decreases as he increases the distance he is to cover. The speed rate decreases as man runs 100 yards, the mile and the marathon, as well as distances intermediate. Table 2-III represents the percentual contribution of both aerobic and anaerobic energy sources, dependent upon the level of maximal intensity which can be sustained for a given time period. Thus, for a 100-meter dash covered in ten seconds, 85 percent of the energy is derived from anaerobic sources. For the marathon, with times approximately 130 minutes, the aerobic energy processes contribute 99 percent.

In summary, the energy sources during activity are derived from diverse sources, which are primarily dependent upon work intensity. Fortunately, in determining the energy expenditure during various types of physical activity, a number of individuals

TABLE 2-111

PERCENTUAL CONTRIBUTION OF AEROBIC AND ANAEROBIC

ENERGY SOURCES DURING VARIENT TIME PERIODS OF

MAXIMAL WORK

Process	Work time, maximal effort							
	10 sec	1 min	2 min	4 min	10 min	30 min	60 min	120 min
Anaerobic								
kcal	25	40	45	45	35	30	20	15
percent	85	65-70	50	30	10-15	5	2	1
Aerobic								
kcal	4	20	45	100	250	700	1300	2400
percent	15	30-35	50	70	85-90	95	98	99
TOTAL	29	60	90	145	285	730	1320	2415

*From Astrand, P. O. and Rodahl, K., TEXTBOOK OF WORK PHYSIOLOGY, 1970. Courtesy of McGraw-Hill Book Company, New York.

have calculated the caloric cost of selected activities and presented the data in the form of generalized statements or graphs and tables.

Energy Expenditure During Physical Activity

The energy expenditure during exercise is dependent upon a number of factors, including the nature of the task, the economy of movement, the speed of muscular contraction in relation to the load, the diet of the individual, his body weight, and the physical condition of the subject (Banister and Brown, 1968). For example, swimming a given distance expends more calories than running the same distance, a heavier individual will burn more calories than a lighter one during a given task, and a beginning swimmer is less economical than one who is more accomplished.

There are several methods available to measure energy expenditure during physical activity. Some institutions possess rather large calorimeters which may accommodate a human. Thus, his heat production may be measured directly during selected physical activities, and the appropriate caloric equivalent of the work task can be calculated. However, the most utilized technique is to measure the oxygen consumption of the subject during work, and calculate caloric consumption on the obtained value. If the RQ is known, the exact caloric equivalent of one liter of oxygen may be obtained. In most cases, an approximation of 5 calories for each liter of oxygen consumed may be satisfactory. In a laboratory situation, the instrumentation necessary for calculating oxygen consumption and carbon dioxide production is available and can be utilized for a variety of work situations. In the field, portable devices such as the Max Planck respirometer, which is relatively light, may be utilized by the subject during diverse activities which may not be performed in the laboratory. Others such as Bradfield (1971) and Skubic and Hodgkins (1966) have described techniques whereby energy expenditure during normal daily activities and athletic activities may be predicted from heart rate. In essence, the relationship between heart rate and oxygen consumption is determined in a number of subjects during a controlled laboratory situation, and a regression equation is established. Then, the heart rate is monitored via telemetry while the subject performs his physical activities, and the oxygen consumption, and hence caloric expenditure, is predicted from the obtained heart rate.

It should be noted that oxygen consumption is directly related to caloric expenditure only during steady state activities, that is, when the oxygen consumption is meeting the metabolic demands of the exercise. If the subject is working anaerobically, then the oxygen debt must be calculated. The oxygen debt represents the anaerobic sources of energy, both lactacid and alactacid, and is measured during the recovery period following the exercise period. Thus, when calculating the energy cost of an activity, both the oxygen uptake during the task and the oxygen debt following the work load must be ascertained. If a subject consumes 3 liters of oxygen/minute while running a seven-minute mile, and has an oxygen debt of 4 liters, his total oxygen cost for that mile is 25 liters. The caloric equivalent would be approximately 125.

The main means of measuring energy expenditure during exercise is by determination of oxygen consumption, and Astrand and Rodahl (1970) advocate the use of oxygen consumption as the means also whereby energy expenditure is expressed. This would appear to be a logical approach, but the use of the calorie and the MET appear to be more popular expressions. Thus, at present, there appear to be several main methods of classifying energy requirements:

(1) METS
(2) calorie/unit time
(3) oxygen uptake/unit time

Calories and oxygen uptake are also expressed per unit body weight and unit time.

The relationship of oxygen to calories was depicted earlier, and both are related to the MET concept. Balke (1974), in establishing values for an international committee on the standardization of physical fitness tests, described one MET as 3.5 ml oxygen/min/kg body weight. This would represent the resting metabolic rate. A 60 kg woman would have a resting MET equivalent to 210 ml oxygen/minute (60 x 3.5). The 210 ml oxygen approximates 1 calorie/minute. Thus, her resting caloric expenditure would be 60 calories/hour. Exercise METS are determined by the

the equation $\dfrac{\text{work metabolic rate}}{\text{resting metabolic rate}}$ or $\dfrac{\text{work oxygen}}{\text{resting oxygen}}$. Since work metabolism is measured by oxygen consumption, a conversion is needed. If an 80 kg man is exercising and consuming 3.36 liters oxygen/minute, his oxygen consumption in ml oxygen/kg/minute is equal to 42 (3360 ml ÷ 80). He is working at 12 METS, since 42 ÷ 3.5 = 12. The MET concept is being used increasingly, as it incorporates body size, age and sex (Banister and Brown, 1968).

However, since the caloric concept is relatively entrenched in the minds of most athletes and coaches, it will be the main means whereby energy is expressed throughout this text.

Calculating Energy Expenditures

A number of means to calculate daily energy expenditure exists. Alfin-Slater and Aftergood (1973) have proposed approximate daily caloric requirements of selected activities above that required for the BMR. After calculating the daily BMR based on an energy expenditure of 1 calorie/hour/kg body weight, the activity levels above the BMR are determined. In values of calories/kg/hour, the following represent the cost of general classes of activities:

- sedentary (sitting, studying)   0.23
- light to moderate exercise (standing to slow walking)   0.27-0.50
- active exercise (fast walking)   0.77
- strenuous exercise (jogging, running)   1.09

To briefly illustrate, a 50 kg woman who jogged for an hour would utilize 54.5 (50 x 1.09) calories above her BMR, or a total of 104.5.

A number of other useful classification schemas for estimating energy expenditure have been developed (Morehouse and Miller, 1971; Passmore and Durnin, 1955; Larson, 1974b). However, one of the more practical of the charts developed relative to occupational and recreational activities is represented in Table 2-IV. The energy expenditure values are expressed in METS, milliliters oxygen per kilogram body weight per minute, and calories per minute based on a 70 kg man. For example, if the reference man

TABLE 2-IV

APPROXIMATE METABOLIC COST OF ACTIVITIES IN

METS, OXYGEN, AND CALORIES*

	Occupational	Recreational
1½-2 METs† 4-7 ml O_2/min/kg 2-2½ kcal/min (70 kg person)	Desk work Auto driving‡ Typing Electric calculating machine operation	Standing Walking (strolling 1.6 km or 1 mile/hr) Flying,‡ motorcycling‡ Playing cards‡ Sewing, knitting
2-3 METs 7-11 ml O_2/min/kg 2½-4 kcal/min (70 kg person)	Auto repair Radio, TV repair Janitorial work Typing, manual Bartending	Level walking (3¼ km or 2 miles/hr) Level bicycling (8 km or 5 miles/hr) Riding lawn mower Billiards, bowling Skeet,‡ shuffleboard Woodworking (light) Powerboat driving‡ Golf (power cart) Canoeing (4 km or 2½ miles/hr) Horseback riding (walk) Playing piano and many musical instruments
3-4 METs 11-14 ml O_2/min/kg 4-5 kcal/min (70 kg person)	Brick laying, plastering Wheelbarrow (45 kg or 100 lb load) Machine assembly Trailer-truck in traffic Welding (moderate load) Cleaning windows	Walking (5 km or 3 miles/hr) Cycling (10 km or 6 miles/hr) Horseshoe pitching Volleyball (6-man noncompetitive) Golf (pulling bag cart) Archery Sailing (handling small boat) Fly fishing (standing with waders) Horseback (sitting to trot) Badminton (social doubles) Pushing light power mower Energetic musician
4-5 METs 14-18 ml O_2/min/kg 5-6 kcal/min (70 kg person)	Painting, masonry Paperhanging Light carpentry	Walking (5½ km or 3½ miles/hr) Cycling (13 km or 8 miles/hr) Table tennis Golf (carrying clubs) Dancing (foxtrot) Badminton (singles) Tennis (doubles) Raking leaves Hoeing Many calisthenics
5-6 METs 18-21 ml O_2/min/kg 6-7 kcal/min (70 kg person)	Digging garden Shoveling light earth	Walking (6½ km or 4 miles/hr) Cycling (16 km or 10 miles/hr) Canoeing (6½ km or 4 miles/hr) Horseback ("posting" to trot) Stream fishing (walking in light current in waders) Ice or roller skating (15 km or 9 miles/hr)
6-7 METs 21-25 ml O_2/min/kg 7-8 kcal/min (70 kg person)	Shoveling 10/min (4½ kg or 10 lbs)	Walking (8 km or 5 miles/hr) Cycling (17½ km or 11 miles/hr) Badminton (competitive) Tennis (singles) Splitting wood Snow shoveling Hand lawn-mowing Folk (square) dancing Light downhill skiing Ski touring (4 km or 2½ miles/hr) (loose snow) Water skiing
7-8 METs 25-28 ml O_2/min/kg 8-10 kcal/min (70 kg person)	Digging ditches Carrying 36 kg or 80 lbs Sawing hardwood	Jogging (8 km or 5 miles/hr) Cycling (19 km or 12 miles/hr) Horseback (gallop) Vigorous downhill skiing Basketball

		Mountain climbing
		Ice hockey
		Canoeing (8 km or 5 miles/hr)
		Touch football
		Paddleball
8-9 METs	Shoveling 10/min	Running (9 km or 5½ miles/hr)
28-32 ml O₂/min/kg	(5½ kg or 14 lbs)	Cycling (21 km or 13 miles/hr)
10-11 kcal/min		Ski touring (6½ km or 4 miles/hr)
(70 kg person)		(loose snow)
		Squash racquets (social)
		Handball (social)
		Fencing
		Basketball (vigorous)
10 plus METs	Shoveling 10/min	Running: 6 mph = 10 METs
32 plus ml O₂/min/kg	(7½ kg or 16 lbs)	7 mph = 11½ METs
11 plus kcal/min		8 mph = 13 METs
(70 kg person)		9 mph = 14 METs
		10 mph = 16 METs
		Ski touring (8+ km or 5+ miles/hr)
		(loose snow)
		Handball (competitive)
		Squash (competitive)

*Includes resting metabolic needs.

†1 MET is the energy expenditure at rest, equivalent to approximately 3.5 ml O_2/kg body weight/minute.

‡A major excess metabolic increase may occur due to excitement, anxiety, or impatience in some of these activities, and a physician must assess his patient's psychological reactivity.

*From Fox, S., Naughton, J., and Gorman, P., Physical activity and cardiovascular health. III. The exercise prescription; frequency and type of activity. *Mod Concepts Cardiovasc Dis.* 41:25, 1972. Courtesy of the American Heart Association.

(70 kg) was doing desk work at 2 METS, this would represent 7 ml O_2 /min/kg, or 2½ calories/min. The caloric cost is based on 490 ml Oxygen (7 ml x 70 kg). One liter (1000 ml) oxygen equals approximately 5 calories. If a lighter or heavier individual wished to determine their caloric expenditure per minute, they would have to base the determination on their body weight. Thus, a 50 kg person doing the same desk work would utilize only 350 ml oxygen, or approximately 1.75 calories. A 100 kg person would expend 3.5 calories. Thus, when doing physical activity, the body weight has a direct bearing on energy expenditure. Mahadeva and others (1953) have noted that the metabolic cost of standardized exercise such as walking is proportioned to body weight. Godin and Shephard (1973) have also substantiated the point that energy is proportioned to body weight when the body is moved. They also noted that inexperience and obesity may further increase the energy cost of the activity.

When interpreting the energy cost in Table 2-IV, several variables which may influence the metabolic cost should be considered. There may be different levels of skill and physical fitness between individuals, and nutritional and environmental conditions may affect the interpretation. However, the reported values are very good approximations, and may be extremely useful in calculating daily energy expenditure for weight control programs, rehabilitation of cardiac patients or other similar purposes. Thus, in summary, the energy cost of physical activity is dependent upon several factors, including type and amount of work done, intensity and body size of the individual.

Walking, Running, and Swimming

Within the past ten years there has been an increasing interest in the value of physical activity to help expend calories and hence lose body fat. The reduced obesity may have important prophylactic value against the development of coronary heart disease. A number of exercising systems have been developed, and one of the more successful is the aerobics program developed by Kenneth Cooper, and popularized in several of his books. Some of the main activities he advocates for exercising the cardiovascular system are swimming, walking and running. Some recent evidence relative to the energy expenditure of these activities has recently been made available, and it appears to be pertinent to include it under this general discussion.

In their excellent book, *Energy, Work and Leisure,* Passmore and Durnin (1967) reported that the relationship between energy and walking speed can be represented by the equation $C = 0.8V + 0.5$ where C = calories/minute and V = speed in kilometers/hour. At a constant speed, $C = 0.047W + 0.02$, where W = body weight in kg. Thus, while walking, energy expenditure is dependent upon both speed and body weight.

Caloric expenditure during running is also dependent upon speed and body weight, and the nomogram presented in Figure 2-2 can be used to calculate the caloric cost of running for a given time period.

Place a straight edge between the speed (km/hour) and grade, which will be 0 if running on the level. A kilometer is about .62 mile. Thus, 16 km/hour equals about 10 m.p.h. A line between 16 km/hour, at 0 level, would intersect the calorie line at approximately 16. If the subject weighted 70 kg, he would utilize 1120 cal/hour at that speed. Portions of an hour could be prorated.

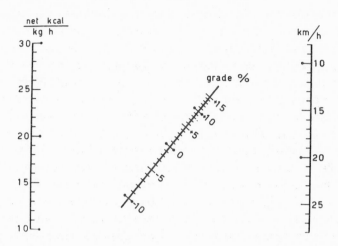

Figure 2-2   Nomogram for calculating the energy expenditure in running at different speeds and inclines. Place a straight edge between the running speed on the right ordinate and grade on the middle, oblique line. Read the net kcal/kg/hr where the straight edge crosses the left ordinate. Add 3 percent if untrained, subtract 3 percent if trained. Multiply by the weight to get total cost per hour (Margaria and others, 1963).

Costill and Fox (1969) derived a regression formula to predict the energy cost of running at different speeds. The equation is $C = 0.001S - 0.026$, where C = cal/min/kg, and S = running speed in meters/min. The formula has been modified slightly by Harger and his associates (1974).

There appears to be a small controversy relative to the differences in energy expenditure between walking or running a given distance. Astrand and Rodahl (1970) have indicated that even though there is a linear relationship between speed and energy expenditure, it should be emphasized that within a wide range of speeds the production of calories per kilometer travelled is practically the same. They contend that the most important factor in burning calories is the distance covered, not the speed. For a given distance, walking at a lower speed or running at a higher speed will utilize equal amounts of calories. Thus, the same number of calories will be expended whether one walks or runs a mile. For the obese individual who does not mind walking a leisurely mile, but dreads the thought of jogging it, this logic is appealing.

When running, Margaria (1971), Harger and others (1974), and Cerretelli (1974), have reported that the energy cost per kilometer covered appears to be constant and independent of speed. The important aspect in burning calories is not the running pace, but distance covered. However, Margaria (1971) notes that walking is much more economical than running in energy expenditure per distance covered. Thus, his viewpoint conflicts with that of Astrand and Rodahl. Margaria contended, based upon his studies, that walking at the most economical speed requires only one half the energy needed for running the same distance. His figures were 0.5 cal/kg/kilometer walking and 1.0 cal/kg/kilometer running. Margaria and others (1963), contended that the lower mechanical efficiency of running compared to low speed walking is probably due to the greater amount of mechanical work done while lifting the body at every step, plus an increase in the energy cost of internal activities such as respiration and cardiovascular adjustments. They did note however, that at a speed of 8.5 km/hr, or approximately 5 m.p.h., running was more economical above this speed, whereas walking was more economical below it.

Using predictions of energy expenditure independent of the two conflicting viewpoints represented above reveals that running a given distance burns more calories than walking it. Passmore and Durnin (1967) project that a 160 pound man walking at a speed of 4 m.p.h. will burn 5.8 cal/min. Using the prediction equation of Costill and Fox (1969) noted above, the equivalent value for running at the same speed is approximately 7.7 cal/min.

In a more recent study, Howley and Glover (1974), conducted an investigation to find the caloric cost of running and walking a mile in men and women. Using a treadmill, eight men and eight women both walked and ran a mile on a treadmill. The speed of walking was approximately 82 m/min, or just slightly faster than 3 m.p.h. The subjects ran at a pace comfortable to them and the average speed was 195 m/min, or roughly 7.3 m.p.h. The results indicated that the net energy cost, or the energy cost above the normal resting level, was significantly higher for running than for walking. In addition, the women used more calories than the men. The net caloric cost, in cal/kg/mile were: males, walking —

0.76 ± 0.07; males, running — 1.43 ± 0.08; females, walking —
0.83 ± 0.08; females, running — 1.53 ± 0.09. These findings
support the viewpoint of Margaria and his associates and may
have important implications for weight reduction programs.
Based on the data of Howley and Glover, a 60 kg woman who ran
a mile/day for a year, instead of walking, would burn 15,330 extra
calories, slightly over four pounds of body weight. Her total caloric expenditure would be 43,507. Males would experience similar beneficial effects of running.

As a general guideline, an individual may calculate the caloric
cost of running a given distance by either one of the following
formulae:

C = 1 cal/kg body weight/kilometer

C = .73 cal/pound body weight/mile

For those individuals who utilize swimming for aerobic exercise, Pendergast and his associates (1974) calculated the energy
cost for swimming a given distance and found that it was, like
running, independent of speed over the velocity range studied (.4 -
1.2 m/sec). The energy expenditure for swimming a given distance is approximately four times the value expended for running
the same distance. They also concluded that women expend less
energy than men per unit distance swimming, which may possibly be attributed to their greater buoyancy.

The latter part of this chapter has centered upon energy expenditure, especially during physical activity; knowledge of these
basic concepts is essential for an understanding of mechanisms of
weight control covered later in Chapter Ten.

CHAPTER **THREE** _____

THE ROLE OF CARBOHYDRATES
IN PHYSICAL ACTIVITY

THE ROLE OF carbohydrates in the diet of the athlete has been of interest to scientific investigators, coaches and athletes for the entire twentieth century. Ever since the classical research studies of Zuntz (1901), Krogh and Lindhard (1920), and Christensen and Hansen (1939) had revealed the beneficial effects of carbohydrates during exercise, man has attempted to incorporate varient types of carbohydrates into the training and competitive diets of the athlete. The results of these early studies were misinterpreted by many in the athletic world and helped create one of the myths about nutrition and athletic performance that is still prevalent today. Many young athletes believe that sugar is a quick source of energy, and that the ingestion of honey, glucose or other forms of sugar are readily utilized by the muscles. A leading company in athletic products markets tablets containing dextrose, with the possible implication of their use as providers of energy. On the other hand, there may be a useful application of a high carbohydrate diet to certain athletic events, and a number of investigators in the Scandinavian countries and in this country are studying the effects of glycogen storage techniques upon endurance capacity. These aspects of carbohydrate effects upon physical performance will be considered following discussion of the metabolic fate of dietary carbohydrate. In addition, a discussion of fuel utilization during exercise will be presented in this chapter.

CARBOHYDRATES: TYPES, SOURCE, DIGESTION

Carbohydrates, one of the basic foodstuffs, are produced when the energy from the sun is harnessed in chlorophyll-containing plants. The carbohydrate is further metabolized to form amino acids, fatty acids, vitamins and other nutrients for the animal world (White, Handler and Smith, 1973). The main function of a carbohydrate is to provide energy. The main forms of carbohydrates include the high molecular weight polysaccharides, the disaccharides and the monosaccharides. The vast majority of carbohydrates which exist in nature are the polysaccharides. The starch found in such plants as wheat, peas, corn and beans is a major source of dietary polysaccharides and may eventually be converted in the body to the animal starch, glycogen. The disaccharides include maltose, lactose and sucrose, with the latter being the most prevalent in nature. Upon hydrolysis, these disaccharides yield the monosaccharides, glucose, fructose and galactose. Sucrose, or cane sugar, yields glucose and fructose; lactose, or milk sugar, yields glucose and galactose; and maltose, malt sugar, yields two parts of glucose. Glucose and fructose also occur abundantly in nature as free monosaccharides; glucose, for example, appears in grapes and fructose in a variety of fruits. However, most of the carbohydrates ingested by man are in the form of starches or the disaccharides. According to Burton (1965), the caloric content of the various forms of carbohydrates varies, with one gram of the following containing the respective number of calories: glucose, 3.7; sucrose, 4.0; starch, 4.1. However, since the average diet contains proportionately more starch, the average caloric value for carbohydrate is 4.0. Man can be maintained on a diet devoid of carbohydrates, but it is the cheapest form of calories and hence is a basic staple of the diet in most of the world.

Although the digestion of carbohydrates may be initiated by the enzyme salivary amylase, its role is minor as it is inactivated in the stomach by the gastric juices. The main part of digestion occurs in the small intestine, where the enzyme pancreatic amylase catabolizes the breakdown process from polysaccharides through disaccharides to monosaccharides. The three monosaccharides are absorbed from the intestinal tract and are utilized for diverse functions within the body. Although the main function is the supply of energy, the basic elements of the carbohydrate, carbon, oxygen and hydrogen, provide the chemical materials for many of the organic compounds of the body, such as steroids, amino acids, lipids and others.

STORAGE AND METABOLISM OF CARBOHYDRATES

The major digestive end-products of carbohydrates are the monosaccharides, principally represented by glucose. Figure 3-1 depicts the central role of blood glucose, which is primarily obtained from dietary carbohydrates.

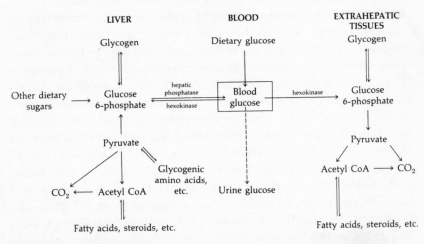

Figure 3-1   Sources and fates of blood glucose. From White, A., Handler, P., and Smith, E., PRINCIPLES OF BIOCHEMISTRY, 1973. Courtesy of McGraw-Hill Book Company, New York.

Blood glucose may also be derived from other sources. In the liver, certain substances may be converted into glucose-6-phosphate which, when acted upon by hepatic phosphatase, may be converted into glucose and released to the circulating blood. Other dietary sugars, such as galactose and fructose, may be converted to glucose-6-phosphate. Through the process of gluconeogenesis, the glycogenic amino acids, such as alanine, may be transformed eventually to glucose-6-phosphate. Lactic acid, the anaerobic end product of glycolysis in the muscle, may be transported to the liver by the blood and reconverted to glucose. Although it is not a simple reversal of glycolysis, it does occur and is energy-consuming. There is no mechanism by which animal cells can effect a net conversion of fatty acid carbon to carbohydrate.

However, in the body, fat is stored primarily as triglyceride, a union of fatty acids with glycerol. The glycerol from the hydrolysis of neutral triglycerides can form glucose through liver gluconeogenesis. Thus, blood glucose can be derived from carbohydrate, protein, and fat. (White, Handler and Smith, 1973).

Figure 3-1 represents the sources and fate of blood glucose. According to White, Handler and Smith (1973), there is only one metabolic fate of blood glucose, and that is the phosphorylation to glucose-6-phosphate. Other dietary sugars are also converted to glucose-6-phosphate. The liver and other tissues of the body cannot store glucose-6-phosphate in that form, and hence it is either converted to and stored as glycogen, or it enters into the glycolytic pathway for the release of energy. If excess carbohydrate is provided beyond the energy needs of the body and the storage capacity for liver and muscle glycogen, the carbon from the carbohydrate may be converted to fatty acids and stored eventually as triglycerides in the adipose tissue of the body. The fatty acids are made from glucose-6-phosphate, primarily in the liver and adipose tissue. As indicated in Figure 3-1, glucose-6-phosphate may also be utilized in the formation of steroids and glycogenic amino acids.

The etiology of fatigue has been associated with two different types of carbohydrate deficiencies in the body, blood glucose and muscle or liver glycogen. Under normal circumstances, the energy requirements of the brain are obtained almost entirely from blood glucose, which is the main energy source crossing the blood-brain barrier at a rate sufficient to sustain normal function. When the blood glucose level drops, resulting in hypoglycemia, the glucose supply to the brain is reduced and cerebral function may be disturbed. There is very little glycogen content in the brain; thus, the blood glucose level is critical to normal activity. According to Newsholme and Start (1973), the glycogen content of the liver can serve as a buffer system, helping to maintain blood glucose levels for up to twenty-four hours. Also, during a fast, the glucocorticoids from the adrenal cortex may facilitate the conversion of glycogenic amino acids to glucose. However, Newsholme and Start contend that if liver glycogen depletion and inhibition of gluconeogenesis occurred during severe exercise, hypoglycemia with attendant malfunction of the nervous system could result. Buskirk (1974b) also noted that hypoglycemia could cause weakness, dizziness and exhaustion in an athlete. It should be noted that this discussion is centered primarily upon acute hypoglycemia in man on a normal diet. The brain may adjust to a diet chronically low in carbohydrates, e.g. the high fat diet of the Eskimos, and utilize ketone bodies for its energy source.

The second condition associated with the etiology of fatigue is depletion of muscle glycogen, one of the major energy sources during high level aerobic exercise. Although not depicted in detail in Figure 3-1, several major energy pathways are presented. As discussed in the last chapter, energy may be provided either aerobically, with oxygen, or anaerobically, without oxygen. The aerobic mechanism is the citric acid cycle, represented in Figure 2-1 by the conversion of acetyl CoA to CO_2. Notice that the source of acetyl CoA, or acetic acid, may be either fatty acids, deaminated protein or pyruvate, the pyruvate being ultimately derived from glycogen. The anaerobic process is glycolysis, represented by the transformation of glucose-6-phosphate to pyruvate in the muscle. The storage form of glucose-6-phosphate is the muscle glycogen. During rest and low level muscular activity, glycogen and fatty acids contribute equally to the energy demands of the muscular tissue (Astrand and Rodahl, 1970). However, during higher levels of exercise, glycogen utilization begins to predominate. During extremely intense levels of exercise, i.e., supermaximal work loads, glycolysis is the main mechanism whereby ATP may be produced. Thus, it is obvious that muscle glycogen plays a key role in the energy processes of actively contracting muscles.

The muscle glycogen store is limited, and it is not readily depleted during fasting, as is the liver, since the resting muscle energy needs for ATP are met by the oxidation of acetoacetate, fatty acids and glucose, all converted to acetyl CoA. However, the almost instantaneous request for large amounts of ATP by contracting muscles is supplied by glycolysis, the massive conversion of glycogen to lactate, and in sustained high level activity the glycogen is converted to pyruvate for entrance into the citric acid cycle, the aerobic process. Glycolysis enables man to produce ATP without the need for oxygen, and thus man may perform supermaximally for a short period of time. However, the capacity of the muscle for glycolysis is limited by the rate of certain enzymic and coenzymic activity and the possible fatiguing effect of accumulating lactic acid (White, Handler and Smith, 1973). Thus, glycogen supply does not appear to be a major factor in fatigue at supermaximal workloads. On the other hand, man may be able to perform at high levels of activity for prolonged periods of time, utilizing mainly muscle glycogen as an energy source. In this case, muscle glycogen stores may be a critical factor in causing exhaustion.

Some important distinctions should be noted between liver and muscle glycogen. Although the concentration of glycogen in the liver is greater, 2 to 8 percent of the wet weight, than in the muscle, 0.5 to 1 percent, the total amount of glycogen is greater in the muscle due to the greater muscle mass. The average man's liver may have 75 g, and the muscles a total of 300 g. An important difference is the presence of the enzyme glucose-6-phosphatase in the liver and its absence in the muscle. Glucose-6-phosphatase converts glucose-6-phosphate to glucose. Thus, whereas liver glycogen may be converted directly into blood glucose, muscle glycogen cannot. (See Figure 3-1) An indirect pathway exists for muscle glycogen reconversion to blood glucose. As muscle glycogen is converted to lactic acid through glycolysis, the lactate diffuses into the blood, is carried to the liver, converted into liver glycogen, which can be released as glucose to the blood.

The following section will discuss current research evidence relative to the role of dietary carbohydrates and the prevention of hypoglycemia and maintenance of high liver and muscle glycogen stores, with special reference to their effect upon endurance capacity.

BLOOD GLUCOSE, HYPOGLYCEMIA
AND PHYSICAL PERFORMANCE

Simonson (1971c), in his monumental analysis of the etiology of muscular fatigue, noted that exhaustion of fuel may be a causative factor only in prolonged heavy work performed near the maximal capacity for a steady state. He noted that it is quite possible that the drop of blood sugar is as important for development of fatigue in prolonged work as the exhaustion of muscle glycogen stores, but that the main site of fatigue under hypoglycemic conditions would be the central nervous system rather than the muscle. This viewpoint was supported by Newsholme and Start (1973) who contended that in prolonged exercise, physical exhaustion may not be due to a changed biochemical state of the muscle, but possibly due to lowered blood glucose levels which affect the nutritive state of the nervous system and adversely affect the neural state of the muscle. This viewpoint is not relatively new, since previous observations have reported rather low blood glucose levels in endurance athletes.

Levine and his coworkers (1924) investigated the blood sugar level of five runners before and after the 1924 Boston marathon. They noted that the winner started with the highest blood glucose level and also finished with the highest. One of their suggestions to runners was to consume sugar during the race.

Best and Partridge (1930) also noted hypoglycemic conditions in three marathon runners following the 1928 Amsterdam Olympic games. However, in a recent report, Maron and others (1975) reported elevated blood glucose levels following a marathon run by six athletes. The elevated glucose may have been due to consumption of glucose solutions throughout the race.

In a more scientific vein, early studies by Christensen and others (1934), Dill (1935) and Christensen and Hansen (1939) all supported the theory that fatigue during prolonged exercise could be attributed to hypoglycemic effects upon the nervous system.

This viewpoint was resubstantiated over thirty years later by Simonson (1971a) and recently in a well-controlled investigation by Pruett (1970). Pruett's study had two major purposes, one of which was to ascertain to what extent a fall in blood glucose levels, represented by available liver glycogen, during prolonged exhausting work of different intensities is a factor limiting endurance. Using intermittant work periods of forty-five minutes, with a fifteen minute rest period, he worked subjects at three different intensity levels: 20, 50 and 70 percent of their maximal oxygen uptake. The 50 and 70 percent workloads elicited a significantly greater decline in blood glucose than did the 20 percent level. The fall was accompanied by central nervous system symptoms typical of hypoglycemia, namely dizziness and partial blackout. However, in experimentation by Bergstrom and his associates (1967) relative to the effect of diet modification upon endurance capacity, they noted that the blood glucose level may be a factor in fatigue, but it was still near 70 mg/100 ml at exhaustion after a high carbohydrate diet. It was only 50 to 60 mg/100 ml at exhaustion after a mixed or high fat-protein diet.

Based upon the relationship of blood glucose to fatigue during prolonged exercise, and the preferential utilization of carbohydrate during exercise of high intensity, it is no wonder that athletes and scientists explored its usefulness in facilitating or increasing physical performance. A number of different approaches have been used, including the consumption of glucose or other carbohydrates immediately prior to and/or during exercise, and the technique of glycogen loading whereby muscle and liver glycogen stores are increased over several days time prior to competition. The subject of carbohydrate intake immediately prior to and during competition will be discussed below; glycogen loading will be examined in a later section.

Carbohydrate Intake Prior to Performance

When glucose or other carbohydrates are administered to an individual within several hours or immediately prior to performance of short or moderate duration, there appears to be a negligible effect. Pampe (1932) studied the effect of the ingestion of 50 to 100 g sucrose upon physical performance capacity. Although the sugar increased the blood sugar level to its highest point thirty minutes after ingestion, there was no influence on the subjects in the tests of short duration. Haldi and Wynn (1945) compared the effectiveness of a high carbohydrate against a low carbohydrate meal, isocaloric in nature and consumed 2.5 to 3 hours prior to swimming a 100-yard dash. No significant difference was attributed to the diets in the short anaerobic work task. In a previous study, Haldi and his associates (1938) conducted a series of experiments with 20 g glucose or fructose, or a 20 g mixture of the two sugars, in order to evaluate their effects upon muscular efficiency. The solutions were ingested thirty minutes prior to the work task. The efficiency was the same as in experiments with water as the placebo. No changes in muscular efficiency were noted after several other experimental conditions, i.e. 50 g mixture of glucose and fructose and a high carbohydrate breakfast. Abrahams (1948), discussing Olympic athletes, noted no effect of sugar given just prior to performance. On the other hand, Keul and Haralambie (1973) reported that 200 g of glucose, taken after a two-hour fasting period, elicited greater cardiovascular efficiency during a two-hour bicycle ergometer ride at approximately 155 watts/min. Based on heart rate data, the watt/pulse, or amount of work per heart beat, was higher after the ingestion of the glucose. However, no maximal tests were conducted.

Karpovich and Sinning (1971) succinctly analyzed the myth relative to sugar serving as a quick source of energy. They drew the analogy between sugar and gas, adding a gallon of gas to a car with a full tank will not make it go faster during a short ride. Moreover, Astrand (1967a) has contended that consumption of excessive quantities of sugar several hours prior to an event may drastically impair maximal work capacity. Darden (1972) supported this contention by noting that excessive amounts of honey, sucrose, dextrose tablets or other concentrated sugars could draw and hold water in the gastrointestinal tract, possibly causing stomach cramps or contributing to dehydration in endurance events.

Carbohydrate Intake and Blood Glucose
Utilization During Exercise

The utilization of sugar compounds during an event may produce different effects than those noted immediately above. Some practical observations, noted as early as the 1920's, were probably ramifications of Zuntz's work in 1901. Based on observations of the victorious Yale University crew team in the 1924 Paris Olympics, Henderson and Haggard (1925) suggested it might be helpful to provide ample sugar in the blood and tissues during any prolonged contest. Gordon (1925), noting low blood sugars in marathoners after the Boston race in 1924, suggested that adequate ingestion of carbohydrates before and during any prolonged endurance activity might be of considerable benefit in preventing hypoglycemia. In a rather uncontrolled study, several runners in the 1925 race were given high carbohydrate meals the day prior to the event, and they were also well-supplied with candy prior to and during various stages of the race. The results showed near normal blood sugar levels at the end of the race as contrasted to 1924, and in general, better times and better physical condition at the end of the race. It was a rather uncontrolled study, but a forerunner of modern laboratory techniques investigating the effect of glucose ingestion during prolonged physical activity.

When considering the effect of exercise on blood glucose level, one must be cognizant of the intensity and duration of the exercise task. In earlier research, Dill and others (1935) have indicated that in strenuous work leading to exhaustion in ten to forty minutes, the blood sugar level may rise above normal, but light work or the early stages of exercise elicited no change from the resting level. Astrand and Rodahl (1970) have noted that during exercise the plasma insulin level falls, thereby limiting glucose entrance into the exercising muscle and hence helping to maintain normal blood glucose levels. Karpovich and Sinning (1971) indicated there would be an immediate rise in the blood sugar level prior to or immediately after the onset of exercise due to the effect of epinephrine upon liver glycogen stores. It would appear that during the early stages of exercise, then, the blood glucose level would either remain near normal or be slightly elevated. As mentioned previously, in prolonged work over an hour duration or so, the blood glucose level tends to fall. Earlier research over thirty years ago has indicated a salutary effect of glucose administration when an individual was in an exhausted state (Boje, 1939; Dill and others, 1935). Henschel (1942) reported there is no evidence that in normal humans fatigue can be delayed or decreased by maintaining a superoptimal blood sugar level. However, he indicated there may be an optimal blood sugar level, at least in long fatiguing work.

In recent years, increased attention has been directed towards the role of blood glucose during physical activity and whether or not glucose supplementation during prolonged endurance work is beneficial as an energy source. At first glance the research appears to be contradictory, but the general consensus appears to support the viewpoint that glucose ingestion may be helpful during the latter stages of endurance activity.

Some evidence is available that blood glucose is not an important source of energy for muscular work. Astrand and Rodahl (1970) indicated that glucose intake into the muscle is inhibited during exercise, and in light exercise at the level of 300 kgm/min for thirty minutes, the results of experimentation by Bergstrom and Hultman (1966) suggest that the essential source of carbohydrates during light muscular exercise in fasting subjects is the muscle glycogen. The blood glucose pool and liver glycogen are not used to any major extent. They studied the arteriovenous difference in blood glucose and found no significant decrease between the arterial and venous glucose levels. Knuttgen (1974) supported this viewpoint, reporting that during high intensity submaximal work, carbohydrates are the prime fuel for energy, primarily the muscle glycogen. He stated the uptake by the muscle of blood glucose is apparently too slow to replenish the rapid metabolism of glycogen. Horstman (1972), citing some Scandinavian research, noted that even when blood glucose concentration was high, on the order of 200 mg/100 ml, muscle glycogen levels were reduced to similar levels during exercise as compared to conditions when no glucose solution was administered, thus suggesting that muscle glycogen is the limiting factor to endurance capacity even in the presence of adequate amounts of blood glucose. Hultman (1967b) investigated the possibility of replacing local glycogen stores by circulating glucose. The subjects were infused with glucose to keep the blood sugar level between 200 and 600 mg/100 ml. The result indicated the muscle glycogen store decreased, even when blood sugar was maintained at the high level. He also noted that circulating glucose produced by the liver plays only a minor role in carbohydrate consumption of the working muscle. However, Hultman (1971) indicated that these conditions were only true during the first thirty to sixty minutes of the exercise period.

Costill, one of the most prolific researchers in this area, and his associates (1973b), agreed that the depletion of endogenous muscle glycogen stores has been shown to be a limiting factor in endurance, but noted that little is known of the effect of oral glucose feeding on carbohydrate metabolism during exercise. Thus, they undertook a study to investigate two factors: (1) the delay between glucose ingestion and its introduction into the blood of resting and exercising man; and (2) the contribution of orally fed glucose to the demands of exercise. Seven male subjects ingested an aqueous solution of glucose, about an 11 percent solution, that was tagged with labeled glucose-C^{14}. The exercise task consisted of a thirty-minute run or cycling before and sixty minutes after the glucose feeding. The exercise was moderate to heavy, constituting 60 to 72 percent of maximal oxygen uptake. The results demonstrated that the exercise had no adverse effect on gastrointestinal absorption of the glucose, as most subjects had small quantities present in their blood serum five to seven minutes after ingestion. The authors noted that it is difficult to determine how much of the ingested glucose must enter the blood in order to significantly contribute to the carbohydrate requirements of exercise, but based on their data, they concluded that it is obvious that any metabolic gain due to the glucose feeding cannot be realized until twenty to thirty minutes postingestion. They also noted that in this study, with exercise duration of only thirty minutes, glucose feedings are of limited importance, since during the final twenty minutes of the exercise the ingested glucose comprised only 20 percent of the total carbohydrate oxidation. However, they did note that the glucose may help prevent liver glycogen depletion during severe prolonged exercise. The general implication of the above reports is that glucose infusion is not beneficial during exercise, but the duration of the work tasks has generally been less than one hour, which may have an important bearing on the results as indicated by several of the investigators.

A number of other investigators have documented the beneficial effects of glucose ingestion during very prolonged work, and some have even indicated the blood glucose becomes available for energy production during the early stage of exercise. Christophe and Mayer (1958) reported that exercise may affect blood glucose utilization due to the increased glucose utilization in the large muscles, or that it may serve as an insulin-type factor. They infer that the glucose enters the muscle cell during exercise and is used as a precursor to rebuild muscular glycogen or phosphocreatine stores. Wahren and his coworkers (1971) noted that as exercise proceeds beyond the first few minutes, blood glucose assumes an increasingly important role as a substrate for muscle oxidation. Reichard and his colleagues (1961), using an isotope trace dose of glucose-U-C^{14} to study glucose metabolism during exercise, noted that stored muscle glycogen represents the immediate fuel for exercise. However, during and after work the muscle increases its uptake of blood glucose, which is compensated by increased output by the liver. The authors concluded that muscular work stimulates glucose uptake.

Whatever the role of blood glucose during the early stages of exercise, it is highly unlikely that it will be a more efficient fuel than the endogenous muscle glycogen. However, recent research indicates that optimal blood glucose levels may be important during very prolonged work, due both to the beneficial effects on the central nervous system discussed previously and as a contributor to the energy demands of exercise.

In extremely prolonged physical work, carbohydrates may be the slightly preferred fuel, as will be discussed in a subsequent section. Young and his associates (1967b) reported an increased rate of production of blood glucose during a 13.5-hour walking task on a treadmill. They reported increased gluconeogenesis from alanine and glycerol. Benade and others (1973) noted an increased RQ following the ingestion of 100 g sucrose during a prolonged aerobic exercise task, indicating the carbohydrates replaced the oxidation of free fatty acids temporarily during this submaximal workload at 47 percent maximal oxygen uptake.

At heavier workloads, Hultman (1971) noted the increasing importance of blood glucose. He reported that during prolonged exercise at 70 percent of the subject's maximal oxygen uptake, glucose uptake by the muscle initially accounted for 10 to 15 percent of the total carbohydrate utilization, and during the last few minutes of work it increased to as much as 50 percent. He indicated that at the end of the prolonged exercise period, the liver glycogen can be an important source of energy for the exercising muscles. Costill (1974), talking about practical applications, reiterated the point that blood sugar levels decline throughout a marathon race, and oral sugar solutions may help alleviate the load on the liver, thus providing for stable levels of blood glucose. Saltin and Hermansen (1967) suggested that the most likely application of oral ingestion of sugar during work is the maintenance of the blood sugar level at a nonexhausted level, for it is impossible to determine whether or not oral sugar can play an important role as a fuel for the muscle during heavy exercise even when the muscle glycogen levels are low. This viewpoint appears to be in conflict with that of Hultman (1971) noted above.

In an experiment to evaluate the effects of oral ingestion of glucose, Brooke and Davies (1972) studied the effects of four dietary treatments upon endurance in prolonged bicycling exercise. In a repeated measures design, eight male cyclists rode to exhaustion under each of the dietary treatments: T_1, glucose syrup; T_2, rice pudding, canned fruit salad and sucrose; T_3, low energy drink with electrolytes, a placebo for T_1; T_4, no dietary supplements. In T_1 and T_2, the energy expended was replaced every twenty minutes; in T_3, a volume of drink equal to T_1 was given. In all treatments, an additional 150 ml of an electrolyte solution was given every twenty minutes. The mean work times to exhaustion, in seconds, were: T_1, 216; T_2, 201; T_3, 180; T_4, 148. A significant difference ($P < .05$) existed between any two pairs, illustrating the beneficial effect of the glucose solution over the placebo. A placebo effect was also realized, and the low energy drink was significantly better than the control.

In a recent unique experiment, Bell and others (1975) studied the effect of glucose ingestion upon the ratings of perceived exertion (RPE), a subjective evaluation of effort, during a three-hour run in trained cross country runners. The subjects received 180 ml of a glucose solution thirty minutes before and 45 ml at twenty minute intervals during the run. An artificially sweetened placebo was used during a control run. The results indicated a significantly lower RPE under the glucose condition, and the authors concluded that glucose ingestion both prior to and during long term work appears to significantly decrease psychophysiological stress. They hypothesized that the effect may be due to the beneficial influence of blood glucose levels upon central nervous system glucoreceptors. Van Handel and his colleagues (1975) investigated the fate of exogenous glucose taken late in prolonged exercise. In the third hour of a bicycle ride at 50 percent of their maximal oxygen uptake, six subjects consumed glucose drinks with either 10 g glucose/400 ml or 42.4 g glucose/400 ml. Based upon their data, they noted that although little of either drink was used oxidatively, the later solution, a 10.6 percent mixture, would provide glucose for a longer period during endurance exercise. It provided 5.8 percent of the total carbohydrate during the last hour of exercise.

In summary, there appears to be sound physiological rationale for the utilization of oral glucose ingestion during the course of prolonged exercise.

Practical Application of Oral Glucose Ingestion

Reviewing the literature dealing with the effects of exercise upon gastrointestinal absorption in humans, the editors of *Nutrition Review* concluded that steady state work does not reduce the absorption of a modest amount of salt and glucose, theoretically enough to replace up to 50 percent of the glucose lost in a sixty-minute exercise period. (Unsigned, 1968). Bergstrom and Hultman (1972) note that in order to prevent hypoglycemia during work, the athlete should consume a flavored isotonic solution of glucose, or glucose and some salt, in small portions at frequent intervals. The fluid should be chilled to about 46 to 53° F. Hypertonic solutions, i.e. those with too much sugar, should not be taken as they may exert an osmotic effect, drawing water into the stomach from the extracellular spaces. The fluid should be isotonic to facilitate gastric emptying. Since the body cannot absorb much more than 50 g of sugar per hour, homemade solutions should not contain more than three rounded tablespoons (50 g) in each hour's supply. Recommended mixtures appear to be 50 g per quart of fluid, or approximately a 5 percent solution. Russian research (Unsigned, 1971a) has indicated that a solution containing sugar alone, apparently sucrose, is not the most desirable, but it should contain glucose and starch as well. They noted that this would intensify the action of the liver and thus possibly increase blood sugar. However, no research data was presented in the brief article dealing with their research in nutrition. Thus, the solution noted above should be adequate for helping to prevent hypoglycemia during prolonged work. Some commercial preparations, such as Gatorade, are available as 5 percent solutions; they also contain other ingredients such as electrolytes, and are discussed further in Chapter Eight.

GLYCOGEN STORAGE TECHNIQUES

Ever since the early work of Krogh and Lindhard (1920) and Christensen and Hansen (1939), investigators have been attempting to ascertain the mechanism whereby carbohydrates, in contrast to fat, increase endurance capacity. With the advent of the needle biopsy technique and analytical micromethods for determination of substrate and metabolic concentration in the muscle during the early 1960's, recent work initiated by the Scandinavians and supplemented by other investigators has begun to unravel the mechanisms involved. As will be revealed in the literature review below, the central ingredients appear to be muscle and liver glycogen stores. It should be emphasized that the size of the glycogen stores are limiting factors primarily in those activities which are of high intensity and long duration, such as long distance running, cross country skiing, bicycle racing and some team sports like soccer and ice hockey (Bergstrom and Hultman, 1972). At these high levels of activity, the oxygen delivery capacity is stressed and carbohydrates are utilized to a higher degree (Horstman, 1972).

A number of studies have been conducted in order to evaluate the fate of muscle glycogen. Hultman (1967b) has noted that a brief fast period up to six hours did not seem to measurably affect the muscle glycogen level, although a week of starvation may decrease it 30 to 40 percent (Hultman, 1971). The glycogen content varies in different muscle groups, and the glycogen in one muscle group cannot be transferred to another. Only the local store can be used during hard exercise. According to Hultman (1971), the only physiological way to empty the muscle of glycogen is by hard prolonged exercise, a finding well-documented in the literature.

The following Scandinavian studies are representative of the early work with the needle biopsy technique. Bergstrom and Hultman (1966) found a significant decrease in muscle glycogen following prolonged exercise. Saltin and Hermansen (1967) had twenty subjects pedal to exhaustion on a bicycle ergometer at approximately 78 percent of the maximal oxygen uptake. Glycogen content in the quadriceps femoris fell progressively as exercise continued for nearly ninety minutes. Hermansen and his colleagues (1967), studying both trained and untrained subjects at 77 percent of their maximal oxygen uptake, reported a close relationship existant between utilized glycogen and combusted carbohydrate; they theorized that at high aerobic workloads, the glycogen stores in the exercising muscles will limit endurance capacity. These are only three of the Scandinavian reports relative to the glycogen depletion effects of prolonged exercise, but the results are supported by others. Using three habitually trained male cyclists, Brooke and Green (1973) noted that the availability of muscle glycogen was important in determining work time to exhaustion on a bicycle ergometer.

Costill and his associates (1971b) noted that the Swedish studies used a bicycle ergometer, and thus isolated the quadriceps muscle group. Therefore, they undertook an investigation to evaluate the effect of a ten mile treadmill run and a continuously run maximal oxygen uptake test, given forty-five minutes after the ten mile run, upon glycogen content in the vastus lateralis, gastrocnemius and soleus muscles. The ten mile run was conducted at about 80 percent maximal oxygen uptake, and the second run was of a shorter duration to exhaustion. The authors noted substantial quantities of muscle glycogen remaining after both tests and noted that glycogen depletion is an unlikely causative agent of fatigue in their investigation. However, the runners did have a lower maximal oxygen uptake when compared to a pretest, and they did not produce as high a blood lactate on the second test as on the pretest. In a subsequent experiment, Costill and others (1971a) noted that muscle glycogen utilization decreased on successive days of a ten-mile treadmill run. Performing on three successive days, the data revealed a decreased carbohydrate metabolism during the second and third runs. The runners were on a mixed diet and apparently had sufficient glycogen storage to complete the run.

In summary, deVries (1974) noted that there is little doubt that in bicycle ergometer work, glycogen depletion is definitely one factor that can set the limits of endurance. However, he noted that other research had questioned this point relative to running. As noted above, Costill and his colleagues (1971b) still found adequate glycogen levels after a ten-mile run and a short run to exhaustion. Thus, is glycogen depletion only important in bicycling as contrasted to running? One may suggest that Costill's run was too short, only approximately one hour for the ten mile run and a much shorter time for the maximal oxygen uptake test. However, even with the earlier bicycle ergometry work, Hermansen and others (1967) noted that the level of glycogen in the muscle at the end of exercise cannot be regarded as the sole determinant of physical exhaustion.

There are possibly two explanations for this latter statement by Hermansen and his associates. First, the liver glycogen store may be important, especially in the prevention of hypoglycemia, and secondly, the depletion of glycogen in the muscle may be selective, decreasing primarily from the slow twitch fibers that function predominantly in the prolonged activity.

Liver Glycogen

Hultman (1971) has noted the average liver weighs 1.5 kg, and stores approximately 44 g glycogen/kg, or a total of 66 g. Pruett (1970) reported that the total glycogen store of the liver ranges between 50 to 100 g and that it could be depleted in the course of a few hours of heavy physical work, provided they are not replaced. As discussed previously, the liver glycogen may be utilized during the latter stages of prolonged exercise, possibly preventing hypoglycemia and allowing for adequate functioning of the central nervous system. These viewpoints have been advocated by a number of authorities in this area. Rowell (1971) indicated that the liver was a significant source of energy substrate, in the form of glucose only, during moderate to heavy exercise. Hultman and Nilsson (1971; 1973), after a review of the available research, concluded that liver glycogenolysis and glucose output can contribute significantly to the energy fuel during the latter stages of aerobic exercise, especially when the muscle glycogen is low. If an athlete is on a low carbohydrate diet, the output from the liver at the end of the exercise will be unable to meet the glucose needs, and hypoglycemia may occur.

Selective Depletion of Muscle Glycogen

In some of the earlier studies, muscle glycogen depletion was questioned as being a causative factor in the development of fatigue during prolonged work because the muscle still contained substantial levels of glycogen. However, the glycogen remaining in the muscles may have been in the fast twitch (FT) rather than the slow twitch (ST) fibers. The FT fibers are high in glycolytic activity, and therefore function primarily in anaerobic, or high speed- and power-type activities. They predominate in such athletes as sprinters and weight lifters. The ST fibers are high in oxidative capacity and are found primarily in the muscles of endurance trained athletes (Piehl, 1974b).

Costill and others (1973a) investigated the depletion of energy substrate in both the FT and ST fibers following a 30 kilometer run. The muscle glycogen concentration decreased 56 percent during the race. The histochemical analysis revealed that the depletion of glycogen was primarily in the ST fibers, thus indicating that these are used most during prolonged running. Although there still was considerable glycogen remaining in the muscle when the subjects were near exhaustion, the results demonstrated that the picture is more complex than simply a direct relationship between total muscle glycogen and the ability to perform long distance running. FT fibers still contained glycogen. The exhaustion is probably due to the extensive use, and therefore depletion, of glycogen in the ST fibers. The authors did note, however, that their results did not completely substantiate the fact that the ST glycogen depletion was the true and only cause of fatigue. On the other hand Costill did note that the depletion of glycogen from the ST fibers is primarily the cause for the distress experienced by marathon runners in the latter stages of the race.

Piehl (1974b) also reported that with normal glycogen levels and in exercise using up to 90 percent of the maximal oxygen uptake, the ST fibers are always the first to be depleted of glycogen. In work exceeding this level, FT fibers were depleted first or at the same level as the ST fibers. Gollnick and his fellow workers (1974) supported Piehl's work, indicating that there is a preferential use of the ST fibers when exercise is performed for a long period of time at less than 100 percent of the maximal oxygen uptake. The FT fibers are used more when the workload is above 100 percent maximal oxygen uptake, and when lower intensity exercise has been conducted for a long period of time and a large number of the ST fibers have become glycogen depleted. They also found that glycogen depletion was faster at higher intensity levels of exercise. Using a bicycle ergometer, they noted that the higher the intensity of exercise, as measured by percentage of maximal oxygen uptake, the greater was the glycogen depletion rate. The ST high oxidative fibers were the first to lose glycogen at all workloads below maximal oxygen uptake. At low intensity workloads, large quantities of glycogen remained even after three hours, but it was almost exclusively in the FT fibers. Thus, the true rate of glycogen utilization by contracting muscle fibers cannot be accurately assessed by measuring changes in the total glycogen of muscle samples. Selective determinations must be made; both ST and FT fibers need be analyzed. It should be noted that similar findings have been noted in animals (Baldwin and others, 1973; Terjung and others, 1974), but this review is centered almost exclusively upon human subjects.

Time Phases for Depletion and Repletion of Muscle Glycogen

Taylor and his associates (1971) studied the time course of glycogen depletion in twenty-seven male subjects of varient fitness levels. Biopsy muscle samples were collected before beginning, every twenty minutes during exercise, at the point of fatigue and ten minutes post exercise. The exercise was a prolonged bout on a bicycle ergometer at 60 to 80 percent of the subject's maximal oxygen uptake. The results indicated a triphasic curve for glycogen depletion. The greatest drop was in the first twenty minutes of exercise, followed by a plateau over a forty to sixty minute period, and then a final decline to exhaustion. They reported near depletion levels at exhaustion. In one part of their study, they noticed a relatively small drop in muscle glycogen when the subjects were exercised to exhaustion during a three to five minute maximal exercise bout.

Relative to the repletion of the glycogen stores, Hultman (1967b) reported that in the experiments whereby the subject exercised to deplete his muscle glycogen, the infusion of glucose, 4 g/kg body weight, produced a rapid resynthesis of muscle glycogen within two hours. In a 70 kg man, this would amount to 280 g glucose infused into the blood stream. In another report, this time using a high carbohydrate diet rather than the apparent direct infusion of glucose, Hultman (1967a) reported that the muscle glycogen was restored within twelve to twenty-four hours. In most cases, the muscle glycogen exceeded the basal level. On the other hand, Piehl (1974a) indicated the preexercise level was not restored until forty-six hours later. He studied the time course for glycogen storage in the muscle after they had been depleted by exercise. Various amounts of carbohydrates were fed during the forty-six hour period following the exercise. Piehl noted a rapid resynthesis, with 60 percent of the total increases occuring in ten hours following depletion, and full restoration in forty-six hours. Thus, with the use of dietary carbohydrate as a means to replenish the muscle glycogen supply following exercise-induced depletion, a time period of twelve to forty-six hours may be sufficient to restore or possibly surpass basal levels. A more rapid repletion may occur if intravenous infusion of glucose is used. However, certain dietary regimens in conjunction with exercise-induced depletion have been developed to create an above average storage of glycogen in the muscle, the so-called overshoot phenomenon. This concept will be covered in the following section.

Diet Modification To Increase
Muscle Glycogen Levels

As is probably obvious by now, there appears to be a decided advantage of establishing and maintaining high blood glucose levels, liver glycogen and muscle glycogen during athletic events characterized by high intensity aerobic work over a prolonged period of time. Thus, glycogen depletion and subsequent repletion techniques have been developed, primarily by Swedish investigators, and have shown to be effective in prolonging endurance time. Observations by Russian investigators (Unsigned, 1971a) on their athletic teams have also indicated that the complex carbohydrate diets are effective in maintaining normal blood sugar levels and increasing total endurance work capacity.

Per Olaf Astrand (1967a), an international authority in exercise physiology and a pioneer in glycogen storage studies, has noted that if an athlete believes in a particular diet, it may help him to win. In attempting to convince an athlete of the value of the following dietary procedures, the athlete should be educated as to the scientific rationale underlying the diet, for it may be difficult for him to undergo a three-day period on a high fat-protein diet.

Bergstrom and Hultman (1972) stated that in order for glycogen repletion techniques to be most effective, it is important that the glycogen stores be maximally depleted through exhaustive exercise. Early research in this area has been characterized by reports from Bergstrom and his associates (1967) and Saltin and Hermansen (1967). The aim of the early research was to determine the extent to which the muscle glycogen content could be altered by varying the diet of the individual following depletion of glycogen. Bergstrom and his colleagues conducted their study over the period of one week. It consisted of one day on a mixed diet, followed by work to exhaustion on the next day and then three days on a high fat-protein diet, followed by work to exhaustion on the fifth day and then three days on a high carbohydrate diet. On the eighth day, the exhaustion test was administered again. The general results were that the fat-protein diet did not help resynthesize the glycogen, as it returned to only about 50 percent of the initial value. However, the high carbohydrate diet raised the value high above the normal range. The results also indicated a high correlation between initial glycogen concentration and work time to exhaustion. They also noted that the blood glucose level was lower on the mixed and the high fat-protein diet than on the carbohydrate diet. The general conclusion of this research emphasized the importance of large glycogen stores prior to heavy prolonged exercise.

Pruett (1970) studied the effect of three different diets upon a number of variables, one being the percentage of energy derived from carbohydrates during exercise at 70 percent of the maximal oxygen uptake. The three diets were all similar in protein and caloric content, with the first being a normal mixed balance of carbohydrates, protein and fat. The other two diets were high fat and high carbohydrate. The subjects were fed one of the three different diets for fourteen days prior to the exercise protocol. The energy derived from carbohydrate on each of the three diets, in percentages, were: mixed, 53; high fat, 50; high carbohydrate, 60. As will be noted in a later section, carbohydrates appear to be a more efficient fuel than fat during exercise, and thus the high carbohydrate diet may be beneficial.

Gollnick and his associates (1972) investigated the storage of glycogen in the different fiber types, FT and ST, of human muscle and its depletion pattern during conditions of normal, elevated or reduced glycogen content as elicited by varient meal patterns. The high carbohydrate diet increased the muscle glycogen content more than the mixed or high fat-protein diet.

Costill (1974) noted that, for distance runners, the muscles appear to be responsive to glycogen storage during the first ten hours after heavy exercise, and therefore, a postevent meal should be primarily carbohydrate. He also noted the diet of distance runners, although it should be well-balanced in reference to protein and the basic nutrients, should also contain a large proportion of carbohydrates as the source of calories expended during high energy activity. On the other hand, Astrand and Rodahl (1970) caution against subsisting on a high carbohydrate diet regularly as this may condition the metabolic processes to a high utilization of carbohydrate fuel rather than free fatty acids. The implication may be that the muscle will not respond as effectively to glycogen storage techniques.

The full technique of glycogen depletion and repletion should be used sparingly, possibly two to three times per year for the really important competition. Zauner and Reese (1973) have proposed a three week preparation program for the key meet. During the first two weeks, the intensity of the workouts should diminish, and the carbohydrate intake should be low with a fat and protein diet predominating during this time period. During the third week, increase the diet carbohydrate in order to get the glycogen storage effect. This is a slight modification of the program developed by Astrand and other Swedish investigators.

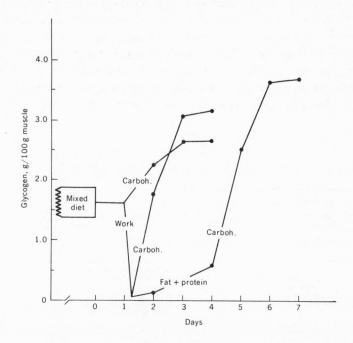

Figure 3-2   Methods for increasing the muscle glycogen content. See text for explanation. From Saltin, B. and Hermansen, L., Glycogen stores and prolonged severe exercise. In Blix, G., (Ed.), NUTRITION AND PHYSICAL ACTIVITY, 1967. Courtesy of Almqvist and Weksells, Uppsala, Sweden.

Figure 3-2 graphically represents the essentials underlying the glycogen enhancement technique developed in Sweden, and has been illustrated by Saltin and Hermansen (1967). There are three different aspects depicted, each one able to increase the glycogen content of the muscle from a resting level of approximately 1.5 g/100 g muscle to values ranging from 2.5 g to nearly 4 g/100 g muscle. *First,* after a period of time on a mixed diet, consumption of a high carbohydrate diet alone may increase the muscle glycogen content. A *second* approach is to deplete the glycogen stores through exercise, and then consume a high carbohydrate diet. As noted in Figure 3-2, the muscle glycogen content attains a higher level than the technique without exercise induced depletion. The *third* approach involves exercise induced depletion of muscle glycogen, a high fat-protein diet for three days, followed by a high carbohydrate diet for three days. This technique will elicit the highest muscle glycogen values, approaching 4 g/100 g muscle. Saltin and Hermansen (1967) have reported values may reach 5 g/100 g muscle under the proper application of this technique.

Table 3-I represents the Astrand dietary regimen for enhanced muscle glycogen technique. A perusal of the table will reveal that

TABLE 3-I

DIETS FOR USE IN THE ASTRAND REGIMEN FOR

ENHANCED MUSCLE GLYCOGEN STORATE

Days 4-6 Before an Event	*Days 1-3 Before an Event*
HIGH ENERGY-LOW CARBOHYDRATE DIET	VERY HIGH ENERGY-HIGH CARBOHYDRATE DIET
Breakfast	
½ grapefruit or ¼ c. grapefruit juice or berries	1 c. orange or pineapple juice
2 eggs	Hot cereal as desired
Generous serving bacon, ham or sausage	Eggs and/or hot cakes
Butter or margarine as desired	Generous serving bacon, ham or sausage
1 thin slice whole wheat bread	Butter or margarine as desired
1 c. whole milk or half and half	2-4 slices whole grain bread
	Chocolate or cocoa as desired
Luncheon and Dinner	
Clear bouillon or ¼ c. tomato juice	Cream or legume soup or chowder
Large serving fish, poultry or liver (>6 oz)	Large serving fish, poultry or liver (>6 oz)
Mixed green (only) salad or 1 c. cooked green vegetable	Added beans or fruits
Salad dressing, butter or margarine as desired	Salad dressing, butter or margarine as desired
1 c. whole milk or half and half	1 c. whole milk, half and half, or milkshake
Artificially sweetened gelatin with whipped cream (no sugar)	2-4 slices whole grain bread or rolls or potato
	Pie, cake, pudding or ice cream
Snacks	
Cheddar cheese	Fruits, especially dates, raisins, apples, bananas
Nuts	More milk or milkshakes
1 slice whole grain bread	Cookies or candy
Artificially sweetened lemonade	

*From Bogart, L. J., Briggs, G. M., and Calloway, D. H., NUTRITION AND PHYSICAL FITNESS, 1973. Courtesy of W.B. Saunders Company, Philadelphia.

the basic difference between the two diets is the content of relatively large amounts of breads, cereal products, and sweets in the diet one to three days before the event, all substances being high in carbohydrate content. A judicious use of the food composition table presented in Appendix A will allow for substitution of diverse foods for those represented in Table 3-I, thus creating variety and meeting the individual food preferences of the athlete.

The rationale for the increased glycogen storage has not been conclusively substantiated, but Hultman (1967a) noted that the factor causing the overshoot phenomenon is located in the muscle cell and not in the circulation. Saltin and Hermansen (1967) hypothesized that a local factor in the muscle, possibly glycogen synthetase, was responsible for the increased storage. This hypothesis has been supported by Brooke and Greene (1973), who noted increased glycogen synthetase activity in the local absence of carbohydrates. However, Piehl (1974b) recently noted that the overshoot phenomenon still awaits explanation.

Astrand and Rodahl (1970) noted one possible drawback to the increased glycogen storage. As an overall bodily energy store, glycogen is not as economical as fat since each gram of glycogen is stored with 2.7 g of water, thus increasing the body weight. In activities where lifting the body weight is important, this could be a disadvantage. Although the distance runner may need to move the extra weight, the benefits from the energy aspects of the increased glycogen should offset the extra water weight. Moreover, if the athlete is working in a hot environment, the extra water content may be beneficial. Each gram of glycogen, upon hydrolysis, will yield the 2.7 g water in addition to 0.6 g water produced by oxidation. Thus, approximately 3.3 g water per gram of glycogen will be available for evaporation and may be helpful in controlling body temperature during exercise in the heat.

Several field studies have supported the application of the glycogen storage techniques. Karlsson and Saltin (1971) indicated that the best performance could be attained following a prescribed diet regimen during the week of an important race. Using a cross over study with ten physical education students, they found that performance in a 30 kilometer (19 mile) race was enhanced if the athlete followed the general diet plan advocated in

Table 3-I. Biopsy measures indicated that the dietary regimen, in contrast to a normal mixed diet, elicited higher glycogen levels prior to and following the race. They noted no difference in speed at the beginning of the race, but as glycogen level dropped in the latter stages, so did speed. Bergstrom and his associates (1973) studied the effect of glycogen storage upon performance in an 85 kilometer (approximately 53 miles) cross-country skiing race. Although the skiiers did have sugared water throughout the race, the authors reported that the high glycogen levels at the start of the race were helpful.

FUEL FOR ENERGY DURING EXERCISE: CARBOHYDRATES AND FAT

Some interesting comparisons of different energy sources in various animals and insects have been made. Drummond and Black (1960) have cited the biochemical unity among animals, and have noted that the processes involved in energy production, i.e. glycolysis, citric acid (Krebs) cycle, phosphorylation coupling to the energy chain, are all quite uniform for different species. They made the observation that humans are not the only animals on whom glucose has been used to increase energy output or relieve exhaustion. They report on various insects, including mosquitos flown to exhaustion, which when fed glucose could resume flight within a minute. In the housefly, glycogen is also a main source of energy, whereas fat is used by the monarch butterfly for flight and many migrating birds also utilize fat for their prime fuel reserve. Although subhuman animal energy is an interesting area in itself, the present concern is with humans.

At one time it was believed that protein was the main source of energy during physical activity. However, since the early part of this century, research has indicated that carbohydrates and fat are the major sources of energy during rest and during exercise in humans. The general energy scheme in the human body was depicted in Chapter Two, but a general overview is represented in Figure 3-3.

All three foodstuffs can serve as energy sources via the different pathways. Carbohydrate may participate in both anaerobic and

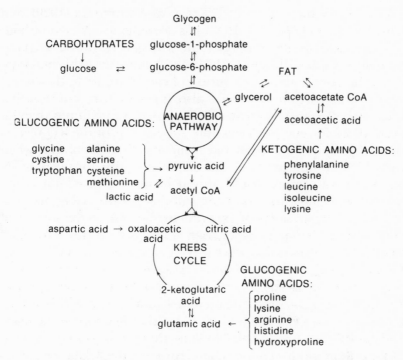

Figure 3-3 Metabolic integration of carbohydrates, fats and proteins as energy sources. From Krause, M., and Hunscher, M., FOOD, NUTRITION AND DIET THERAPY, 1972. Courtesy of W. B. Saunders Company, Philadelphia.

aerobic reactions, including glycolysis whereby glycogen breaks down to lactic acid under anaerobic conditions and pyruvic acid under aerobic conditions; the pyruvic acid is then converted into acetyl CoA and is completely oxidized in the Krebs cycle. Neutral fat may be hydrolyzed to glycerol and fatty acids, the glycerol entering the glycolytic pathway and the fatty acids being converted eventually to acetyl CoA and subsequent oxidation in the Krebs cycle. Protein catabolism can provide either ketogenic or glycogenic amino acids which may eventually be oxidized either by conversion to one of the intermediate substrates in the Krebs cycle, or conversion to pyruvic acid or acetoacetic acid and eventual transformation to acetyl CoA. During prolonged starvation, protein catabolism may become an important source of energy.

Early work by Zuntz (1901), Krogh and Lindhard (1920), and Christensen and Hansen (1939) has documented the use of both fat and carbohydrate as energy sources. In general, however, it has been reported that the closer the individual works to his maximal level, the greater the contribution of carbohydrate to the energy source. The early research has also supported the concept that muscular efficiency is greater when more carbohydrates than fat are utilized for energy derivation. An analysis of the RQ reveals that 5.047 calories are derived from one liter of oxygen when carbohydrates are oxidized; the respective value for fat is 4.686. Thus, carbohydrates would appear to have approximately a 7 percent advantage in producing calories per liter oxygen.

In their classic series of experiments relative to the sources of energy for muscular energy, Krogh and Lindhard (1920) reported that all series agreed that work was more economical when carbohydrate was the source of energy. They noted that when fat was used as a source of energy, instead of carbohydrates, there was an 11 percent decrease in efficiency. Marsh and Murlin (1928) studied the effects of high fat and high carbohydrate diets upon efficiency, and agreed with Krogh and Lindhard that carbohydrates are 11 to 12 percent more efficient than fat. However, their data appears to reflect only a 5 to 6 percent advantage. Bierring (1932) studied efficiency during one-half hour of exercise and reported an 8.3 percent advantage for carbohydrates. Two early reviews of the completed literature (Carpenter, 1931; Gemmill, 1942) support these general findings. As early as 1931 Carpenter's summarizing statement still holds true. He noted that in extremely light work, carbohydrates and fat are both used for fuel and that as the work load is increased, carbohydrates are increasingly used. As work continues in duration, fat becomes a prevalent source.

The vast majority of this chapter has championed the superiority of carbohydrates over fat as a fuel for muscular exercise. However, it is hoped that the point has been accentuated that carbohydrates are not the only fuel during all levels of intensity. Welch (1973) has indicated that the skeletal and cardiac muscles can utilize a wide variety of substrate for energy production during rest and exercise, including glucose, pyruvate, fatty acids, amino acids and ketone bodies. A number of recent studies have further documented the role of fat. Issekutz and his associates (1963) noted that at light work loads fat can play a large part in the energy sources of work metabolism. Costill and his associates (1971a) reported that as carbohydrate utilization decreased on the second and third days of three successive ten-mile runs, fat utilization increased accordingly. In a subsequent study, Costill and others (1973a) noted that after a 30 kilometer (18.7 mile) run, the triglyceride content in the muscle was reduced 30 percent. In an exceedingly long duration race, a six-day Tour de Israel, Jung (1972) reported that the main source of energy was glycogen and trylycerides.

Although the next chapter will discuss fats in more detail, it was deemed important to refer to their participation in the energy scheme at this particular point in the text, since they are integrated with carbohydrates in the production of energy during exercise.

There appears to be two important sources in the body that can contribute fat to energy production during exercise. These include the locally stored triglycerides in the muscle cells, and the free fatty acids (FFA) that are derived from the triglycerides in the adipose tissue. The FFA are delivered to the muscle cells via the circulation.

In prolonged exercise, Newsholme and Start (1973) contended that most of the energy demand in man can be met by increased mobilization and utilization of fatty acids from the adipose tissue. Costill and his associates (1973a) support this point of view, noting that although the intramuscular triglycerides are used during running, in this case a 30 kilometer race, the results of their research indicate that the major contributor of lipid substrate during distance running appears to be the extramuscular sources, probably enhanced lipolysis in the adipose tissue. Simonson (1971a) stated that during exercise, 50 percent of the fat-derived energy came from each of the two sources, the muscle triglycerides and the FFA.

Simonson (1971a) reported that although the storage supply of FFA in adipose tissue is practically inexhaustible even for prolonged exercise, at higher workloads and energy expenditure the ability of the blood to supply FFA to the muscle in prolonged performance may be one of the main factors limiting work capacity and endurance. Some support for this theory was presented by Pernow and Saltin (1971b) in a well-designed study to investigate the role of substrate upon the capacity for prolonged heavy exercise in man. They found that when the glycogen stores are reduced, prolonged work can still be performed on submaximal tasks, less than 60 to 70 percent maximal oxygen uptake, provided that the supply of FFA is adequate. However, when the subjects were in a state of low muscle glycogen levels, the investigators administered nicotinic acid to them in order to block the release of FFA from the adipose tissue. Thus, the muscles were deprived of both muscle glycogen and FFA, and the endurance capacity was reduced below the level when either one of those compounds were available.

At very intense energy output levels, Astrand (1967b) noted that glycolysis is the main mechanism for the anaerobic supply of energy and indicated fat cannot take part in the anaerobic process. Part of the rationale may be that lactic acid has been reported to suppress FFA mobilization (Gollnick and King, 1969), although Saltin and Hermansen (1967) noted that it is not known why fat is not used during high intensity exercise. Pernow and Saltin (1971b) noted that there is a controversy concerning whether or not the intramuscular triglyceride pool is utilized as an energy source during strenuous exercise in man. The most likely explanation, as advanced by Gollnick and his associates (1974), is that when energy needs to be supplied quickly the rate of oxidation of intramuscular triglycerides and/or the rate of entry of plasma FFA into the muscle cell may be insufficient to satisfy exercise energy requirements.

In summary, fat does have a central role in energy supply during certain phases of exercise, ranging from prolonged low intensity to prolonged moderate intensity. However, the available opinions appear to support the conclusion that fat is not utilized extensively during strenuous anaerobic work or high intensity aerobic work, at least to any appreciable degree. The inherent mechanisms of glycolysis, with appropriate coenzymes to facilitate the rapid transportation of electrons, provides the main means for what has been termed supramaximal work.

Effect of Training Upon Utilization
of Energy Sources

Taylor and his colleagues (1971) noted previous reports of increased aerobic and glycolytic enzyme activity in the muscle following training, thus contributing to enhanced deposition and utilization of glycogen during heavy submaximal aerobic workloads. Piehl (1974b) also reported higher muscle glycogen levels are related to training. Referring back to the discussion concerning muscle glycogen and endurance capacity, the advantages of this training effect should be evident.

At submaximal exercise levels, the effect of training has been reported to improve capacity for fatty acid oxidation and thus reduce dependancy upon blood glucose and muscle glycogen (Newsholme and Start, 1973; Lewis and Gutin, 1973). After a period of seven months training, Karlsson and his associates (1972) noticed several changes relative to substrate utilization and deposition in the musculature. At a standard submaximal workload, a lesser utilization of both phosphagens and glycogen occurred, and muscle lactate was significantly lower at both the same absolute and relative submaximal workloads. In a subsequent study, Karlsson and others (1974) studied the effect of two months training upon the utilization of muscle glycogen during prolonged aerobic tasks of 90 and 120 minutes duration. Following training, less carbohydrates and more fat were oxidized at the same workload. The authors hypothesized that the decreased glycogen consumption was probably due to enhanced oxidative capacity in the muscle, which led to a greater capacity to oxidize fat. Holloszy (1973) provided credence to their hypothesis. He measured the RQ and the rate of C^{14}-labelled fatty acids to CO_2 [14] and found that physically trained individuals oxidize more fat and less carbohydrates than untrained persons during submaximal exercise. The capacity of the mitochondria to oxidize fatty acids was increased following training. In addition, endurance exercise training appeared to produce adaptations which result in a greater rate of release of fatty acids from adipose tissue. These two increases probably act synergistically to explain the trained subjects greater utilization of fat as an energy source during submaximal exercise, thus sparing carbohydrate utilization.

CHAPTER FOUR

THE ROLE OF FAT
IN PHYSICAL ACTIVITY

THERE ARE A variety of functions of fat in the body and in the diet. Body fats serve to protect various body organs, are main constituents of some bodily structures, and are the major source of stored energy in the body. Dietary fats are important conveyors of essential fatty acids and the fat soluble vitamins. Also of interest is their role in the energy processes of the body during exercise. The fact that fats do participate as a source of energy during exercise has been known for most of this century. Zuntz (1901) noted that fat was essentially the only fuel for muscular energy when man was on a high fat diet. A comparison of the relative roles of carbohydrates and fat as energy sources during exercise was presented in the last chapter. This chapter will briefly cover the metabolic aspects of fat, a summary of its role in exercise and the relationship of dietary fat to coronary heart disease. The role of exercise in reducing serum triglycerides and cholesterol will also be discussed.

SOURCE, TYPE AND DIGESTION

According to the National Research Council (1974), dietary fat is important as a carrier for fat soluble vitamins, such as A, D, E and K, and also provides certain essential fatty acids. Aside from these needs, which can be met by approximately 15 - 25 g of appropriate food fats, there are no specific requirements for fat as a nutrient. It can be synthesized in the body from excess carbohydrates and proteins. White, Handler and Smith (1973) have noted that lipids are a heterogeneous group of structures, and they offer the following classification schema:
1. fatty acids
2. lipids containing glycerol

    a. neutral fats such as the mono-, di- and triglycerides
    b. phosphoglycerides such as phosphotidates
3. lipids not containing glycerol such as steroids
4. lipids combined with other classes of compounds such as lipoproteins and lipopolysaccharides

Fatty acids are one of the components of fat; they are chains of carbon and hydrogen atoms and vary in the degree of saturation with hydrogen. A saturated fatty acid contains a full quota of hydrogen ions; unsaturated fatty acids may absorb more hydrogen and may be further classified as monounsaturated, capable of absorbing two additional hydrogen atoms, and polyunsaturated, capable of absorbing four or more additional hydrogen atoms. In typical animal fats, palmitic is the most abundant fatty acid, with stearic ranking second. These fats are usually solid at room temperature. Oleic, linoleic, and palmitoleic are the common unsaturated fatty acids in animals and are normally liquid at room temperature. Most fatty acids may be synthesized in the body, but according to the National Research Council (1974), linoleic and arachidonic fatty acids must be supplied in the diet.

Dietary fats consist almost entirely of triglycerides, which are fatty acid esters of glycerol, a clear colorless syrupy liquid. Figure 4-1 represents the basic formula for a triglyceride. These neutral fats are the most abundant group of lipids in nature. Prominent food sources of fat include oils and shortenings, mayonnaise, milk, nuts, peanut butter, margerine and butter. The percentages of fat in each vary, with the cooking oils being 100 percent fat. Animal fats are generally saturated fats, whereas unsaturated fats are usually liquid and generally derived from vegetable sources. Some examples of unsaturated fats include corn, soybean, cottonseed, safflower and peanut oils. The role of dietary saturated and unsaturated fats in relationship to coronary heart disease will be discussed in a later section. The bulk of body lipid is also in the form of triglycerides, predominately esters of palmitic, stearic, oleic, linoleic and palmitoleic fatty acids. The composition of body fat varies as to the percentage of each of the above fatty acids.

Although there are a number of different forms of fat, two others are of interest for the present discussion, namely cholesterol and lecithin. Cholesterol is a fatlike pearly substance found

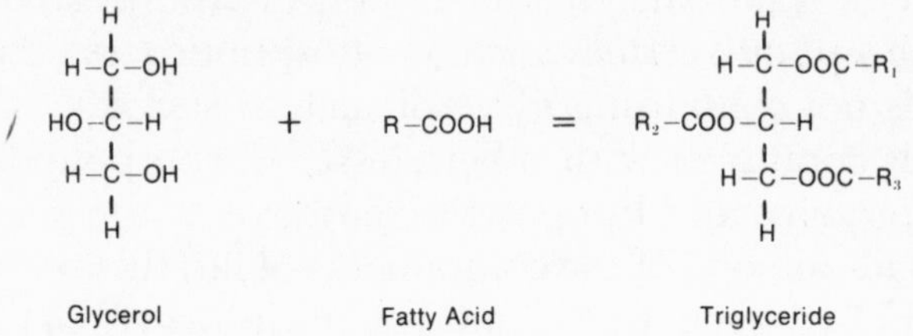

```
       H                                    H
       |                                    |
   H-C-OH                              H-C-OOC-R₁
       |                                    |
 /  HO-C-H      +    R-COOH    =     R₂-COO-C-H
       |                                    |
   H-C-OH                              H-C-OOC-R₃
       |                                    |
       H                                    H


   Glycerol            Fatty Acid            Triglyceride
```

Figure 4-1 Formation of triglycerides from glycerol and fatty acids. From Krause, M., and Hunscher, M., FOOD, NUTRITION AND DIET THERAPY, 1972. Courtesy of W. B. Saunders Company, Philadelphia.

in animal tissues, essential for the formation of various body compounds such as the adrenal and gonadel hormones.

Since all animal tissues contain cholesterol, the diet is a major source; in addition, it is synthesized in the body from acetyl CoA, and therefore can be formed endogenously from carbohydrate and fats. Since plaques forming on the intima of the arteries have been found to contain cholesterol, there has been some interest in reducing serum cholesterol levels as a prophylactic measure against the development of atherosclerotic heart disease. This topic, and the effect of exercise on cholesterol levels, will be discussed.

Lecithin, found mainly in the yolk of eggs, is a colorless crystalline compound bound to fatty acids, and is also known as a phosphatide. Lecithin, and compounds of similar chemical composition, are said to have the therapeutic properties of phosphorus. Lecithin has been utilized as an ergogenic food and the relevant research is discussed in Chapter Nine.

The major dietary source of lipids are the triglycerides. In the gastrointestinal tract they are hydrolyzed by the pancreatic lipases (fat enzymes) to fatty acids and glycerol. The major site of digestion is in the small intestine. The resultant fat droplets are emulsified by the bile for transportation through the intestinal wall. The fatty acids are absorbed into the intestinal lymph and transported via the lymphatic system. The glycerol is absorbed via the portal route.

STORAGE AND METABOLISM

The general schema for the storage and metabolic fate of fat is presented in Figure 4-2. Following absorption of fat from the gastrointestinal tract, the fat is present in the lymphatic system as chylomicrons, which are eventually released into the blood stream. Although there is a rise in the blood serum lipid level following a meal, these chylomicrons may be transported to the liver, heart, adipose tissue or muscle cells (Newsholme and Start, 1973), where they are eventually converted to energy or stored for future use.

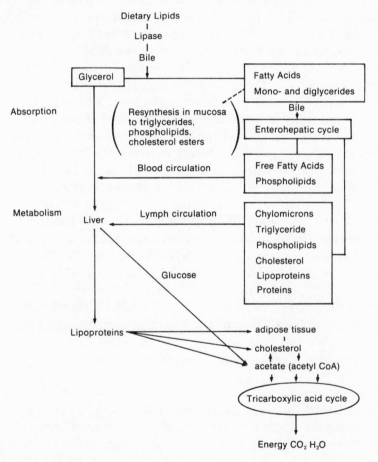

Figure 4-2 Brief summary of fat metabolism. From Krause, M., and Hunscher, M., FOOD, NUTRITION AND DIET THERAPY, 1972. Courtesy of W. B. Saunders Company, Philadelphia.

The average blood lipid level is approximately 700 mg/100 ml blood and is composed of varient fat compounds (Guyton, 1971):

	mg/100 ml of plasma
Cholesterol	180
Phospholipids	160
Triglycerides	160
Lipoprotein protein	200

The blood lipids represent a very small portion of the total body lipids, as the vast majority of fat is stored as triglyceride in the organs and adipose tissue. More than 99 percent of the body fat is in the form of triglycerides, and the composition is similar throughout the body, irregardless of anatomical location (White, Handler and Smith, 1973). As mentioned previously, the fat depots are used as vast reservoirs of energy. Fat is stored in a relatively water free state, in contrast to glycogen, and hence is a much more concentrated form of energy. Newsholme and Start (1973) have indicated that fat is nine times more efficient than carbohydrates as an energy store. During exercise, the fat in the adipose tissue may be mobilized and transported via the blood stream to the muscle cells for utilization as an energy source.

Following the metabolic pathways in Figure 4-2, it is evident that both glycerol and the fatty acid breakdown products of the dietary fat can be utilized eventually as energy sources. The glycerol may be converted into acetyl CoA and enter the tricarboxylic acid cycle (the Krebs or citric acid cycle). White, Handler and Smith (1973) have noted that glycerol can be converted to glycerol-3-phosphate, which may further be transformed into triose phosphate for entrance into the glycolysis process. The fatty acids eventually are converted to acetyl CoA, used for the formulation of other bodily compounds, or stored in the adipose tissue.

The present view of the adipose tissue is that of a highly metabolically-active tissue regarding the uptake and release of fat. The adipose tissue assimilates carbohydrates and lipids for fat synthesis and storage, and when needed later, mobilizes the lipids as free fatty acids and glycerol (White, Handler and Smith, 1973). Any substance capable of producing acetyl CoA can generate fatty acid synthesis and subsequent deposition in the cells. This process is called lipogenesis. If the total calories in the diet are restricted and become insufficient to maintain body weight, the rate of lipogenesis will fall considerably. On the other hand, when excess protein, carbohydrates or fats are consumed, they may all contribute to the deposition of fat in the adipose tissue. The etiology of obesity, and the role of exercise, are discussed in Chapter Ten.

The fat stores in the adipose tissue are constantly being mobilized, for the resting muscle consumes only small amounts of glucose; muscle depends mainly on oxidation of fatty acids for resting energy (White, Handler and Smith, 1973). During exercise, increased mobilization occurs. The fat is hydrolyzed to glycerol and fatty acids. Both appear in the blood, with the free fatty

FATTY ACID CYCLE

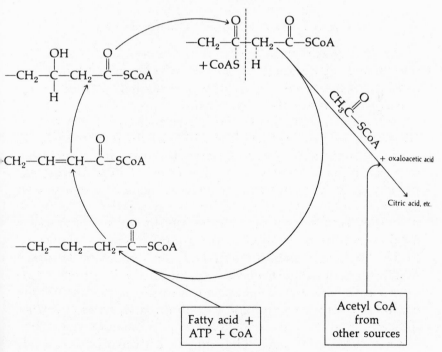

Figure 4-3   Relationship of fatty acid degradation to the citric acid cycle. From White, A., Handler, P., and Smith, E., PRINCIPLES OF BIOCHEMISTRY, 1973. Courtesy of McGraw-Hill Book Company, New York.

acids being transported bound to albumin. The glycerol, as previously mentioned, is glucogenic and may enter the glycolytic pathway. The fatty acids are oxidized in the mitochondria to acetyl CoA, which has a number of metabolic fates including entrance into the Krebs cycle.

Figure 4-3 illustrates the relationship of fatty acid degradation to the Krebs cycle. According to White, Handler and Smith (1973), the mechanism of mobilization of depot lipid is unknown, but various hormones such as epinephrine and the adrenal steroids do affect it.

White, Handler and Smith (1973) have stated that man is unable to convert fatty acids into carbohydrates because the formation of acetyl CoA and carbon dioxide from pyruvate is irreversible.

Fat as an Energy Source During Exercise

Exercise appears to increase mobilization of fat from the adipose tissue, and although the role of fat as an energy source was contrasted to carbohydrates in the preceding chapter, several summarizing points are discussed below.

Young and his associates (1967a) have attested to the fact that it is common knowledge that plasma FFA arising from the adipose tissue are important sources of energy for muscular contraction, and that trained athletes use higher levels of FFA. During extremely prolonged low intensity exercise, characterized by sixteen hours of walking, 88 percent of the energy was derived from the oxidation of fat. Carlson, (1967a; 1967b), in several reviews dealing with lipid metabolism and muscular work, summarized the role of the various lipids in the body during exercise. He noted that fats can contribute to energy expenditure in the muscle, as the muscle cells have the enzyme systems necessary to oxidize the long chain fatty acids to water and carbon dioxide. Carlson further indicated that the fatty acids for energy production may come from a variety of sources. They may be delivered to the muscle from the plasma by any of the three major lipid transport mechanisms, namely the chylomicrons, lipoproteins and FFA. In addition they may also be derived from local storage pools, either the intercellular triglycerides and phospholipids, or the extracellular lipid pools in the adipose tissue between the muscle fibers.

During exercise Carlson (1967b) has indicated an initial fall in plasma FFA during the early stages, probably due to an increased uptake by the muscle cells. There was a subsequent rise in the plasma FFA, due to increased lipolysis in the adipose tissue, resulting in greater mobilization of fatty acids from this source.

In summary, the advantage of fat as an energy source is that of a very concentrated form, which can be utilized during prolonged low intensity work. However, as discussed in the previous chapter, carbohydrate is the preferred fuel during sustained high level activity. Therefore, a high fat diet is not a recommended diet for athletes. Asmussen (1965) has offered several hypotheses whereby high fat diets may adversely affect endurance capacity. First, resultant low blood sugar levels may deteriorate performance through effects on the central nervous system. Secondly, there is a higher energy cost, or oxygen demand, per calorie of energy when fat is oxidized. Finally, the intermediate metabolites formed when fat is metabolized, such as acetoacetic acid and betahydroxybutyric acid, may create a condition of acidosis which may prove detrimental.

As has been noted in the previous chapter, the endurance athlete should have a diet well-balanced in the basic nutrients, but also relatively high in carbohydrate content in order to meet his energy needs and replenish his muscle glycogen stores.

DIETARY FAT, EXERCISE AND CORONARY HEART DISEASE

One of the major causes of death in the United States involves disorders of the cardiovascular system. According to the most recent statistics from the American Heart Association, 53 percent of the deaths in America over a one-year period of time are associated with the heart or vascular system. Although rheumatic heart disease, hypertensive heart disease and congenital conditions accounted for some of these deaths, the majority may be attributed to atherosclerotic disease of the coronary arteries. Arteriosclerosis has been utilized as the popular term to describe the development of coronary heart disease, and it does reflect a condition marked by loss of elasticity, thickening and hardening of the arteries. However, it includes a variety of conditions which cause the arterial walls to thicken and lose elasticity. Atherosclerosis is a specific form of arteriosclerosis, when the inner layers of the artery wall, the intima, develop a buildup of yellow plaques of cholesterol, lipid material, neutral fat and lipophages. The internal channel narrows and the blood flow is reduced considerably. When this condition develops in the small arteries of the heart, a decreased blood supply to a portion of the heart may cause myocardial infarct resulting in a heart attack with symptoms ranging from mild angina to death. Plaque development in the brain may cause an impeded blood supply and a resultant stroke, with possible development of paralysis.

Since disorders of the cardiovascular system have become the prominent cause of death in most industrialized countries, it is little wonder that a great deal of research has been conducted in an attempt to discover cause and effect relationships, with hopes of developing a preventative or curative technique. Thus, over the years, a number of risk factors have been associated with coronary heart disease. However, as Hursh (1974) has indicated, a risk is simply a statistical expression of probability and is not to be associated with a cause. Nonetheless, Bajusz (1965) has identified a number of factors that have been statistically associated with an increased incidence rate of coronary heart disease. These risk factors include such items as diet, serum lipids, cholesterol, physical inactivity, obesity, hypertension, age, heredity, liver function, smoking, stress, neuroendocrine function, hormones and electrolyte metabolism. Hursh (1974) has identified the three major risk factors as high blood pressure, smoking and high blood cholesterol levels.

Given the number of risk factors above, one can surmise that the difficulty of determining whether or not one factor is solely responsible for an increased chance of developing coronary heart disease. Indeed, Mueller (1974) has stated that the cause of atherosclerosis is unknown, even though many factors are statistically related to its severity, and hence to its genesis; Bajusz (1965), discussing the nutritional aspects of cardiovascular diseases, accentuated the multiple causality aspect. Nevertheless, certain factors relevant to the present discussion, namely diet, serum lipids, cholesterol, obesity and physical inactivity, have been associated with the development of coronary heart disease. Needless to say, a wealth of literature exists covering these subjects. The scope of this presentation is limited, and no thorough review is to be presented. The reader is referred to Bajusz (1965) and Naughton and Hellerstein (1973) for a more detailed coverage. However, the salient points are presented as assimilated from relevant review articles and experimental studies.

Role of Diet in Coronary Heart Disease

According to anthropologists, man's arborial ancestors were primarily vegetarians, but as he descended to the plains, he became a hunter, thus a carnivore rather than a herbivore. With the onset of agriculture about 8000 years ago, civilized man became a carbohydrate eater, and today he is beginning to consume more meat and hence more fat. Albrink (1965), after a review of the dietary habits of mankind, suggested that the cause of atherosclerotic vascular disease in affluent countries is due to an increase in total calories rather than in dietary fat. Thus, although Albrink may rate obesity ahead of diet composition as the main dietary factor associated with the development of coronary heart disease, cholesterol and saturated fats may be important considerations as potential risk factors. Obesity will be covered in Chapter Ten, and the present discussion will center upon the role of cholesterol and saturated fats.

There appears to be some controversy relative to the importance of dietary fat to the development of atherosclerosis and resultant coronary heart disease. Connor (1970) has indicated a close relationship between serum lipids and atherosclerosis when the cholesterol level was over 220 mg percent, or when serum triglycerides were above 150 mg percent. Doyle (1970) has noted that above certain concentrations of blood fat the disease of atherosclerosis is almost inevitable. Mueller (1974) has stated that this is a point of agreement among most authorities. He noted marked elevation of serum cholesterol levels is clearly associated with accelerated atherosclerosis; similar associations exist between accelerated atherosclerosis and the serum lipid components such as beta-lipoproteins and low density lipoproteins. However, Mueller also noted that all public health authorities do not agree on the preventive role of diet in relation to the development of atherosclerosis. Thus, while high serum lipids are definitely associated with atherosclerosis, the effect of dietary fat upon these blood lipid levels is still somewhat controversial.

Some authorities have implicated dietary fat as an etiological factor in atherosclerotic heart disease. Keys (1953) implicated that the total fat content of the diet, while Mayer (1967) and Doyle (1970) cited the potential dangers of excessive saturated fat intake. In a review of diet and coronary heart disease (Unsigned, 1967a), the need to restrict the diet in both cholesterol and saturated fatty acids was stressed. In one of the few long term clinical studies, the results favored a reduction of dietary cholesterol. Miettinen (1972), in a twelve-year crossover experiment, placed patients in two mental hospitals on either a cholesterol lowering diet or a normal diet. The results indicated that males on the cholesterol lowering diet experienced a significantly lower mortality from coronary heart disease. In women, the mortality rate was lower on the experimental diet, but not significantly so.

On the other hand, Mueller (1974) notes that although a strong case has been made for establishing a causal relationship between saturated fatty acid dietary intake and the incidence of coronary heart disease, based on world wide epidemiological data not all authorities agree with the findings. Most authorities probably feel, as does Bajusz (1965), that there is no reason to believe that any of the common cardiovascular diseases, such as hypertension or atherosclerosis, are caused solely by the diet. According to Hursh (1974), the current trend is to investigate the possible interaction of nutritional factors with other risk factors.

Those who state that cholesterol and saturated fatty acids in the diet have not been conclusively substantiated as causative factors in the etiology of coronary heart disease in man are essentially correct. As Bajusz (1965) has noted, no exact conclusion may be made relative to the effect of any specific nutrient upon the maintenance of normal cardiovascular health. That viewpoint, made approximately a decade ago, has been reiterated recently by Mueller (1974) and Speckmann (1975), who stated that there is no absolute proof that dietary modification of any individual or group will provide protection against coronary heart disease. Indeed, in relation to the dietary intake of children, the Committee on Nutrition of the American Academy of Pediatrics has noted there is no evidence as yet that the prevalence or severity of atherosclerosis can be diminished by limiting the intake of cholesterol beginning early in life. The Committee on Nutrition of the American Heart Association has recommended against a radical reduction of saturated fats in the diets of all children until much more is known about the benefits versus possible adverse effects. Hursh (1974) has indicated these statements have been supported by the National Research Council Food and Nutrition Board and the American Medical Association Council on Foods and Nutrition.

While there is no conclusive cause and effect relationship established between dietary fat and atherosclerosis, the same authorities who advance the positions in the preceding paragraph also note that dietary modification may affect blood serum lipid levels. Bajusz (1965) stated, as a general rule, and under conditions of constant daily intake of dietary fats (about 40% of total calories, the normal American percentage), diets high in saturated fats such as animal fats and hydrogenated vegetable oils are more likely to elicit higher serum lipid levels than those diets high in unsaturated fats. Hursh (1974) has also indicated that compared to each other, certain saturated fats tend to elevate blood cholesterol levels, monounsaturated fats have no effect and polyunsaturated fats tend to lower the blood cholesterol levels. Thus, there appears to be general agreement that dietary modification may reduce blood lipid levels.

Although a cause and effect relationship between dietary fat and coronary heart disease has not been conclusively established, the statistical relationship between high blood levels and coronary heart disease has some implications. Analogies may be noted between smoking and lung cancer; no definite cause and effect relationship has been substantiated, but there is a statistical relationship between number of cigarettes smoked and the incidence of lung cancer. In the latter case, the prudent individual should cease or restrict his level of smoking; in the former case, dietary fat intake should be limited. Indeed, this is the recommendation of most authorities.

In summary, it would be prudent for the average individual to reduce his blood lipid level. This may possibly be accomplished by two means, dietary modifications and exercise, both of which are discussed in the following sections.

Dietary Modifications To Reduce Blood Lipids

In his excellent book on the *Nutritional Aspects of Cardiovascular Diseases,* Bajusz (1965) indicated that although atherosclerosis appears to be a disease of multiple causality, there appears to be enough evidence to justify the prophylactic measure of reducing blood serum cholesterol and lipid levels. Mueller (1974) concluded, on the basis of existing scientific data, that reducing dietary saturated fat and cholesterol is likely to retard progressive atherosclerosis.

The Committee on Nutrition of the American Heart Association (1974), in a statement prepared for physicians and other health professionals, made the following five general dietary recommendations. Their recommendations and discussion are supplemented by information from other sources, particularly the major report by the British Committee on Medical Aspects of Food (1975) concerning diet and coronary heart disease.

1. The caloric intake should be adjusted to achieve and maintain ideal body weight. Correction of obesity may often reduce serum lipid levels and blood pressure. A more detailed discussion of obesity is presented in Chapter Ten.

2. There should be a reduction in total fat calories, achieved by a substantial reduction in dietary saturated fatty acids. The normal American diet derives 40 to 45 percent of its total calories from fat. This value should be reduced to no more than 35 percent. Less than 10 percent should come from saturated fats, 10 percent from polyunsaturated fats and the rest should naturally come from monounsaturated sources.

If Americans would shift their diets in the direction that prudent scientific thoughts indicate, Mueller, (1974) noted that in all candor, the milk, egg and meat industries would be seriously and adversely affected. These products should not be eliminated entirely from the diet. However, animal fats should be restricted. Animal fats differ from vegetable oils in that they contain a larger variety of fatty acids including a high concentration of saturated fatty acids. Of the three different kinds of fat in the diet — saturated, monounsaturated, and polyunsaturated — the saturated fats have been labelled as the villain. All three are usually present in any single food fat, but in varying proportions. Thus, one should choose foods high in unsaturated fats.

As practical guidelines, one should eat less butter, fatty meats, whole milk, cheeses, eggs, gravies, creamed foods or desserts made with animal fats. Eat more fish, poultry, fruits and vegetables, bread and cereal products, lean meats and vegetable oils, which are high in polyunsaturates. Use low fat milk and substitute sherbert and ice milk for ice cream. Margarines predominately composed of liquid oils, such as safflower, corn, soybean or cottonseed, should be utilized instead of butter or hydrogenated vegetable oils. Meats should be baked, broiled or roasted rather than fried. Excess fat should be removed from meats, and fat-free gravies, sauces and salad dressings may be prepared. These are only a few suggestions, but the general idea is to be conscious of dietary sources of fat, particularly animal fat, and reduce its intake.

3. A substantial reduction in dietary cholesterol should be achieved. Although a major proportion of cholesterol is synthesized from other dietary components in the liver, dietary cholesterol still contributes a substantial amount to the serum cholesterol level. White (1974) has indicated that the lowering of blood cholesterol is achieved with some difficulty and requires expert medical counseling and guidance. Bajusz (1965) also indicated the need of reducing saturated fats as they are related to cholesterol formation. Nonetheless, the Committee on Nutrition of the American Heart Association has recommended an average daily intake of 300 mg. Connor (1970) recommended a slightly lower value, 100 to 150 mg/day. The cholesterol content of most foods is represented in some nutritional tables.

Connor (1970) has indicated that there is no cholesterol in plant foods. In general, the principle sources of cholesterol in the American diet are in meats, poultry, fish, eggs and dairy products. Meats of all kinds contain cholesterol, and the content is higher in organ and glandular meats such as liver, brains, kidney and heart. Egg yolks are extremely high in cholesterol. An excellent reference on the cholesterol content of foods has been written by Feeley and others (1972).

One should consult appropriate nutritional tables to determine the cholesterol content of various foods. Adhering to the advice presented relative to the reduction of saturated fats in the diet should help to reduce blood cholesterol levels, as cholesterol is associated with animal products and saturated fats may serve as precursors for the endogenous production of cholesterol. Hopefully, most food manufacturers will adhere to the Food and Drug Administration's food labeling regulations, which permit the listing of fat and cholesterol content of the food on the label. Saturated and polyunsaturated fat in grams per serving, as well as the total fat content as a percentage of the total number of calories may also be listed (Hursh, 1974).

4. In relation to dietary carbohydrate, an increased amount will be necessary since the proportion of the total calories from fat is to be reduced. It is preferable to obtain the additional calories from foods containing complex natural carbohydrates, such as vegetables, fruits and cereals, rather than from empty carbohydrates such as refined sugar, soda pop and other sweets. The rationale is that the complex carbohydrates contain additional nutrients. Bajusz (1965) has also noted that there is no evidence that protein or carbohydrate intake variation have any significant etiological role in the development or genesis of atherosclerotic heart disease.

5. Salt intake should be partially restricted, as data from experiments from both human and animal studies suggest salt intake may be related to the development of hypertension. Bajusz (1965) has cited international epidemiological survey findings that whenever sodium intake is high in the diet, hypertension and arteriosclerosis are also high even if fat consumption is relatively low. He indicated that an enhanced dietary intake of sodium chloride elevates the blood pressure, especially in hypertensive

patients.

In summary, the above five recommendations are advisable means to reduce the dietary risk factor associated with coronary heart disease or hypertensive heart disease. The Committee on Nutrition of the American Heart Association noted that most individuals with high blood lipid concentrations will respond to diet modification.

Eating patterns are familial and cultural. Thus, in order to modify dietary habits, early education is essential. Mueller (1974) noted that adolescence appears to be an especially critical stage in the natural history of atherosclerosis, with an acceleration of the process during the period of growth and development, particularly in the male. Therefore, the concept of dietary modification may be stressed at this time during health education classes. In addition, the beneficial effect of exercise may be stressed during health and physical education classes.

Exercise Effects Upon Blood Lipids

As indicated in the previous section, it would be prudent action to modify the diet in order to reduce blood lipids. Another action which may help prevent coronary heart disease would be the initiation of an exercise program stressing aerobic endurance activity. Bajusz (1965) concluded that a causal link between habitual physical inactivity and the increased incidence of coronary heart disease with myocardial degeneration and necrosis seems to be well-established.

The mechanisms whereby habitual physical activity may prevent coronary heart disease have been enumerated and discussed in the October, 1972 issue of the *Physical Fitness Research Digest*, a publication of the President's Council on Physical Fitness and Sports. Another excellent source of information on the role of exercise in the rehabilitation and prevention of coronary heart disease may be found in the book edited by Naughton and Hellerstein (1973).

Some of the beneficial effects of exercise may include, among others, reduced body fat and obesity, decreased blood pressure in hypertensive patients, increased collateral circulation and capillarization in the myocardium, increased fibrinolytic activity and reduction of blood cholesterol and triglycerides.

The literature is not in complete agreement relative to the effect of exercise on the reduction of blood lipid constituents. The evidence appears to support the effectiveness of exercise in lowering serum triglycerides, but cholesterol levels have not consistently been lowered.

Cantone (1964) reported that exercise performed immediately after the ingestion of high fat meals caused a significant reduction in hyperlipemia and plasma lipoproteins. He indicated lipid metabolism is increased in muscular exercise, and some of the lipid in the blood may be used for energy production. Carlson (1967b), after a review of lipid metabolism during muscular work, also noted that training reduces the content of plasma triglycerides. Oscai and Holloszy (1969) reported that both running three to four miles, and strenuous weight-lifting were effective in lowering serum triglycerides. These normal subjects exercised thirty minutes daily for four consecutive days. The triglyceride level was lowered significantly following one day of exercise, and the effect was cumulative as a greater reduction was noted following the four-day trial. A finding of interest was the fact that individuals with initially low serum triglyceride levels, in the range of 90 mg percent, did not show a consistent reduction in triglyceride levels in response to exercise. Lampman and others (1975) studied the effect of either diet, exercise or a combination of the two upon men with Type IV hyperlipidemia. The data showed that triglyceride levels were significantly reduced with the training program, but that a greater decline occurred with a low fat diet. However, the combination of training and diet tended to produce a greater change than training or diet alone. The above studies were concerned with triglycerides alone, and all found significant reductions associated with exercise.

The following studies evaluated the effect of exercise upon both triglyceride and cholesterol level. While triglyceride levels were uniformly lowered, cholesterol was not. Carlson and Mossfeldt (1964) reported a significant decrease in the concentration of plasma triglycerides and phospholipids following a ski race of eight to nine hours duration. No significant changes were noted in cholesterol content. Holloszy and his associates (1964) studied the effect of a six-month training program, two to three miles per day for three to four days per week, upon blood lipids. There was a statistically significant decrease in serum triglycerides, but not in cholesterol. Goode and his associates (1966), although using a different experimental design, reported similar results following a daily running program, five m.p.h. for twenty-five minutes, for fourteen days. In a review of several studies dealing with the effect of a distance running program upon serum lipids, a significant reduction of serum triglycerides was noted, with no change in cholesterol level. However, the effect was acute, occurring about two hours after exercise and lasting about two days (Unsigned, 1967b). Giese and Corliss (1974) recently reported that a combined effect of exercise and diet normalized blood triglyceride levels, and although cholesterol levels were reduced by high caloric expenditure exercise in their study, the results were not statistically significant. From the above reports, it may be concluded that exercise programs characterized by rather prolonged aerobic exercise will reduce serum triglycerides, but have relatively little effect upon serum cholesterol.

On the other hand, a number of reports have indicated the effectiveness of exercise in lowering blood cholesterol. Rochelle (1961) reported active exercise such as running two miles per day/five days per week for five weeks elicited a significant decrease in blood plasma cholesterol. Campbell (1965) compared the effectiveness of different types of exercise, namely golf, tennis, gymnastics, weight training, wrestling, cross-country running, with a control group, for reducing cholesterol levels. The cross-country running elicited serum cholesterol levels significantly lower than all other groups except tennis, supporting the contention that activity needs to be vigorous and continuous in order to reduce serum cholesterol. This contention was also supported by the research of Tooshi and Cureton (1971). They involved middle aged men in a continuous walking, jogging and running program five days a week. Four groups were established with a control group being compared with the three experimental groups who exercised, respectively, fifteen, thirty or forty-five minutes per day. Only the forty-five minute group experienced a significant reduction in serum cholesterol. Campbell (1968) studied the effect of a ten week running program, thirty minutes per day for three day per week, upon cholesterol levels in men of three different body compositions — slim, muscular or obese. The experimental protocol elicited a decrease only in the obese subjects. Several recent reviews (Unsigned, 1969b; Unsigned, 1970a) noted that while it is not clear exactly how cholesterol oxidation might be enhanced by muscular activity, the evidence in its favor is rather persuasive. However, they noted that more research is needed to explore the relationship between muscular activity and the degradation of cholesterol. Some research is available. Malinow and Perley (1969), using a rather unique approach to study the role of exercise on cholesterol metabolism, injected some labeled, 26-C^{14}, cholesterol into four healthy male volunteers and then exposed them to a twenty minute exercise task at 460 kgm/min on a bicycle ergometer. After analysis of gas samples, the authors suggested that exercise increases the rate of cholesterol oxidation in man. Results from the studies in this paragraph would tend to support an exercise induced lowering of serum cholesterol. However, due to the conflicting results of other studies, more research is definitely advised, perferably with the effect of prolonged aerobic activity.

To conclude this section, one may wonder about the relative effectiveness of dietary techniques as contrasted to exercise as a means of reducing blood lipids. Schaefer (1974) suggested that sustained physical activity may outweight dietary factors in the control of blood lipids and obesity. Noting the difference between Eskimo hunters and their counterparts who settled in a larger community, both consuming similar diets, Schaefer indicated the lower levels of serum cholesterol and obesity in those individuals eighteen to thirty-nine years of age was due to the physical activity of hunting. There may be some problems associated with the interpretation of the data in this retrospective study, and Schaefer observed that both diet and physical activity are both practical means to control obesity and blood lipid levels. The previous report by Lampman and others (1975) indicated that a combined diet and exercise program was more effective than diet or exercise alone as a means to reduce blood lipid levels.

Thus, the prudent informed individual should incorporate this advice into his daily life style. Control the caloric, fat, cholesterol and salt content of the diet and initiate or continue an exercise program stressing endurance activity such as running. This may be even more important for ex-athletes, who as Mayer (1975) has contended, remain on high atherosclerotic-producing diets even after the cessation of training.

CHAPTER FIVE

THE ROLE OF PROTEIN
IN PHYSICAL ACTIVITY

O F THE THREE basic foodstuffs, protein has persisted throughout the years as the food of the athlete. The proclamation by Liebig over 100 years ago that protein is used during exercise was probably one of the reasons for the consumption of meat as a main ingredient of pregame meals. Wishart (1934) claimed that endurance athletes, from ancient times, have always placed great emphasis on the inclusion of an ample supply of protein in the diet. Even though it has been shown that protein is not a major source of energy during exercise, there are those who advocate massive dosages of protein in the diet based on the association of protein to muscle tissue, and the implications for strength and power.

Fleming (1968), in his book *Super Food for Super Athletes,* has indicated that high protein natural food is the magic pill that will do wonders for athletes. Astrand (1967a) noted that the consumption of thousands of protein tablets is the result of smart advertising, i.e. taking advantage of the protein-strength association. One recent advertisement has attributed virtually unlimited value to protein, indicating that its products had been university-tested with the implication that their use would improve athletic records. The advertisement attempted to capitalize on the magic of the word *protein,* using it as a prefix for their diverse products, including weight gainers, powerizers, slimmers and energizers. The products were advertised to help the athlete gain weight, keep that winning edge, and have a source of quick energy. Although the advertisements noted that the products were university tested, perusal of the reports revealed they would not meet acceptable standards of research with dietary supplements (General Health and Fitness Corporation Report, no date).

Yet, many authorities in the area of nutrition for athletes

indicate an increased need for dietary protein when the athlete is in training, especially during the developmental years and in weight training programs designed to increase muscle mass. The purpose of this chapter is to briefly discuss the nutritive aspects of protein and its role in the diet of the athlete.

SOURCE, TYPE AND DIGESTION

Proteins serve a central position in the functioning of living matter. They have large molecular weights, and are actually a collection of various amino acids linked together in a particular formation specific to the nature of the tissue or compound they form. In the human body, proteins may serve two functions. Their main role is to serve as the basic structure of most body tissues, including also such bodily substances as enzymes, hormones, and oxygen carriers such as hemoglobin and the cytochromes, genes and antibodies. The DNA in the genes determines the nature and amount of proteins that are synthesized in any given cell or tissue. The secondary role of protein is to serve as an energy source, and it may be oxidized directly or converted into carbohydrates or fat for energy use or storage. If adequate amounts of carbohydrates and fats are not available, protein is utilized for energy purposes since energy takes priority over tissue building in metabolism. The emaciation of prisoners of war who are kept on low calorie rations is an example of protein catabolism for energy purposes; the musculature served as a reservoir of protein energy. Other subsidiary functions of protein include maintenance of normal body pH and osmotic equilibrium. Man does not need protein per se, but rather a balanced amino acid mixture in order to construct protein in the body.

Dietary protein comes from both plants and animals. White, Handler and Smith (1973) have noted that plants, living in symbiotic relationships with microorganisms of their roots, are able to produce amino acids by reducing nitrogen and sulfur, and bind these compounds to intermediate products derived from the photosynthetic fixation of carbon dioxide and water to carbohydrates. The twenty major amino acids are found in Table 5-I. In plants and animals, the principal fate of the amino acids is synthesis into proteins specified by the DNA of the particular cell.

TABLE 5-1

ESSENTIAL AND NONESSENTIAL AMINO ACIDS

Essential Amino Acids	*Non-Essential Amino Acids*
Methionine	Alanine
Threonine	Serine
Isoleucine	Glycine
Valine	Asparagine
Leucine	Proline
Lysine	Ornithine
Phenylalanine	Cystine
Tryptophan	Tyrosine
Histidine	Glutamic Acid
Arginine	Glutamine

Animals can synthesize some of the amino acids in their bodies, but cannot synthesize others. The amino acids man cannot synthesize in his body are called the essential amino acids. Thus he must get these from his diet. In the normal interpretation of the word essential, all amino acids are essential and necessary to the optimal maintenance of body growth and function. The utilization of the term in association with amino acids is to distinguish between those which can be produced in the body out of other substances and those which cannot.

Vegetable proteins are nutritionally inferior to those of animal origin. They exist in smaller concentrations in plant materials and are lower in lysine, methionine and tryptophan content. However, a strict vegetarian may be able to obtain all the necessary amino acids from plants. For example, Incaparina®, made from sorghum, corn, cottonseed meal, and yeast, is similar to cow's milk and is a biologically sound protein compound. (White, Handler and Smith, 1973).

The amino acids in the diet are present as proteins, and must be released through the process of digestion. In the stomach, the gastric juice and pepsin initiate hydrolysis of protein at the peptide bond. In man, the main function of pepsin is to hydrolize proteins to polypeptides. As these pass into the small intestine, the pancreatic enzymes, the proteases, produce the final hydrolysis to amino acids. The amino acids are absorbed through the intestinal villi and travel via the portal route to the liver.

In man, the requirement for protein represents a dual need; essential amino acids and amino nitrogen must be provided. Simonson (1971b) noted that the minimum nitrogen intake to maintain equilibrium is 0.0548 g nitrogen/kg body weight/day, amounting to 0.34 g protein/kg body weight/day. He does note, however, that minimal nitrogen balance is an exceptional situation, and perhaps there should be a reserve built into the diet of the normal person. The National Research Council (1974), in the Recommended Dietary Allowances, noted that high protein diets which exceed the RDA are often desirable, since low protein diets usually contain only a small amount of animal products and thus may be low in important trace elements.

The RDA for protein has dropped over the years, from a value of 1.0 g protein/kg body weight/day prior to 1968, to 0.9 g in 1968, and 0.8 g in 1974. The current RDA protein allowances are based upon an average need of 0.47 g/kg; an allowance is made for the fact that there is individual variability in the need for protein, with a 30 percent coefficient of variation increasing the values to 0.6 g/kg. Since protein intake only has a 75 percent efficiency of utilization, the allowance is increased to 0.8 g/kg/day. Thus, the protein requirement for an average man weighing 154 pounds, or 70 kg, would be 56 g/day (0.8 X 70 kg).

Mayer (1974) had indicated that the only readily available natural form of pure protein is egg white, being albumin, a basic protein. One of the basic protein foods in the diet of children is milk, which contains about 1 g protein/ounce. Mayer noted that meat and fish rank just below cow's milk in biological value. Thus, animal foods are the best source of protein, for they are more concentrated in protein content and contain the essential amino acids. Alfin-Slater and Aftergood (1973) reported that the following amounts of food contain the same amount of protein:

3 ounces meat
3 ounces fish
3 ounces poultry
3 ounces cheese
3 ounces peanut butter
3 eggs
.75 cup cottage cheese
1.25 cups baked beans
1 pint milk

Discussion of the protein needs of athletes is covered in a later section of this chapter.

STORAGE AND METABOLISM

The general metabolic fate of dietary protein is presented in Figure 5-1. Following digestion and absorption, the amino acids

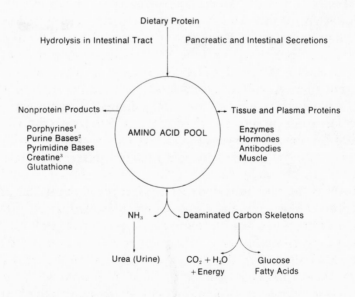

Figure 5-1   General metabolism of protein. From Krause, M., and Hunscher, M., FOOD, NUTRITION AND DIET THERAPY, 1972. Courtesy of W. B. Saunders Company, Philadelphia.

are transported to the liver, which serves to catabolize and synthesize the amino acids needed for the body. The liver synthesizes a balanced amino acid mixture for the various tissue and plasma proteins. Thus, as indicated previously, the main metabolic fate of protein is conversion into bodily tissues and functional compounds.

Proteins may also be channeled into pathways of carbohydrate and fat metabolism, and the liver is the main organ where this transformation occurs. Glycogenic amino acids are transformed via a deamination process to pyruvic, oxaloacetic and alpha-ketoglutaric acids, making possible a net glucose formation. Ketogenic amino acids may be transformed to acetoacetic acid and eventually converted to fat. These pathways are illustrated in Figure 3-3. Surplus protein cannot be stored as amino acids, but it is not wasted. Most of the carbon of the amino acids is transformed eventually to carbohydrate or fat.

Approximately 12 to 17 percent of the nitrogen in dietary protein is not oxidized, and is converted to ammonia and then eliminated from the body as urea.

Protein breakdown and synthesis is a constant process in the human body. During the growing years, there is a positive nitrogen balance, indicative of the need for increased synthesis of bodily tissue as the child grows and develops. In muscle-building programs, there is also a positive nitrogen balance, the increased protein being assimilated in the muscle tissue. During some conditions associated with athletics, there may be a negative nitrogen balance, as in the wrestler or boxer who undertakes a starvation program to make a certain weight class. In general, however, in the adult on a normal diet, the synthesis and breakdown of bodily protein appears to be exactly balanced. White, Handler and Smith (1973) have indicated that the factors regulating the rates of protein synthesis and degradation are not fully understood, but apparently the supply of amino acids is not the rate limiting factor. This may be true for the normal individual, but may not apply to the athlete training for increases in muscle mass, especially if done in conjunction with the utilization of anabolic steroids.

One other aspect of protein metabolism deserves some

attention in this discussion, as some have contended that knowledge of the specific dynamic action (SDA) of protein may be useful in the design of a weight reducing diet. Berland (1974) has noted that following a meal, the metabolic rate rises, and that it rises in relationship to the composition of the foodstuff ingested. Fats and carbohydrates elevate the metabolic rate approximately 4 to 6 percent, while protein elevates it approximately 30 percent. This is the SDA of food. Although it is not clear as to why protein has such a high SDA, Burton (1965) hypothesized that it may be due to the additional energy needed to deaminate the amino acids to form urea or convert them to carbohydrate and fat in the liver. The role of the SDA in dieting will be discussed in Chapter Ten.

ATHLETIC TRAINING AND PROTEIN NEEDS

As indicated previously, the RDA for the average adult is 0.8 g/kg body weight/day. For a boy or girl going through the developmental years, the RDA is higher, being about 2.0 g/kg during the very early years, to 1.0 g/kg during the ages eleven to fourteen. During the ages fifteen to eighteen, the value approximates 0.9 g/kg. Thus, during the years when an individual might be undergoing serious athletic training, the normal protein requirement, as specified by the National Research Council, approximates 1 g/kg body weight.

Some authorities recommend increased allowances of protein during athletic training, while others believe the RDA approximation of 1 g/kg body weight is sufficient. Although the National Research Council (1974) notes that vigorous activity may elicit substantial losses of nitrogen through the skin, and small amounts of protein may be required for the development of muscles during conditioning, there is little evidence that muscular activity increases the need for protein, especially in light of the margin of safety built into the RDA protein allowance. Moreover, experts in the area of work physiology have contended that as long as the diet is adequate and varied, the protein requirements of the body during training may be met. Additional amounts of protein tablets or extreme meat diets do not stimulate an increase in muscle mass (Astrand and Rodahl, 1970).

Those who recommend increased protein intake during athletic training have cited some rather cogent rationales. The increased protein has been theorized to facilitate the development of muscle mass or to prevent a condition called sports anemia or protein anemia. Darden and Schendel (1971) cited several reports whereby protein intake of 3 g/kg or higher has been recommended for weightlifters in training. Reports of Russian research (Unsigned, 1971a) have indicated recommendations of 2.5-3.0 g/kg for athletes engaged in moderate exercise for prolonged periods, due to the fact that nitrogen losses are increased and may lead to negative nitrogen balance. The same report recommended 2.4-2.5 g/kg for those athletes training for speed and strength. Enriching the diet with protein during the rest period following exercise has been theorized to contribute to increased muscle protein synthesis after the catabolic effects of exercise. Buskirk and Haymes (1972) noted that in some athletic events where trauma may occur, such as in football or wrestling, the developing athlete might need 2.5 g protein/kg/day due to the need for the repair of damaged tissue and synthesis of new tissue. They also noted that protein intake as high as 20 percent of the ingested calories might be appropriate for the growing athlete. It should be emphasized that Buskirk and Haymes are referring to the growing athlete, not the mature individual.

Other studies and reports corroborate these recommendations. According to Bogart and her associates (1973), there is an increased need for protein during training on the order of 2 g/kg/day, for they note that muscle tissue as well as the plasma proteins and the iron-containing muscle and blood proteins must be built. Celejowa and Homa (1970) conducted a study of weightlifter's diets during training, and recommended a daily protein requirement of 2.0-2.2 g/kg. Travers and Campbell (1974) indicated that whenever an individual trains to develop strength and power, the daily intake of protein must be increased from an approximate normal value of 70-120 g/day. They also cited the need for an increased rate of repair following the increased rate of breakdown of muscle tissue caused by the increased work. Yamaji (1951a) in one of the earlier studies dealing with protein metabolism in hard muscular exercise, noted that positive nitrogen retention occurs as training continues, and that dietary protein supplements should be used daily during hard training. In general, the reports cited above recommended increased protein intake due to its effect on enhancing muscle tissue growth and repair.

Others have recommended extra protein because prolonged exercise has been associated with a condition called sports anemia. In an early study, Yamaji (1951b) reported that at the beginning of training, red blood cells (RBC), hemoglobin and serum protein, as well as other blood parameters, decrease regardless of the amount of protein intake. If protein intake is in the range of 1 to 1.5 g/kg/day, the decrease in hemoglobin and serum protein cannot be easily recovered even a month after training. Yamaji explained the decrease, noting that the muscle needs protein during training and it receives it at the expense of the blood proteins. A remarkable anemia develops due to the loss of blood protein, probably due to increases in muscle myoglobin. Thus, Yamaji recommended protein supplementation for a month or so during the early stages of training. Yoshimura (1970), in a review of studies by his Japanese colleagues, documented the fact that increased destruction of RBC's during exercise has been known for over sixty years. He indicated the mechanism involved the release of a hemolyzing factor from the spleen during exercise, probably initiated by adrenalin. Thus, the protein hemoglobin which is released is utilized to produce muscle protein and new RBC's. Yoshimura further suggested that the destruction of the RBC's is one of the adaptive reactions of exercise which promotes hypertrophy of the muscle. He concluded that dietary protein at the level of 2 g/kg body weight was required to prevent an athlete in training from developing sports anemia.

Several other rationale for dietary supplementation of protein have been advanced by Russian investigators (Unsigned, 1971a). They noted that physiological studies have shown that foods rich in proteins increase the excitability of the nervous system, enhance reflex activity, and increase the speed of reaction and ability to concentrate. Vegetable oils rich in methionine, an amino acid, have been recommended because it may contribute to the rise in efficiency of prolonged exercise.

Although it has been recommended by a number of professionals that protein intake be increased during athletic training, there is not very much objective experimental evidence to support these contentions, especially in the trained, mature athlete. In relation to sports anemia, Consolazio and Johnson (1972) have reported there is no conclusive evidence at the present time that indicates that muscular activity results in an increased destruction of cellular protein in individuals on a normal diet. However, Mole and Johnson (1971) found that exercise may increase protein catabolism. They noted that the mechanisms underlying the increased protein loss, measured by excretion of both nitrogen and sulfur, are not fully understood, but may be due to the catabolism of proteins that have leaked out of the muscles during exercise.

In a relatively controlled study, to directly study the problem of sports anemia, Rasch and his colleagues (1969a) utilized officer candidates as subjects, and evenly matched an experimental and control group based upon physical fitness scores. Using a double blind experimental design, each subject received one tablet/kg body weight. The tablet for the experimental group contained 0.69 g protein, consisting of milk powder, casein, soya protein and gelatin. It had all the essential amino acids except arginine. The control group received a placebo. Thus, all subjects undertook the same training program at a Marine Corps training center, which could be construed as hard physical training; the only basic difference was the protein supplementation to the experimental group. The blood analysis to check for sports anemia consisted of tests for RBC count, hematocrit, hemoglobin and reticulocyte count. Some of the tests at the end of three days training were suggestive of sports anemia as described by Yoshimura. There was a drop in hemoglobin and hematocrit, but the authors attributed this to the dilution effect of expanded plasma volume rather than an anemic effect per se, i.e. destruction of RBC's. However, it should be noted that the plasma volume was not actually measured. Nonetheless, the authors hypothesized that if the RBC's are destroyed, the reticulocyte number would increase; this did not occur. Another interesting point was that the tendency towards the sports anemia occurred in the experimental group who were receiving the protein supplementation. On the basis of their findings, the authors concluded there was no evidence of sports anemia after three days of hard training. Rasch and his associates noted that the difference between the findings of their investigation and that of Yoshimura may have been due to the choice of subjects. Yoshimura used dogs, whose spleen has a different role as compared to man.

In relationship to strength and power development the results of the limited number of studies are contradictory relative to the effect of protein supplementation. In an early report, Kraut and Muller (1950), using two undernourished subjects, studied the effect of vigorous muscular training at two different levels of protein intake — 55 g and 100 g. No increase in muscle strength was noted during the first four weeks while on the lower protein intake, but their strength gradually increased during the following four weeks while on the high protein level. The authors concluded that high protein intake was necessary for maintenance of high muscle strength. In a subsequent report, Kraut and his associates (1953) found a doubling of strength over a three-month period when two subjects received 2 g protein/kg/day in conjunction with heavy training. They studied the same two subjects over an additional 4.5 months with lower levels of protein in the diet. They concluded that protein supplementation and heavy exercise were necessary for increased muscle tissue and strength. The nature of these experiements, with a very limited number of subjects and an ineffective control condition, precludes a valid generalization relative to the effectiveness of protein supplementation on strength development. Travers and Campbell (1974) cited two recent experiments, both double blind, wherein the effects of supplemental protein increased the strength of college students engaged in a training program to a greater extent than other students in either a control or placebo group. However, no other data or references were provided beyond this statement, and thus the details of the experiments could not be explored.

In the only two studies uncovered which reported the experimental methodology, no significant effects of protein supplementation on strength or power were noted. In the report by Rasch and his associates (1969a) concerning sports anemia, discussed previously, tests of strength, power and local muscular endurance were also administered to the experimental and control groups. Although significant increases were noted in these tests of physical performance, they were attributed to the physical training since there was no significant difference between the control group and experimental groups. Thus, they concluded that protein supplementation had no effect on physical performance.

In an earlier study, Rasch and Pierson (1962) evaluated the effect of a protein supplement on muscular strength and hypertrophy. Thirty male adult subjects were matched on strength scores and assigned to either an experimental or control group. The experimental group received 10 tablets/day of a protein dietary supplement; the total protein content was 25 g/day. The control group received a placebo in this double blind study. All supplements were taken daily during the six weeks of training. Although both groups made significant gains in strength on the four isotonic lifts, there was no difference between the groups. Thus, the authors concluded that the protein supplement was not effective in increasing strength or hypertrophy during training. One possible limitation to this study was the amount of protein, only 25 g/day total, which would average about .33 g/kg for a 75 kg adult.

The role of protein supplementation in promoting gains in body weight has not been completely elucidated. If one consumed extra protein, which resulted in extra caloric intake, theoretically the extra protein would not be utilized by the body to synthesize muscle tissue, but would be converted to carbohydrate or fat for utilization or storage in the energy scheme. Few studies have been uncovered which have adequately assessed the role of protein supplementation upon body weight gains. Since body fat is not much of an advantage in many sports, analysis of body weight gains should involve the determination of body composition to insure that the accumulated weight is lean body mass, i.e. muscle tissue, rather than adipose tissue. Furthermore, to provide an adequate stimulus for the deposition of the protein supplement as muscle mass, a proper training regimen should be followed. As progressive resistive exercise (PRE) training with weights or other tension producing devices has been shown to hypertrophy muscle mass, a training program stressing some form of weightlifting should be utilized. As PRE is anabolic in and by itself, the protein supplementation, in conjunction with a PRE program, should be compared with a PRE program with no supplementation, or a placebo to mimic the protein.

In the study previously reported by Rasch and Pierson (1962), the protein supplementation, on the order of 25 g/day, did not augment the PRE effect. As a matter of fact, neither the PRE program with or without protein supplementation significantly increased the body weight. On the other hand, several other reports did report significant body weight gains when protein supplementation was used. Sims (1970) used twenty male high school students as subjects, placing ten each in a control and experimental group. The experimental group consumed one 12.5 ounce can of Nutrament® daily, with a composition of 25 g protein, 44 g carbohydrate and a total of 375 calories. The control group had a 12.5 ounce serving of a chocolate flavored placebo containing one calorie. All subjects were on the same exercise program, which consisted of weight training and conditioning exercises. Over the period of study, the experimental group gained 11.1 pounds compared to 3.7 for the controls. Greater chest and arm girths were also noted for the experimental group. However, no statistical analysis was used and the nature of the body weight gain was not determined by body composition analysis; the weight gain may have consisted mainly of body fat although the increased arm and chest girth measurements would provide some evidence that the gain was in musculature. In addition, although the author did not state he was evaluating protein supplementation per se, it would be difficult to determine whether the weight gain was due to the protein or to the calories in the supplement. Would the replacement of the protein by 25 g carbohydrate elicit the same effect?

In a similar study, Blanchard (1972) evaluated the effect of a high protein-calorie liquid food supplement upon the prevention of body weight loss during early preseason football practice at Stanford University. There were forty subjects, twenty each in an experimental and control group. The experimental group consumed a 10 ounce can with a weight gaining formula, one at each meal for the two week study. Each can contained 675 calories, with 35 g protein, 50 g carbohydrate, and 37 g fat. No placebo mixture was reported for the control group. Although no statistical analysis or body composition analysis was noted, the experimental group gained an average of 3.9 pounds, and the control group lost 4.6 pounds. No physical performance data was collected.

Crooks (1975) recently offered some suggestions for high school and college athletes relative to the use of protein supplementation in weight gaining programs. First. the athlete should ascertain whether or not increased weight will benefit performance in his sport; in football it might, but in gymnastics and cross country running it could be a disadvantage. If the answer is yes, Crooks suggests the following:

1. Set a reasonable target goal.
2. Keep careful and exacting measurements of body weight, height, body fat and muscle girths at standard reference points. He notes that reference points should include the neck, upper and lower arm, chest, abdomen, thigh and calf.
3. Use a protein with a high biological value, such as 65 percent utilizable protein. He noted that there are a number of protein tablets and powders on the market which will meet this requirement. They usually average about 15 g/heaping tablespoon, whereas an egg contains about 6 g protein. If you use a 90 percent protein powder supplement, he recommended it should also contain a natural enzyme to aid digestion. Flavored powders and protein candy bars are also available.
4. The dose should be about 45 g protein/day, in three separate doses at 15 g.
5. Caloric supplementation is also needed so the protein may be used for tissue building, not as an energy source.

Although Crooks recommended this program, he offered no scientific data to support its effectiveness, although personal experiences were cited. In the growing athlete, maybe caloric supplementation alone would be effective in increasing body weight, as extra protein would be a natural constituent of the foods he would eat for extra calories, if selected judiciously.

Several reports are available relative to the effect of protein deprivation upon physical performance. Darling and his colleagues (1944) classified twenty-four subjects into three equal groups of eight each. One group received a normal diet, and the other two had a high protein and low protein diet, respectively. The dietary phase of the experiment was eight weeks in duration. The criterion measure for physical performance was a thirty-minute step test. The authors noted no deleterious or beneficial effects on the physical vigor or efficiency of men on low or high protein diets. The high protein diet contained 160 g protein/day, while the low diet had 50-55 g. Although this study is over thirty years old, the 50-55 g protein ratio would not be construed as deficient in the normal male today. In a more contemporary report, Rodahl and others (1962) compared the effectiveness of four different diets upon maximal oxygen uptake and maximal endurance capacity. The four diets were mixtures of normal and low caloric content and normal and low protein. After base line data was gathered on the normal diet (3000 cal, 70 g protein), the subjects were studied for ten days on each of the other diets. The normal calorie-low protein diet (3000 cal, 4 g protein), low calorie-normal protein diet (1500 cal, 70 g protein), and the low calorie-low protein diet (1500 cal, 4 g protein) had no deleterious effects upon the maximal performance tests when performed at normal temperature. However, the low calorie and low protein diets, when coupled with a prolonged cold stress at 8°C, elicited a decrease in physical working capacity within a few days. The results of this study indicate that short term restriction of calorie or protein intake exerts no adverse effect upon maximal endurance capacity. There may be some implications for wrestlers who must control body weight through dietary restriction.

In man, protein synthesis is affected by the male hormone, testosterone. In recent years, certain drugs called anabolic steroids have been developed to elicit the protein synthesis, or anabolic, effect of testosterone. A review of their effectiveness on body composition and strength changes has been presented elsewhere (Williams, 1974). In order to elicit increased muscle mass and strength, the ingestion of anabolic steroids must be accompanied by PRE training and adequate calorie and protein supplementation. When these conditions have been met, a number of studies have reported increased strength levels and muscle mass although other studies have not found such increases. However, the vast majority of these experiments were designed to evaluate the effectiveness of anabolic steroids and did not compare protein supplementation per se with a control group. Thus, no generalization about protein supplementation per se may be made.

Is protein supplementation, in the form of high protein commercial products or high meat diets, necessary for the attainment of increased muscle mass during a training program? The general answer is no. During a weight gaining program, the athlete may need some slight additional protein in order to assure the necessary amino acids for muscle synthesis. Many authorities, including Buskirk and Haymes (1972) advise dietary protein intake approximating 2 g/kg body weight/day for the developing athlete or one who is on a muscle building weight training program. However, they also note that the mature athlete can subsist and maintain protein balance on 1 g/kg/day. Darden and Schendel (1971) have also noted that once an athlete achieves desired weight, he can maintain that level with 1 g protein/kg/day. Moreover, Horstman (1972) concluded that the normal diet in western industrialized countries provides adequate protein intake, and during heavy training, if the diet increases, the protein intake should automatically increase also.

The average weight for a male between the ages of fifteen to eighteen approximates 60 to 70 kg, or 132 to 154 pounds. The average caloric intake is 3000 calories. If the protein content of his diet is normal, about 15 percent, then 450 calories are derived from protein sources. This would represent approximately 110 g protein, or 1.8 g/kg for the 60 kg body and 1.6 g/kg for the 70 kg boy. If the boy becomes active in athletic training, his caloric intake would naturally increase to meet the increased energy demands of physical activity. If the caloric intake increased to 4000, and the percentage of protein remained stable, 600 calories would be derived from protein, the equivalent of 150 g. Thus the 60 kg and 70 kg males would be receiving 2.5 g and 2.1 g protein/kg respectively. This represents the recommended protein content for those in active training. Buskirk and Haymes (1972) have recommended that the protein content of the diet be increased to 20 percent in developing athletes. This would increase the grams of protein/kg even greater.

The general conclusion, based upon the available evidence and theoretical considerations, is that protein supplementation during athletic training is or should be met by increased caloric consumption in the normal diet. Commercial protein supplements may have some usefulness if the athlete is not assured of adequate protein in his diet, but they are relatively expensive in relation to natural sources of protein and are not highly recommended.

One other aspect of protein's role in the diet of the athlete deserves consideration, and that is the protein content of the pregame meal. This topic is discussed in Chapter Eleven.

CHAPTER **SIX** _____

THE ROLE OF VITAMINS
IN PHYSICAL ACTIVITY

$\mathbf{V}$ITAMINS REPRESENT A number of relatively unrelated organic substances that are found in small amounts in
many foods. They are essential for the optimal functioning of a
number of diverse bodily functions, and since some of these physiological functions are important during increased levels of physical activity, some authorities have contended that vitamin
supplementation is necessary in order for the athlete to maximize
his potential. One recent advertisement displayed the all purpose
vitamin selected for use by the United States Olympic team, the
implication being that its use was associated with superior athletic performance.

To be sure, there is a necessity for a certain amount of selected
vitamins in the diet of man. Lack of a certain vitamin may cause a
deficiency disease. This was a main cause of many disorders in the
past, and vitamin deficiency diseases still persist in some parts of
the world today. However, in a modern industrial society with a
well-balanced diet, outright deficiency diseases are rare.
Nevertheless, in a review of studies of vitamin and mineral nutrition in the United States from 1950-1968, Davis and his associates
(1969) concluded that a significant proportion of the population
examined had intakes below the RDA and some of the biochemical indices were in the deficient range. They noted also that the
dietary habits of Americans have become worse since 1960. Thus,
a number of vitamin and mineral supplements have been on the
market for years, and vitamin production is a main function of
many drug companies.

Vitamin supplements fall into various categories according to
their potency. Prescription vitamins are classified as a drug and
may only be prescribed by a physician. Over-the-counter vitamin
pills include the therapeutic or high potency vitamins, sometimes
called megavitamins, and the regular vitamin supplements that

supply the daily requirements found essential to man. However, except for persons with special medical needs, the Food and Nutrition Board of the National Research Council has indicated there is no available scientific justification for recommending the routine use of vitamin supplements. They noted that vitamins and minerals are supplied in abundant amounts by commonly available foods.

Tatkon (1968), in his excellent analysis *The Great Vitamin Hoax,* indicated the American public is being defrauded, for manufacturers and advertisers are implying that our diets are inadequate in vitamins when in truth they are not. He has severely criticized the vitamin industry, noting that vitamin supplements have been suggested as cures for medical problems ranging from gall bladder difficulties to gray hair, and that advertisers have perpetuated the myth that many diseases stem from a faulty diet; hence, the conclusion to be inferred is that you are not getting all the vitamins you need.

As vitamins are in almost everything one eats or drinks, the individual on a well-balanced diet will receive the RDA, the amount recommended to maintain a good nutritional state in all healthy individuals. This value is usually larger than the minimal daily requirement (MDR), that amount needed to prevent vitamin deficiency. Many foods today, such as milk and bread, are also fortified with vitamins, thus helping to insure vitamin sufficiency. The measurements for the RDA are usually expressed as IU (International Units), or USP (United States Pharmacopia units); both standards are related to the biological activity of the vitamin. Only prolonged exposure to an inadequate diet will cause any of the vitamin deficiency diseases.

According to Tatkon (1968), there are several misconceptions about vitamins of which the general public should be cognizant. Contrary to popular belief, vitamins can be harmful, especially overdosages of the fat soluble A and D which may accumulate in the tissues over a period of time. Secondly, taking vitamins will not make up for a skipped breakfast, for they have no caloric value. Relative to purchasing vitamin supplements, a brand name does not mean a better vitamin. Thus, the cheapest brand should be purchased. In addition, there is no essential difference between a synthetic and natural vitamin, the only difference being the manner of production.

In summary, Tatkon (1968) concluded that vitamin supplements appear to have little or no practical value for the average American, much less for the athletic performer. However, the use of numerous vitamins and minerals as potential ergogenic aids still persists among many world class performers, as well as the local high school athlete.

USE OF VITAMINS BY ATHLETES

A number of recent reports have indicated widespread use of vitamin supplementation in the athletic world. One contributing factor may be the fact that while many drugs are illegal, vitamin and mineral supplements are not since they are considered to be foods. Thus, the athlete searching for an ergogenic aid may believe that a particular vitamin or mineral will provide the needed ergogenic effect. Van Huss (1974) cited a report that 84 percent of Olympic athletes used vitamin supplements. In a report to a United States Senate subcommittee studying the role of drugs in athletics, a team physician for the 1968 United States Olympic team reported the widespread use of various food supplements, including multivitamins, vitamin B_{12} and vitamin E. He also noticed some athletes consuming as much as 10,000 mg vitamin C in one day, and receiving injections of 1000 mg vitamin B_{12} an hour before competition (United States Senate, 1973). Novich (1973) reported that weight lifters, in conjunction with anabolic steroids, consumed prodigious amounts of vitamin B_{12}, iron, vitamin C and other vitamins in the B complex family. Talbot (1974), the assistant coach of the Canadian national swim team, indicated he was not aware of a hard training distance athlete who could be successful without vitamin supplementation or some forms of mineral supplements. He did note that his comments were based upon personal observations. In an interview with Jim Ryan, a world record holder in the mile run, Maddox (1974) reported that the runner's diet was rather normal, although he did take vitamins C and E.

Some rather authoritative reports have recommended the

utilization of vitamin supplements by athletes in training. Even as early as 1922, Sherman and Smith (1922) noted that athletes may require additional quantities of vitamins A, B and C in order to elicit full stimulation of all body secretions and to prevent nervousness. Although Marrack (1948) indicated that it is doubtful that athletic performances are improved by vitamins, more recent comments in sports medicine books and athletic journals may imply otherwise. Klafs and Arnheim (1973) noted that extremely demanding endurance activities may increase the normal requirement for vitamin B, vitamin C and others as much as fifteen times, an apparent misinterpretation of the available research. They do note however, based on their own research and others, that vitamin supplementation will not markedly improve performance unless a deficiency exists. Cureton (1969a) also noted that during hard training, the work stress can deplete a number of critical body nutrients, such as vitamins B and C, which should be replaced.

In a translation of Yakovlev's book on Russian experimentation with nutrition and athletic performance, recommendations for increased levels of vitamins B_1, B_6, C, and E were stressed. The Russian researchers indicated that the most effective enrichment of the body included a complex of vitamins: A, B_1, B_2, B_5, B_6, B_{12}, C, D, E, and PP (Unsigned, 1971a). This viewpoint was recently reiterated by Yakovlev and Rogozkin (1975). Other European reports (Prokop, 1965; Scheunert and Grafe, 1961; Nocker, 1970) have recommended vitamin supplements for athletes in different sports. Table 6-I represents the vitamin dosage recommendations of Nocker and Glatzel (1963) for different sportsmen. *PP* is the pellagra preventing vitamin known as niacin, nicotinic acid or nicotinamide.

The utilization of vitamin supplements by athletes may have some rationale. In 1972, the United States Department of Health, Education and Welfare completed a ten-state survey and found some problems with several nutrients, mainly deficiencies in iron and several vitamins (White, 1974). Williams (1962) indicated that evidence exists that vitamin C and some of the B complex vitamins are not present in sufficient quantities in the normal diet, and Klafs and Arnheim (1973) suggested some athletes may suffer

TABLE 6-1

VITAMIN DOSAGE RECOMMENDATIONS FOR DIFFERENT

ATHLETES IN MG/DAY

Vitamin	Non-Athletes	Power and Strength Athletes	Endurance Athletes
A	1.5	2	2
B_1	1.5	4-6	6-10
B_2	2	3	4
PP	20	25	25-30
C	75	100-200	100-300
D	2	2	2
E	5	7	10

*From Nocker, J. and Glatzel, H., DIE ERNAHRUNG DES SPORTLERS, 1963. Courtesy of Nationales Olympisches Komitee fur Deutschland.

trom a vitamin shortage of sufficient degree to lessen their effectiveness. Thus, if the athlete is not on a well-balanced diet, vitamin supplementation may be advisable. However, vitamin supplements are consumed by athletes who are on sound diets, with the thought that physiological functions will be improved. Some implications have been suggested by exercise physiologists. Buskirk and Haymes (1972) indicated that if the number of mitochondria in the muscle cells increases with physical conditioning, then additional vitamin cofactor linkages may be necessary to support the increased mitochondria enzymatic reactions. Some of the B vitamins play important roles in the energy schema in the muscle cell mitochondria. Zauner and Updyke (1973) stated that most endurance athletes take large daily dosages of vitamin C in an effort to stimulate myocardial and skeletal muscle capillarization, with the theoretical beneficial effect of increasing physical efficiency.

Although some contend that vitamin supplementation will enhance athletic performance capacity, the available objective experimental evidence appears to be rather limited. In the remainder of the chapter, each vitamin will be discussed in relation to the theoretical physiological application to athletics and the available experimental evidence.

Although vitamins are usually identified by names descriptive of their chemical nature, e.g. ascorbic acid, the old terminology persists and thus will be discussed in alphabetical order with the chemical name or names in parentheses.

VITAMIN A (RETINOL)

Vitamin A is an unsaturated alcohol and exists mainly in mammals and saltwater fish as preformed vitamin A, or retinol. Carotene, notably beta-carotene, is found in many fruits and dark green and yellow vegetables; carotenes are readily converted into vitamin A in the human body. Vitamin A deficiency has a profound effect on virtually every organ, and deficiency has been associated with skin lesions, cessation of skeletal growth and night blindness. However, the store of vitamin A in the liver may meet the demand for years in one who has been well fed. Although vitamin A is associated with a number of bodily functions, except for its role in the visual process, its exact metabolic functions are unknown (White, Handler and Smith, 1973).

Vitamin A is one of the fat soluble vitamins and hence may be stored in the body for considerable periods of time in contrast to the water soluble vitamins. Overdosages over a period of time may cause a condition known as hypervitaminosis A, characterized by loss of appetite, loss of hair, enlargement of the liver and spleen, swelling over the long bones and general irritability (Tatkon, 1968). White, Handler and Smith (1973) noted possible limitations to motion with hypervitaminosis A. The 1974 RDA varies by age, but the daily values for the average male are 1000 retinol units or 5000 IU; female values are, respectively, 800 and 4000. Bair (1951) cited a case of vitamin A poisoning in a child who received 240,000 IU daily for three months.

The application of vitamin A supplementation to athletics

does not appear to be substantiated upon theoretical or practical bases, although Russian research (Unsigned, 1971a) has suggested that in sports requiring considerable eye alertness and stress, extra vitamin A is needed. One early experiment relative to vitamin A deficiency upon maximal endurance capacity was uncovered. Wald and his associates (1942) placed five subjects on a vitamin A deficient diet for six months, and then placed them on a vitamin supplement program for six weeks. Physical performance was tested on a treadmill, with a fifteen-minute warm-up followed by a run to exhaustion. Measures of heart rate, oxygen uptake, lung ventilation and blood lactate were monitored. For thirty days prior to the initial test, the subjects received a diet with a high level of vitamin A, thus starting the experiment with a high baseline level. In general, during the six months of the vitamin A deficiency, no significant decrements were noted on physiological functions during submaximal or maximal exercise. Endurance capacity was not compromised. However, the authors noted that the plasma vitamin A maintained its initial level throughout the entire experimental deprivation period. In addition, no significant effects were elicited during the six weeks of supplementation.

It would appear that vitamin A supplementation is not necessary in athletes on an adequate diet. Bodily stores are available for short term deficiency periods. There is also the possibility of some pathological disorders due to prolonged overdosage.

THE B VITAMINS

There are a number of different organic compounds that help regulate diverse metabolic functions which have been categorized as the B vitamins or the vitamin B complex. White (1974) has noted that the expression vitamin B complex is less frequently used as more is learned about the individual B vitamins. Thus, the terms vitamin B_1, B_2, B_3 are not utilized in the scientific literature since they are known by other names, thiamine, riboflavin and niacin. The B vitamins are thiamine, riboflavin, niacin, pyridoxine, pantothenic acid, folic acid, cyanocobalamin and biotin. Although the following are not known as vitamins in the strictest sense of the word, they have been historically grouped with the B vitamins: choline, inositol and para-aminobenzoic acid. The B complex term is useful, however, since many of the factors in it are found together in nature. The B vitamins are water soluble, hence their storage in the human body is not significant.

Although Olson (1958) has characterized the B complex vitamin as the "great American placebo," the use of vitamin B supplementation in athletics has been advocated by several authorities due to the diverse roles of the B vitamins in energy metabolism. Keys (1943) noted that the capacity to perform physical work is obviously hindered by the development of vitamin deficiency states, and since thiamine, riboflavin and niacin function in the enzyme systems basic to energy production, an increased need may occur during exercise. Bourne (1948) reported that the vitamin requirement for the B complex may be increased four to five times during exercise, and he posed the question whether an athlete attempting to attain an Olympic standard could fulfill his vitamin requirements from the food he normally eats. Bourne concluded that, on the whole, the literature supports the view that added vitamins have a beneficial effect on muscular exercise. Although Mayer and Bullen (1960b) have noted that water soluble vitamin supplementation does not appear to convey an additional advantage to the athlete, there is a paucity of evidence available. Thus, during hard exercise, increased demands for these vitamins may be made by the body. Relative to the psychological aspects of sports, Watson (1972) has noted that vitamin B deficiency may affect brain metabolism, and hence alter psychic behavior.

Each individual vitamin in the B family which has been studied in relationship to physical performance is discussed below. In those studies where two or more vitamins in the B complex were investigated, they are grouped under the heading "B complex." Other studies which combined the B complex with other vitamins are covered in a later chapter.

Vitamin B_1 (Thiamine)

Thiamine, vitamin B_1, plays an important role in energy metabolism and the nervous system. It is a water soluble vitamin, a deficiency of which leads to beriberi, a condition rarely seen in the Western world except in cases of chronic alcoholism. Thiamine is found in the outer layers of seeds, and in other good sources, including animal tissues such as meat, fish and poultry, eggs, milk, cheese, whole grain, enriched breads and cereals, dried beans and peas and all vegetables.

Early and Carlson (1969) indicated that thiamine may modify physiological processes in order to deter fatigue. Thiamine plays an important role in the oxidative decarboxylation of pyruvate to acetyl CoA for entrance into the Krebs cycle and subsequent oxidation to ATP. If the thiamine level was deficient, the increased demand for acetyl CoA during physical activity would not be met; hence, more pyruvate would be converted to lactic acid, and possibly fatigue would develop. Early and Carlson also noted thiamine deficiency could result in inadequate amounts of succinate, a coingredient of heme. A deficiency in heme would limit the oxygen carrying capacity of the blood. Brozek (1962), analyzing the research reports emanating from the Institute of Nutrition of the U.S.S.R. Academy of Medical Sciences, noted the relationship of thiamine to glucose metabolism, glucose being essential for the optimal functioning of the central nervous system.

The need for thiamine replenishment would appear to be dependent upon the daily loss. As related to exercise, the National Research Council (1974) noted that the need for thiamine is dependent upon energy expenditure and is influenced by carbohydrate intake. Nijakowski (1966) studied the changes in thiamine content of twelve athletes and twelve nonathletes after two work tasks. One was a short submaximal exercise of 900 kgm/min for six minutes, while the second was a four hour skiing excursion of 12 kilometers with a 1500 feet incline. His results indicated a drop in the thiamine content after the four hour exercise in the athletes, but no change after the short term exercise. The nonathletes did not experience any drop in thiamine, a rather confusing finding.

Some older sports medicine books have implied that athletes may need fifteen times the amount of thiamine in heavy training as at rest. This recommendation is based on an erroneous interpretation and application of the research by Bicknell and Prescott (1953). They reported that the thiamine requirement is proportional to the metabolic rate, and physical exertion can elevate the metabolic rate fifteen times. However, this is not to imply that the athlete needs a fifteen-fold increase in his daily thiamine requirement. It is probably just proportional to the time spent in physical activity. The National Research Council (1974) has reported that as energy expenditure is increased during physical activity, the increased needs for thiamine, or any other nutrient, should be met by the larger quantities of foods consumed, provided that they are well selected. Nevertheless, Vytchikova (1958) has indicated that the usual content of thiamine (1.5-2.0 mg/day) in food rations of athletes is considered inefficient, and that medical observations recommend approximately 10-20 mg daily supplementation.

Since the role of thiamine in energy metabolism has been known for over thirty years, it has been one of the most studied vitamins in relation to physical performance. Even so, the total number of relevant studies is limited. Many of the studies with thiamine were conducted in association with riboflavin and niacin and are covered in a later section. The following represents the available research dealing with the utilization of thiamine alone.

After reviewing the pre-1939 studies, Boje (1939) contended that there is no value to extra amounts of thiamine. Throughout the 1940's, several conflicting reports were published. In most cases, experimental methodology was inadequate to validly assess the role of thiamine. With little detail available, Gounelle (1940) reported that the supplementation of diets of bicyclists with vitamin B_1 improved their performance during the Tour de France race in 1939. McCormick (1940) suggested that increased thiamine intake would improve oxygen uptake and sustained physical performance. In an experiment with no controls, no statistical treatment, and tremendous potential for placebo effect, he reported significant gains on an endurance arm-holding test after one week of B_1 supplementation. Karpovich and Millman (1942) replicated McCormick's study with better controls, using pre- and post-test scores as well as a control placebo group. The thiamine supplement was 5 mg/day for one week. There was no significant effect of the thiamine on the arm endurance test.

Several other studies during the 1940's were centered around the effect of thiamine deficiency upon physical performance. Keys and his colleagues (1943), in four series of complex experiments each ten to twelve weeks long, studied the effect of controlled thiamine intake upon a number of performance parameters, including strength, and responses during brief exhausting work and prolonged severe work. There were four subjects in each series of experiments, and the average thiamine intakes in the four series were 0.63, 0.53, 0.33 and 0.23 mg/1000 calories. The results indicated, for the period of time studied, no benefit of any kind upon the physical performance parameters was produced by an intake of more than 0.23 mg/1000 calories. Since the diet was normal except for thiamine control, and consisted of 3000 calories/day, the lowest level of thiamine intake for a ten to twelve week period was 0.69 mg/day. For the males used in this study, this value would be approximately half of the RDA. One possible limitation would be the fact that the subjects did not appear to work to exhaustion in all tests, and apparently maximal performance capacity was not assessed.

In a later study by Archdeacon and Murlin (1944), three persons were subjected to a moderate exercise workload and a workload to exhaustion on a bicycle ergometer during a period of thiamine deprivation. The subjects were restricted to thiamine intakes of 0.27 mg/day on one diet and 0.15 mg/day on another. The general results reflected a decline in muscular endurance within ten to fourteen days on the deficient diet, increasing back to normal when the vitamins were restored. However, they also noted that the inclusion of B complex vitamins in a diet already adequate in these vitamins did not result in increased muscular endurance. In another study relative to thiamine deficiency in the diet, Tuttle and his colleagues (1949a) reported that those subjects who received 2500 calories/day for 45 days, but were getting only .14 mg or less thiamine/day, suffered an increase in reaction time. In this latter case, the results would indicate an adverse effect upon the nervous system rather than the energy-producing aspects.

In the most recent revelation concerning the role of thiamine in the diet of the athlete, Steel (1970) noted that a group of Australian Olympians who gained places in the finals and some winning medals, were found to have higher thiamine intakes when compared to another group whose thiamine intakes were lower than the suggested allowances. Although not a controlled study, Steel recommended that the athlete should pay particular attention to his thiamine intake.

Although it appears that thiamine plays an important role in some metabolic processes associated with energy metabolism and central nervous system functioning, there is no conclusive evidence to support the contention that thiamine intake above and beyond normal RDA will enhance physical performance. Extra amounts are probably not harmful, as they will be excreted from the body. However, the expense and the creation of a belief in the mind of the athlete that thiamine is a magic ingredient are two reasons for recommending against thiamine supplementation.

Vitamin B₂ (Riboflavin)

Riboflavin, vitamin B_2, functions as a coenzyme for a group of flavoproteins concerned with biological oxidations, the most common one being flavin adenine dinucleotide (FAD). Riboflavin is found in liver, yeast, wheat germ, milk, cheese, meats, eggs and green leafy vegetables. Its role in man appears to be central to the oxidative reactions occurring in the energy schema of the mitochondria. The RDA for riboflavin has been computed at 0.6 mg/1000 calories for all persons. The average adult male, with a 3000 calorie diet, would need 1.8 mg/day. Since the National Research Council (1974) reported that there is no evidence that riboflavin requirements are raised when energy utilization is increased, the allowances are intended for individuals engaged in normal activity.

No research has been uncovered which has studied the role of riboflavin individually during physical exertion. However, it has been studied in conjunction with thiamine and niacin intake, and those studies are reported in a later section dealing with the B complex.

Vitamin B₃ (Niacin)

Niacin, vitamin B_3, is also known as a nicotinic acid, nicotinamide or the antipellagra vitamin. In the foreign literature it is ofttimes represented by the symbol *PP* or *pellagra preventive* vitamin. Niacin is widely distributed in plant and animal sources, being most abundant in poultry, meats, organ meats, fish, grain products, peanuts and peanut butter. Milk and eggs are almost completely empty of niacin. White, Handler and Smith (1973) have indicated it is difficult to assess the niacin requirement of man, as it may be synthesized in the body from tryptophan. The RDA is 6.6 mg/1000 calories.

The major function of niacin is to serve as a component of two important coenzymes concerned with glycolysis, fat synthesis and tissue respiration. Nicotinamide adenine dinucleotide (NAD) and nicotinamide adenine dinucleotide phosphate (NADP) serve as hydrogen acceptors in the energy schema. According to White, Handler and Smith (1973), no serious impairment of oxidative reactions have been demonstrated in tissues of niacin deficient animals. On the other hand, Bialecki (1962) observed an increase in niacin in the blood of man after a short exhausting exercise. He noted that these results suggest increased demand for niacin in physical exertion. With the role that NAD plays in glycolysis, it might be theorized that increased niacin levels might lead to increased anaerobic capacity.

An early report suggested an ergogenic effect of niacin, primarily in an anaerobic exercise task. Frankau (1943), although primarily studying the effects of multiple vitamin preparations upon physical performance, did conduct some experiments with niacin alone. The performance task was an agility test similar to a shuttle run with blocks. Subjects were tested 1.5 to 3 hours after taking 50-200 mg niacin. Highly significant improvements in shuttle run times were noted and Frankau concluded that niacin, given to fit young men, could result in increased efficiency in severe tests involving coordination and physical effort. It should be noted, however, that no statistical analysis was run on the data, and the explicit experimental methodology was not noted. In a later study, Hilsendager and Karpovich (1964) studied the effect of niacin, and glycine in combination with niacin, upon endurance capacity of eighty-six subjects as measured by performance on either a bicycle ergometer or forearm ergometer. The dosages consisted of either 750 mg glycine, 75 mg niacin, or a combination of the two. A double blind placebo experimental design was used with a double repeated measures application. The data from this well-designed experiment revealed no significant effect of the treatments upon the endurance task. The results of these two experiments are contradictory, but the more appropriate experimental design of the Hilsendager and Karpovich study lends support to the neutral effect of niacin.

In experimentation to investigate the acute effect of niacin, Carlson and Oro (1962) found that the plasma-free fatty acids (FFA) decreased within fifteen to thirty minutes following administration of niacin. After sixty to ninety minutes, the plasma FFA rose again. Since plasma FFA are a source of energy during prolonged submaximal work, there may be implications relative to niacin supplementation. In a subsequent study, Carlson and his associates (1963) reported that niacin greatly decreased mobilization of FFA into the blood at both rest and during exercise. The rise in the RQ and the fall in the plasma concentration of glucose following the administration of niacin suggests that increased combustion of carbohydrates occurred in association with the decreased availability of energy from FFA. However, the investigators noted that niacin had no effect on the efficiency of work. Jenkins (1965) also noted an increased RQ in subjects exercising for a prolonged period of time following the administration of niacin. Although the plasma FFA levels were changed little during exercise following the niacin, they did not rise as in the control trial; FFA normally rises during exercise. Therefore, the niacin blocked FFA mobilization from the fatty tissues in the body. However, Jenkins noted no difference in energy consumption as calculated from the RQ and oxygen uptake.

Some have contended that the reduction in plasma FFA could contribute to the development of fatigue, since muscle glycogen would be used at a faster rate during prolonged exercise. Bergstrom and his associates (1969) studied the effect of niacin on muscular endurance capacity in two series of experiments. The niacin blocked the release of FFA, thus the muscle used glycogen for its main source of energy. The ability to perform either short term near-maximal work or prolonged submaximal work was unchanged after administration of niacin. However, the subjects experienced the work after administration of niacin as heavier and more fatiguing. Thus, although glycogen was utilized to a greater degree during exercise, and theoretically has a greater efficiency ratio than the oxidation of fats, the objective evidence did not support a beneficial effect of niacin while the subjective evaluation of the work task suggested a detrimental effect.

Based upon current viewpoints, the use of niacin as an ergogenic food supplement is contraindicated. There is no substantial evidence to support a detrimental effect upon energy metabolism during a deficiency state, and supplementation above normal RDA has not increased endurance capacity.

Vitamin B$_6$ (Pyridoxine)

Vitamin B$_6$ is not a single substance, but rather a collective term for three naturally occurring pyridines — pyridoxine, pyridoxal and pyridoxamine — which are all metabolically and functionally related. Best sources for vitamin B$_6$ are meats, poultry, fish, potatoes, whole grain products, yeast, eggs and seeds. The adult RDA is 2 mg/day. Although White, Handler and Smith (1973) reported that there is no specific disease syndrome associated with a deficiency of B$_6$ in the diet, the National Research Council (1974) noted that depression and confusion may occur in adults, and other disorders, such as anemia, occur in children. Vitamin B$_6$ plays a central role in the biochemical reactions whereby a cell converts nutrient amino acids into the particular amino acid necessary for the cell's own activities. Buskirk and Haymes (1972) reported that vitamin B$_6$ is important in the formation of hemoglobin, myoglobin and the cytochromes, all compounds essential to the oxygen transportation and utilization processes in the body. Although one might theorize that B$_6$ would be helpful in endurance-type activities, no research has been uncovered relative to this point. In man, the requirement for B$_6$ also appears to increase when high protein diets are consumed, a finding which may have some implications for athletes on high protein diets. Since B$_6$ is found in meats and other animal products, it may be sufficiently provided if these foods are the source of the high protein diet.

Vitamin B_{12} (Cyanocobalamin)

Cyanocobalamin, vitamin B_{12}, is present in all body cells and appears to be essential for optimal functioning. Cobalt is part of its structure. It is found mainly in animal products, meats, cheese, organs, milk and eggs. One important point is that B_{12} is not found in plant foods, an observation which should be heeded by strict vegetarians. The RDA is 3 μg/day. The average diet contains 5-15 μg/day. Although the deficiency of B_{12} may cause several disorders, including some dysfunction of nerve cells, the main effect is pernicious anemia. White, Handler and Smith (1973) noted that pernicious anemia results not from an inadequate ingestion of B_{12}, but rather from an inadequate amount of gastric secretion of the intrinsic factor, which is known to facilitate absorption of B_{12} from the intestinal lumen.

Anemia in an athlete would adversely affect his endurance capacity, since the decreased amount of circulating RBC's and hemoglobin would restrict his oxygen-carrying capacity. There are a number of different causes of anemia, ranging from a lack of iron in the diet to bone marrow diseases. Iron deficiency anemia has been reported in athletes, especially females, and appropriate iron therapy may help ameliorate the condition. Pernicious anemia, or macrocytic anemia, is of a different cause, mainly lack of the intrinsic factor in the gastric juice and may be helped by B_{12} therapy techniques. The normal individual is more likely to have iron deficiency anemia rather than pernicious anemia. Thus, B_{12} will not benefit the normal athlete; yet, Hirata (1973) indicated that vitamin B_{12} injection is a common practice throughout the athletic world. Some athletes have been reported to receive 1000 mg an hour or so prior to competition. The belief probably persists that if a little B_{12} can prevent anemia, a lot will do something magical to increase capacity. Russian researchers (Unsigned, 1971a) have indicated a need for more research into the application of B_{12} to athletics, but Montoye has presented some useful evidence over twenty years ago. His experimentation was the only research uncovered relative to the ergogenic application of B_{12}.

Montoye and his colleagues (1955) studied the effect of B_{12} supplementation upon performance in a half mile run. Fifty-one boys, ranging in age from twelve to seventeen, who were residents of a state institution, served as subjects. Three groups were formed, the experimental group receiving 50 μg B_{12} daily; a placebo and control group were also included in the experimental design, a double blind study. The subjects were matched on their ability to run the half-mile. The experiment was conducted over a seven-week period. During this time, all boys in the experimental and placebo groups trained one hour daily in their regular physical education class and also ran the half-mile three times/week. Although both groups improved significantly in the half-mile run due to the training program, no significant differences were noted between the groups. In another report, Montoye (1955) noted that in normal young men, B_{12} supplementation had no effect on grip strength, heart rate recovery after submaximal exercise, or maximal performance capacity on a bicycle ergometer. He concluded that there is not sufficient evidence to recommend vitamin B_{12} supplementation as a general practice among athletic teams.

Although vitamin B_{12} may be useful as a medical treatment for pernicious anemia, it does not appear to convey any extra benefit to the normal athlete.

Pantothenic Acid

Pantothenic acid is a factor of the vitamin B complex, and in the body it is found as a component of acetyl CoA, the intermediate metabolite of carbohydrate and fat metabolism leading to energy release and other essential reactions. It is found in all animal products, eggs, yeast and whole grains. Its richest source, one of the so-called ergogenic foods, is royal jelly, the nutrition for the queen bee. The RDA is 5-10 mg/day.

Although White, Handler and Smith (1973) have noted that the nutritional role of pantothenic acid for man has not been determined, its central role as a component of acetyl CoA suggests it may be involved in the energy schema in man. Nijakowski (1966) reported a statistically significant higher level of pantothenic acid in athletes, in contrast to controls, probably due to the fact that it is bound to acetyl CoA and is needed in aerobic activities of athletes. He also reported a decrease in pantothenic acid following an intense short duration exercise, with no decrease following four hours of moderate exercise. However, the short, intense exercise was only 900 kpm/min, rated by many as a submaximal workload. Early and Carlson (1969) reported that a multiple vitamin supplement helped reduce exercise fatigue in a hot climate and theorized that part of the effectiveness could be attributed to pantothenic acid. They suggested that a deficiency in pantothenic acid, which might occur through excess sweating, could possibly decrease the availability of substrate for the Kreb's cycle, thus shifting the energy production to glycolysis, which is less efficient. However, since there were five other vitamins in their supplement, an ergogenic effect may not be attributed to pantothenic acid per se. The Russian investigators (Unsigned, 1971a) suggest more research is needed with this vitamin.

Although some reports are suggestive of a beneficial application of pantothenic acid to physical activity, the objective data is not available to support this suggestion.

Folic Acid (Folacin)

Folic acid, or folacin, is involved in growth processes, since it is related to DNA synthesis. Its best source includes organ meats, green vegetables, dry beans and whole grains. A deficiency may lead to growth failure and anemia. Theoretically, a deficiency in folic acid could handicap an endurance athlete due to anemic effects upon oxygen transport, but no experimental evidence has been uncovered to support this statement. Moreover, the effect of folic acid supplementation on physical performance has not been found in the literature.

Other B Complex Vitamins or Factors

Although several other vitamins and related factors in the B complex appear essential to man, such as biotin and para-aminobenzoic acid, there is little theoretical or experimental evidence to support their use as supplements to the diet of the athlete.

Vitamin B Complex Supplementation

In many of the older reports, due to the close association of many of the vitamins in the B complex, the effect of deprivation or supplementation with selected vitamins in the complex were studied together. As the three principal vitamins in the complex — thiamine, riboflavin and niacin — are all associated with the energy schema during exercise, they were the primary vitamins investigated as a group.

The effect of a prolonged dietary deficiency in the B complex results in a decreased capacity for endurance exercise. Egana and his associates (1942) studied the effect of a B complex deficient diet upon the exhaustive work capacity of seven healthy physicians. The deficiency was created over a four-week period, and the criterion test of endurance was a run to exhaustion on a treadmill. Although other physiological parameters were measured, the main finding was that a shorter run to exhaustion occurred during the period of deficiency, although the scores were not treated statistically; the subjects also experienced a subjective sensation of fatigue during this period. When brewers yeast, high in vitamin B, was included in the diet, the fitness levels returned to normal.

Keys and his colleagues (1945), in a complex study over a 161-day period, reported similar results with eight conscientious objectors. There were several phases to the study, but following the phase where the diet was almost completely devoid of the B complex vitamins, yet adequate in calories and other nutrients, the subjects experienced deterioration in endurance capacity. Criterion tests involved heart rate measurements during a sixty-minute walk and a ninety-second run, as well as during performance on the Harvard Fatigue Laboratory test. Strength was also measured during the experiment, and no changes were noted. When thiamine supplementation was administered near the end of the experiment, endurance capacity was restored to normal.

Berryman and his coworkers (1947) conducted similar experimentation with seven subjects. Their main purpose was to study the rate of change in physical and psychomotor performance associated with restricted intakes of thiamine, riboflavin, niacin, and other lesser known B complex vitamins. The experiment was conducted in several phases over the period of a year, with the various criterion tests being administered periodically. The criterion test for endurance was a double work period to exhaustion on the bicycle ergometer and treadmill. Psychomotor tests included body sway and hand steadiness. The authors concluded that vitamin B complex deficiency created a definite decrease in endurance capacity; the changes in the psychomotor tasks were less clear. Following return to supplementation, the improvement in physical performance returned gradually rather than immediately. There was no indication that any vitamin supplement conveyed an ergogenic effect. Although their number of subjects was small, the improvement was more rapid in those subjects who received full supplementation rather than stepwise addition of the nutrients. Friedman and Ivy (1947) reported that in a five to seven month period of time, subjects maintained on a dietary intake of 0.95 mg riboflavin and simultaneously, for two to five months on an average intake of 0.85 mg thiamine, remained in good health without any evidence of physical deterioration on a wide variety of physical tasks at ground level or at a simulated altitude of 15,000 feet. However, they noted that although the intake of thiamine and riboflavin was low, it was above the accepted minimal level. It should be noted, however, that the levels did not meet current RDA, which of course are not minimal levels.

In general, it may be concluded that a deficiency of the B complex vitamins over a period of time, a few weeks at the most, may lead to decreased endurance capacity. The athlete on a sound diet is not likely to encounter this deficiency. However, there are those who advocate B complex supplementation to the diet of the athlete. The research is contradictory relative to the effectiveness of B complex supplementation.

In an early study, Csik and Bencsik (1927) reported an increase in the working capacity of two subjects who received vitamin B extract over a six-month period. The criterion tests consisted of performances on dynamometers and a treadmill. Karpovich and

Sinning (1971) have criticized the study, indicating a training effect could have confounded the results. Two later studies evidenced no significant effect of vitamin B supplementation on muscular work.

Simonson and his colleagues (1942) studied the effect of vitamin B surplus upon the capacity for dynamic muscular endurance, maximal strength and other such tests involving function of the central nervous system. An experimental group consumed 8 tablets/day of Betolake®, each tablet containing 0.75 mg thiamine, 10 mg niacin, 1 mg riboflavin and 0.03-0.04 mg B_6. The tablets were taken over a six-week period. In comparison to a control group, no difference was noted for the muscular performance tests. However, the investigators did note favorable effects of the vitamin preparation upon tasks involving fatigue of the central nervous system, such as the fusion frequency of flicker test. Foltz and others (1942) utilized a double work period to exhaustion as a criterion measure for endurance to study the ergogenic effects of a number of the B complex vitamins. Five young men who were on a controlled diet, which was adequate in B vitamins, received intravenous injections over a total of forty-three trials. Twenty of the trials involved 25 mg thiamine, seven trials were conducted with a combined dosage of 30 mg thiamine, 100 mg niacin, 3.3 mg riboflavin, and 10 mg pyridoxine, four trials involved 10 mg cocarboxylase, and twelve trials contained 1.25-10 mg riboflavin. In none of the cases was the total work output greater following administration of the vitamins than it was in the control or placebo series. The authors concluded that vitamins do not act promptly in facilitating recovery.

In a more recent report, Early and Carlson (1969) concluded that vitamin supplementation reduced fatigue which could be induced by loss of vitamins through exercise-induced sweating in a hot environment. They matched eighteen high school boys, and assigned them to an experimental and placebo group. The criterion test was a series of ten dashes, with a thirty-second rest period in between; this test was administered on days one, nine and fifteen of the experiment. During days one through nine, no vitamin supplement was given, and all boys underwent heavy training to induce sweat losses. During days nine through fifteen, the experimental group received a supplement including 100 mg thiamine, 8 mg riboflavin, 5 mg pyridoxine, 25 mg cobalamin, 100 mg niacin, and 30 mg pantothenic acid. Using a sophisticated ANOVA technique with trend analysis, they concluded that the degree of fatigue of the experimental subjects was less than that of the placebo group on the days of vitamin supplementation. They theorized that thiamine and pantothenic acid were the active substances, due primarily to their roles in oxidative metabolism, as discussed previously.

B Complex and Other Vitamins

Several investigators have studied the effect upon physical performance of multivitamin supplementation and deprivation. Barborka and his associates (1943) reduced the thiamine, riboflavin, vitamin A and vitamin C content, as well as calcium, phosphrous and iron, in the diet of four men for two months. The endurance capacity, as tested by a double work test to exhaustion on a bicycle ergometer, decreased during the deficiency phase of the experiment. Upon restoration of the vitamins via yeast extract in tomato or lemon juice, a definite increase in work output was noted within forty-eight hours of administration, and within four weeks of supplementation all the subjects had increased their work output back to normal levels. Again, a deficiency of vitamins appears to adversely influence physical working capacity.

Keys and Henschel (1941) investigated the effect of vitamin supplements upon physiological parameters during a standardized fifteen-minute exercise task on a treadmill with full pack. A placebo and experimental group were utilized, with the experimental group receiving 100 mg niacin, 5 mg thiamine and 100 mg ascorbic acid over a four-week period. There was no effect on the physiological responses to exercise. In a subsequent experiment, Keys and Henschel (1942) studied the influence of vitamin supplementation upon physiological and biological responses to standard exercise tasks in twenty-six soldiers, involving a total of 256 experiments. The supplements were classified as large, and included 5-17 mg thiamine, 100 mg niacin, 20 mg calcium pantothenate, 10 mg riboflavin, 10-100 mg pyridoxine, and 100-200 mg ascorbic acid. The supplements were administered over periods of four to six weeks, alternating with placebo periods of the same duration. The investigators concluded that in neither a short anaerobic exercise nor in prolonged hard physical work of an aerobic nature did vitamin supplementation exert any beneficial effect.

On the other hand, Frankau (1943) reported some beneficial effects of multiple vitamin preparations upon performance in a task involving coordination and anaerobic capacity. The criterion test was a 300 yard shuttle run. Frankau cited a series of his experiments. With ten subjects in both a placebo and experimental group, he reported a beneficial effect of a compound containing 8000 IU vitamin A, 1200 IU vitamin D, 2 mg thiamine, 4 mg riboflavin, 100 mg ascorbic acid, and 40 mg niacin administered daily over a three-day period. A similar beneficial effect was noted in another experiment with twenty-two subjects in each of the placebo and experimental groups. The supplement included 5 mg thiamine, 5 mg riboflavin, 50 mg niacin and 100 mg ascorbic acid over a four-day period. Although Frankau reported a significant effect of the vitamin supplement in each case, no statistical analysis was utilized to evaluate the data. The explicit experimental methodology was also not delineated.

In another report, although not dealing specifically with increases in physical performance, Barnes (1961) reported that the use of a multiple vitamin tablet once each day for seven weeks was helpful in maintaining overall health of high school athletes and nonathletes. The experimental group had a much lower incidence of colds than the control group. Although the number of subjects in the study was small, Barnes suggested that all high school students, especially during the strenuous athletic season of fall and winter, need vitamin supplements.

Although there appears to be some evidence to support the viewpoint that supplementation with the B complex vitamins and multivitamins may be helpful in some situations, the evidence is extremely limited and there are also reports that do not substantiate an ergogenic effect of these compounds if the individual is on a sound diet. B complex vitamins are important in the energy metabolism of exercise, but supplementation would be advised only when their intake does not accompany the increased caloric intake necessary to sustain energy expenditure replacement.

VITAMIN C (ASCORBIC ACID)

Ascorbic acid, or vitamin C, is a dietary essential to man. Although some animals can synthesize vitamin C from blood glucose, man somehow lost this ability. Vitamin C is present in fresh fruits and vegetables, primarily the citrus fruits such as oranges, grapefruit, lemons and limes. Other good sources are tomatoes, white potatoes, broccoli, green peppers and greens. As vitamin C is heat labile, it is destroyed in the cooking process. The body can accumulate a pool of vitamin C which, according to Baker and his associates (1966), is about 2-3 g in the young healthy male. The National Research Council (1974) has indicated that 30 mg/day is sufficient to replenish that used, while 45 mg/day will maintain an adequate body pool and thus is the RDA. The normal range for plasma ascorbic acid is 0.7-1.2 mg/100 ml. The most prominent development of vitamin C deficiency is scurvy, whose symptoms include weakness, anemia, impaired wound healing, spongy gums and arrested skeletal development. The anemia may be due to impaired ability to utilize stored iron, and the other changes are associated with impaired formation of collagen, the main supportive protein of skin, tendon, bone, cartilage and connective tissue.

According to Shaffer (1970), ascorbic acid is one of the most perplexing vitamins with regard to its mechanism of action. The National Research Council (1974) noted that the total role of vitamin C has not been completely elucidated. However, it is known to function in the synthesis of collagen, in the metabolic reactions of amino acids and in the synthesis of epinephrine and the anti-inflammatory corticoids of the adrenal gland. Thus, vitamin C is essential to a variety of biological oxidative processes in the body. However, according to Lamb (1974) some faddists have indicated that massive dosages of vitamin C can cure a diverse array of disorders including arthritis, diabetes, ulcers, allergies, heart disease and viral infections, as well as prevent fatigue. Stone (1967) has indicated that research is needed to ascertain whether vitamin C supplementation may increase the life span, help maintain a youthful appearance and increase resistance to infectious diseases. Although not a topic central to the theme of this book, it should be noted relative to the last statement by Stone, that the National Research Council (1974) does not feel the claims are justified regarding the preventative aspects of vitamin C supplementation as a means of preventing the common cold.

As will be discussed below, many athletes, as well as others, utilize massive dosages of vitamin C in attempts to prevent fatigue or increase performance capacity. Recent evidence has indicated some possible dangers. Lamb (1974) reported large amounts may irritate the bowel and cause diarrhea. Herbert and Jacob (1974) suggested vitamin C supplementation may increase biochemical reactions in the body that destroy vitamin B_{12}, essential for prevention of anemia.

Hanley (1968) and others (United States Senate, 1973) have reported athletes using dosages of vitamin C ranging from 2500-10,000 mg/day, even though the RDA is only 45 mg. The Russians were reported to have attributed their success in the 1960 Olympics to increased intakes of vitamin C (Van Huss, 1966), and other authorities in the area of exercise physiology or sports medicine have advocated dietary supplementation of vitamin C due to certain of its physiological properties. Baker (1967) has cited claims that the damaging effects of heat may be alleviated by administering large doses of ascorbic acid. Cureton (1969b) recommended that vitamin C supplementation be increased in athletes during training as research indicated it was effective in lowering the oxygen debt. Horstman (1972) noted that vitamin C, added to *in vitro* solutions of blood, shifted the oxygen dissociation curve to the right. If this would occur *in vivo*, it could facilitate oxygen release at the cell level, thus increasing the amount of oxygen available to the cell. Van Itallie (1968), citing L. Prokop, an international expert in sports medicine, noted that vitamin C may influence oxidation-reduction phenomena in the cells. He hypothesized that if oxidative processes are adversely affected during exercise, and if vitamin C can favorably influence oxidation, then it may benefit performance. In relation to the role of the vitamin C in cellular energy metabolism, Horstman (1972) has indicated that it functions in the electron transport chain between DPNH (NADH) and one of the cytochromes. Lamb (1974) has indicated that although the RDA is only 45 mg/day, stress may increase the need three-fold, or 135 mg/day. Boddy and his associates (1974) noted that a two-hour training session involving vigorous exercise resulted in a drop in ascorbic acid in the white blood cell. Thus, they indicated stress such as exercise may reduce vitamin C content in the body.

Thus, there appears to be some theoretical basis for the utilization of vitamin C supplementation in athletes undergoing training or competition. Since vitamin C has been known for some time, and since one of the deficiency symptoms is weakness, its effect upon physical work capacity has been studied intermittantly over the past forty years. The following section reviews those studies which have been uncovered relative to supplementation or deficiency upon physical performance.

Not too much evidence is available relative to the effect of vitamin C deficiency upon physical performance, although one of the symptoms is general weakness, which would appear to deter performance. Horstman (1972) stated that vitamin C deficiency, ranging from two to four months, could cause decrements in work performance, and Hettinger (1961) observed that hypovitaminosis C would adversely affect the trainability of the muscular system.

Regarding the effects of vitamin C supplementation, the results are rather contradictory. Older reports and more contemporary research are both in disagreement as to the ergogenic merits of vitamin C. This review will center first upon those reports signifying a beneficial effect of increased levels of dietary vitamin C followed by those revealing no significant change. As is expected, the experimental methodology was more controlled in the contemporary studies.

Vitamin C appears to be utilized during physical exertion. As reported previously, Boddy and his colleagues (1974) noted a decrease in blood ascorbic acid during a prolonged session involving vigorous exercise. Wachholder (1951) reported increased muscular extraction of ascorbic acid during training; however, his study did not actually show that vitamin C increased work performance, only that more was used during exercise. Namyslowski (1956) studied the quantitative relationship between the intensity of physical exertion and the vitamin C requirement of young athletes. Using physical education students undertaking normal activities in the Academy of Physical Culture and later undergoing exhaustive ski training, he noted that increased activity depleted vitamin C. Therefore, he recommended 200-250 mg/day while training in ski camp, and 100-150 mg/day while in physical education training. Namyslowski suggested more research is necessary, since only four to thirteen subjects were used in this investigation.

A number of early reports indicated an ergogenic effect of vitamin C. Bourne (1948) cited reports in the 1930's by Sobecki and Rugg-Gunn that large dosages of vitamin C had a beneficial effect upon muscular exercise. However, the details were not available. Brunner (1941) reported beneficial effects of 200 mg vitamin C/day upon men in training, while Basu and Ray (1940) noted that 600 mg vitamin C daily for three days elicited an increase in resistance to fatigue on a finger ergograph. However, when the subjects were removed from the vitamin supplement, the fatigue curve did not return to normal, indicative possibly of a training effect which may have confounded their study. In a brief report, DuPain and Loutfi (1943) also noted that vitamin C increased efficiency and delayed fatigue. Hoitink (1946a; 1946b) reported that the oral administration of vitamin C for a certain period of time would increase working capacity on a bicycle ergometer, and thus recommended that an increase above the saturation level be maintained continuously in order to increase physical working capacity. In a more recent article, Rasch and others (1962) indicated that most of these earlier German and French studies lacked the proper experimental design.

However, in more contemporary research, some reports favorable to vitamin C are also available. Baker (1967) cited the work of a medical research council special report in 1953 that in tests of physical fatigue, statistical analysis favored a group of subjects receiving 70 mg vitamin C/day as compared to a group receiving 10 mg/day. The 10 mg/day group, however, is below the RDA. Van Huss (1966) cited numerous reports from Russian and central

European countries attesting to the value of vitamin C supplementation to athletes. The Russian investigator Yakovlev suggested, based on his studies, that speed or strength athletes need 75 mg/day while endurance athletes require 300 mg/day.

Hoogerwerf and Hoitink (1963) suggested that the effect of vitamin C supplementation resembles the effect of athletic training. In a rather well-controlled study, they evaluated the effect of vitamin C upon mechanical efficiency. They pretested thirty subjects and assigned fifteen each to an experimental and control group. The experimental group received 1 g vitamin C/day for five days in the form of Redoxon®. Efficiency was computed for ten minutes at a workload of 120 watts. The C vitaminization caused a pronounced rise in the vitamin C content of the blood, and elicited a significantly greater rise in efficiency in the experimental group as compared to the placebo group. The efficiency of the experimental group increased from 21.47 to 23.63 percent. The investigators concluded that adequate C vitaminization increases the working capacity, and in some respects there is a resemblance between the conditions of training and vitamin C saturation. However, it should be noted that the work was submaximal, and not to exhaustion. Would the same dietary routine increase maximal work capacity? Spioch and his associates (1966) conducted a similar study on mechanical efficiency. They measured cardiovascular and metabolic responses to a five-minute step test, patterned after the Harvard Step Test, and calculated mechanical efficiency. They used a repeated measure design where thirty subjects undertook a control test, and then took the experimental test the following week. Thirty minutes prior to the experimental trial the subject received 500 mg vitamin C injected intravenously. The results revealed a significant reduction in oxygen consumption, pulmonary ventilation, oxygen debt, total energy cost and heart rate. The mechanical efficiency increased by 25 percent from 22.4 to 28.1 percent. The authors reiterated the statement by Hoogerwerf and Hoitink that vitamin C mimics the training effect. However, a training effect could have occured in this study, since the order of administration of treatments was not counterbalanced. Any systematic error in the data collection could have biased the results.

Namyslowski (1960), in contrasting reports from various parts of the world, noted that the German, Russian and Central European studies have indicated a beneficial effect of vitamin C on physical fitness levels, whereas the studies from western Anglo-Saxon countries do not find such increases. He believes the contrasting findings may reflect the baseline values of vitamin C in the different athletes, noting that central European athletes may have had low vitamin C levels to begin with, and possibly a deficiency was being removed. He cited previous research with over 100 Polish physical education students whose vitamin C saturation was low.

Although the preceding material favored vitamin C as an ergogenic aid, other studies find no beneficial effect. Boje (1939), after reviewing the pre-1939 literature, contended there is no value of extra vitamin C in the diet of athletes. Jetzler and Haffter (1939) reported very little effect of 300 mg vitamin C daily upon the endurance performance of five subjects in a 50 kilometer ski race. Two separate but similar reports revealed no beneficial effect of a 40 mg vitamin C/day supplement to workers on relatively low daily intakes. Using the shotput, 100-yard dash, and one mile run as performance tests, Jokl and Suzman (1940) found no effect after a seven-month period of supplementation. Fox and his colleagues (1940) used the same vitamin C supplementation and performance tests on nearly 2,000 workers. The normal daily intake was approximated at 12-25 mg/day; therefore, the 40 mg supplement would bring the workers to the RDA. Other than the fact that the control group experienced twelve cases of scurvy and the experimental group had only one mild case, no significant differences were noted between the groups relative to physical performance. The same criticism which was leveled at the early research producing beneficial results could also be applied with the above research showing no effect, as adequate controls were not maintained.

In three series of experimental studies on forty-four young men under rigidly controlled conditions of diet, physical work and environment, Henschel and his coworkers (1944) studied the effects of 20-40 mg and 520-540 mg vitamin C/daily upon cardio-vascular dynamics and performance on standard physical work tasks, as well as other psychomotor tasks, in a hot environment. In general, all subjects were on the same diet, with the exception that the experimental group received 500 mg vitamin C daily. Placebos were used for the control group. In general, during exercise there were no significant changes in cardiovascular responses or rectal temperature that could be attributed to the vitamin C supplementation. The tests of strength and psychomotor performance also were not affected. However, the cardiovascular performance tests were not maximal, and thus no conclusions relative to maximal performance may be made. Relative to strength, however, Hettinger (1961) also observed that hypervitaminosis C does not affect strength.

In a field study, Rasch and his associates (1962) conducted an experiment with the entire cross-country team of Long Beach State in California. The whole team trained for three weeks while receiving a placebo. They were then tested on a distance run and assigned to matched groups based on their times. The experimental group received 500 mg vitamin C/day while the control group continued to receive the placebo. No control of diet was otherwise undertaken. This procedure was continued throughout the season, and a post-test at the end of the season on the same course revealed no significant effect of the vitamin C supplementation. The authors concluded that the normal American diet contains sufficient vitamin C. In a study of the acute effects of vitamin C, Margaria and others (1964a) administered 250 mg to the subjects approximately ninety minutes prior to a run to exhaustion; the treadmill test was designed to elicit exhaustion in less than ten minutes. The results showed no significant effect on time to exhaustion or maximal oxygen uptake.

Van Huss (1966) also studied the acute effects of vitamin C upon several performance tests. One test involved the evaluation of various physiological changes during moderate work on a treadmill, 6 m.p.h. at zero grade. A second task involved the determination of maximal oxygen uptake and endurance time to exhaustion on a treadmill at 10 m.p.h. and 8 percent grade. The subjects were ten well trained males involved in this repeated measures study; all subjects were tested one, two and three hours following the ingestion of four experimental beverages: (1) orange juice in which all but 15 mg vitamin C was destroyed; (2) reconstituted orange juice with 2.98 mg vitamin C/kg body weight; (3) synthetic orange juice with 2.98 mg vitamin C/kg body weight; and, (4) a beverage with no vitamin C. The results indicated, for a single performance, no enhancement of physical performance; however, the vitamin C did aid in faster recovery as subjects returned to normal physiological values, i.e. heart rate, blood pressure and oxygen consumption. One possible shortcoming was that during the phase of the experiment involving determination of maximal oxygen uptake and maximal endurance time, not all subjects took all experimental beverages.

Grey and his associates (1970), in a double-blind placebo experiment, evaluated the effect of twelve weeks of vitamin C supplementation upon aerobic endurance capacity. Prior to the beginning of training, 286 male officers with a mean age of twenty-eight years, were tested on a twelve-minute run for distance. The subjects were then assigned to either a placebo or experimental group, the latter receiving 500 mg ascorbic acid/day. There was no attempt to control diet, but all officers lived in the same general environment. The daily physical activities included general physical conditioning for the first three weeks of the experiment, followed by nine weeks of team sports such as soccer, volleyball and flickerball. At the conclusion of the training period, the twelve-minute run test was readministered. No significant differences were noted between the experimental and control group.

Lamb (1974) has cited reports contending that cigarette smoking may destroy vitamin C in the body. With this premise in mind, Bailey and others (1970) studied the physiological response to exercise of smokers and nonsmokers exposed to vitamin C supplementation. Heart rate, minute ventilation, oxygen uptake and oxygen pulse were evaluated during a nine-minute treadmill run. Forty subjects were involved; ten in each of the four groups comprised of smokers and non-smokers with supplemental vitamin C and no supplement. The supplemental groups received 2 g/day for five days. A double-blind placebo experimental design was used. The results indicated no significant difference between the groups, and the authors concluded that five days of vitamin C supplementation had no effect upon respiratory adjustments or oxygen utilization before, during or after exercise in either smoking or non-smoking subjects. This study evaluated only physiological responses to submaximal exercise, not maximal performance. Although the daily dosage was relatively large, the duration of the experiment may not have been optimal.

Even though the above studies reveal no significant effect of vitamin C supplements on physical performance, one should not accept this as conclusive evidence. In some of the studies, only the acute effect of vitamin C was studied, with little attention to building up the vitamin C body pool. Other studies may have been limited in duration. On the other hand, the two studies by Rasch and his colleagues (1962) and Grey and his associates (1970), with substantial supplementation over an adequate period of time, provide some evidence against the blanket recommendation of vitamin C for athletes in training.

Nevertheless, based upon his review of the literature and his own research, Van Huss (1974) reported that it would be prudent for the athlete to utilize approximately 3-5 mg/kg body weight daily, especially during the developmental years. For an average athlete of 70 kg body weight, this would represent 210-350 mg vitamin C/day. Baker (1967) has concurred that there is a definite need for an increased requirement for ascorbic acid in all forms of stress, including physical exertion. However, he noted that there is insufficient knowledge relative to the absolute or quantitative levels of the increased requirement. It is highly recommended that further controlled research be conducted in this area since some apparent disagreements exist relative to the efficacy of vitamin C as a potential ergogenic food.

One other potential role of vitamin C for athletes involves its effect upon muscle soreness or wound healing. Staton (1952) studied the effect of ascorbic acid saturation on the degree of localized muscular soreness resulting from strenuous muscular activity. He subdivided 103 subjects into three groups: control, experimental and placebo. Throughout the thirty-day preparatory period prior to the trial, the experimental subjects ingested 100 mg ascorbic acid daily. Staton induced muscular soreness by a maximal repetition of sit-ups test. The test was administered again twenty-four hours later, and the criterion of soreness was the decrement in performance in the second test. Although the author postulated that the addition of liberal amounts of vitamin C to the normal diet may be of value in minimizing local muscular soreness, the insignificant difference between the experimental and placebo group did not support this theory. Schwartz (1970), in a review of studies relative to vitamin C and wound healing, reported that a relationship had been established between minimum tissue stores and/or dietary intake of vitamin C in order for adequate wound healing to occur. Although there may be some implications for athletic injuries, data relating dosage to quality of healing are not conclusive.

VITAMIN D

Vitamin D represents any one of several related sterols which promote calcification in the bones. According to the National Research Council (1974), the main role of vitamin D is to regulate calcium and phosphate metabolism. White, Handler and Smith (1973) have noted that vitamin D promotes calcium absorption from the intestine, and the physiological results of vitamin D deficiency are mainly derived from a lack of calcium. In reference to humans, Vitamin D exists in two forms. D_2, ergocalciferol, is the result of the irradiation of ergosterol. D_3, cholecalciferol, is the naturally occurring compound in the skin, formed by exposure to sunlight. Vitamin D is known as the sunshine vitamin and is present in fish liver oil and milk fortified with vitamin D. Sunlight activates the natural compound in the body. It is also known as the antirachitic vitamin, since it prevents the development of rickets, a bone disorder. DeLuca (1971) has suggested that vitamin D should not be visualized as a vitamin, but rather as a hormone due to its role in bone mineralization.

The RDA is 400 IU; deficiency results primarily in the development of rickets. Since vitamin D is fat soluble, overdosages may lead to increased storage in the body, and pathological results have been reported. Tatkon (1968) reported hypervitaminosis D leads to loss of weight, vomiting, nausea, lethargy and loss of muscle tone. Calcium may be released from the bones to be deposited in the soft tissues such as the wall of the blood vessels and kidneys. White, Handler and Smith (1973) reported that over-dosages of vitamin D may produce demineralization of bones, and multiple fractures may occur even from minimal injury. Dr. John Boyer (United States Senate, 1973) indicated that the combination of large amounts of vitamin D, plus prolonged exposure to ul-traviolet light, increases the hazard of vitamin D intoxication. A case of vitamin D poisoning has been reported in a medical journal (Weinstein, 1953). Seelig (1970) reported more severe pos-sible consequences. He noted that high levels of calcium in the blood, attributed to excess amounts of vitamin D, are associated with damage to the brain resulting in mental retardation, and injury to the heart and blood vessels. He noted that one form of mental retardation and one form of congenital heart disease may be related to hypervitaminosis D in pregnant women. Thus, as with vitamin A, there appear to be sound medical reasons not to utilize vitamin D supplementation with healthy individuals.

Application of vitamin D supplementation to athletes appears to have no theoretical basis. The limited research which has been conducted substantiates this statement. In a German report, Seidl and Hettinger (1957) studied six subjects over a two-year period. Although their results indicated an improvement of physical per-formance through the systematic utilization of ultraviolet rays, the oral administration of vitamin D_3 did not improve per-formance on the bicycle ergometer. Berven (1963) studied the effect of vitamin D daily supplementation upon the physical working capacity of sixty schoolchildren, ages ten to eleven. Over a period of two years Berven administered 1500 IU of vitamin D at different time periods to some of the subjects and placebo pills to the others. During another phase of the experiment, he gave a single massive dose of 400,000 IU to some of the subjects. The criterion test of physical performance was the PWC-170 test, a submaximal performance test. His results indicated no signifi-cant beneficial effects of either the daily supplementation or the single massive dosage of vitamin D.

It would appear that vitamin D supplementation is unneces-sary in athletes, and may be potentially hazardous if prolonged overdosage occurs. It should be noted, however, that in Berven's study, season variations did occur. Some investigators have reported ergogenic effects of ultraviolet radiation, while others have not. In light of the interaction of sunlight and body sterols in forming vitamin D, this topic may need further investigation.

VITAMIN E

Vitamin E is a fat soluble vitamin; activity is derived from a series of tocopherols and tocotrienols of plant origin. There are at least four forms of the tocopherols. The most active of these is alpha-tocopherol, which has the highest biological potency, although delta-tocopherol is considered to be the best antioxidant (Alfin-Slater and Aftergood, 1973). Good sources of vitamin E include wheat germ oil, salad oils, margarine, green leafy vegetables, legumes and nuts. Although vitamin E deficiency causes a number of disorders in rats and other animals, such as muscular dystrophy, the reported signs of tocopherol deficiency in cases of defective fat absorption or transportation are the only evidence that vitamin E is required by humans. Tissues of vitamin E deficient animals, particularly cardiac and skeletal muscles, consume oxygen more rapidly than do normal tissues. The increased oxygen consumption appears to relate to peroxidation of unsaturated fatty acids (White, Handler and Smith, 1973). White (1974) noted that it is generally agreed that vitamin E functions primarily as an antioxidant, preventing unwanted oxidation of polyunsaturated fatty acids in the body and in foods. However, in their review of the literature, Green and Bunyan (1969) reported that the antioxidant theory of vitamin E remains to be substantiated. The antioxidation role of vitamin E has been associated with its labeling as the antiaging vitamin. However, no scientific information is available to support this claim.

White (1974) also reported that vitamin E is probably involved in certain synthetic activities in the body, such as the formation of red blood cells. According to the Food and Nutrition Board of the National Academy of Sciences, the apparent absence of vitamin E deficiency in the general population suggests the amount of the vitamins in foods is adequate (White, 1974). The RDA for males is 15 IU/day, and for females, 12 IU/day. Tocopherols are generally considered relatively nontoxic to man; however, in view of recent reports relative to toxicity in animals, and the known toxicity of vitamins A and D, other fat soluble vitamins, caution is indicated whenever consumption of large doses of vitamin E for a long period of time is contemplated (National Research Council, 1974).

Of the various food supplements that have been claimed to be ergogenic in nature, vitamin E has been one of the more controversial. According to one recent advertisement in *Scholastic Coach,* a compound named Energol® has been noted as being particularly rich in vitamin E, and necessary in building energy and endurance. Since vitamin E is a natural constituent of wheat germ oil, some have claimed the theoretical ergogenic effect of wheat germ is due to the vitamin E content. The physiological rationale underlying the theoretical ergogenic effect of vitamin E is apparently related to oxygen utilization and energy supply, although other rationale have also been reported. Bourne (1968) noted that Dr. Jyunichi Aoki, in a 1967 meeting of the Japan Society for Sports Medicine, suggested that vitamin E facilitates the utilization of oxygen by athletes and reduces the accumulation of lactic acid in the blood. Percival (1951), in a report for the Shute Foundation for Medical Research, noted that the alpha-tocopherol in wheat germ oil is purported to reduce oxygen requirements of the tissues, improve collateral circulation, stimulate muscle power, and supply fatty acids for energy utilization during aerobic workloads. Since some animals have been shown to achieve greater resistance to hypoxia after vitamin E intake, a possible beneficial effect to athletes was extrapolated (Unsigned, 1971b). Thus, since vitamin E prevents unwanted oxidation of fatty acids, supplementation has been theorized to increase this preventative role, thereby possibly increasing the oxygen supply for other purposes, such as energy production in the citric acid cycle, and also increasing the fatty acid supply for energy. Hence, vitamin E should be effective in endurance activities. These are theoretical viewpoints, however, and no objective evidence appears to be available to substantiate these effects during an exercise situation.

There are several reports available which support the viewpoint that vitamin E is an effective ergogenic aid, but they are limited. Cureton, from the University of Illinois Physical Fitness Research Laboratory, has conducted a number of studies over the years with wheat germ oil as an ergogenic aid. However, although his research supports the use of wheat germ oil in athletics, he does not attribute the beneficial effect to vitamin E. The research dealing with the effects of wheat germ oil upon physical performance is discussed in Chapter Nine. Nevertheless, Cureton often used vitamin E as a placebo in his research. In one report (Cureton, 1955), he indicated a significant effect of vitamin E supplementation in cottonseed oil, in contrast to a control group, on increasing treadmill running time to exhaustion in a group of wrestlers. However, the vitamin E in this study was used as a placebo, whereas the control group received nothing. Therefore, a placebo effect could have been created.

Clausen (1971), in an unpublished report, studied the effect of three treatments upon cardiorespiratory endurance; the treatments were aerobic training and vitamin E, aerobic training and placebo, and vitamin E with no training. Subjects were tested for maximal oxygen uptake at the beginning of the experiment, and after five and nine weeks the aerobic exercise and vitamin E treatment produced an increase (p < .10) in maximal oxygen uptake during the period of pretest through the fifth week, while the other treatments did not. Clausen concluded that aerobic exercise and vitamin E appear to be effective when combined, but not when used separately. There are several apparent problems with the study, which was only a brief report. The level of significance used is unconventional, and apparently the improper statistical techniques were utilized to analyze the data.

Several Russian reports are available favoring vitamin E supplementation. Sakaeva and Efremov (1972), noted that during intense athletic training in cyclists and skiers, the blood serum level of vitamin E tended to decrease. They reported that supplemental doses of 50-300 mg tocopherol increased the blood serum vitamin E level and performance of the athletes. Since the activity of naturally occurring alpha- and delta-tocopherol is 1.49 IU/mg, the Russian dosages would have been about 33-200 IU. In a subsequent report (Efremov and Sakaeva, 1973), the English translation was rather confusing. Although the investigators noted that the incorporation of 600 mg vitamin E in the daily diet for a period of three weeks produced a significant increase in the blood serum vitamin E level, a reduced performance capacity of the athletes was noted toward the end of the training period. However, the title of the article involved the importance of vitamin E during intense physical training of athletes, thus implying a beneficial effect of vitamin E.

There are several reports, including some very recent findings from well-controlled studies, that supplemental vitamin E exerts no effect on physical performance capacity. One of the most cited reports relative to the ineffectiveness of vitamin E is a masters thesis by Thomas. Though this author was unable to locate the original document, supposedly completed in 1957 at the University of Southern California, the results were rather fully reported by Mayer and Bullen (1959). Thomas used thirty young male students, assigning fifteen of them 450 IU alpha-tocopherol acetate daily for five weeks, and then a placebo for five weeks. The other fifteen students simply reversed the procedure, taking the placebo the first five weeks, and then the vitamin E. Thomas reported no significant effect of the vitamin E supplementation upon speed sit-ups, vertical jump or cardiorespiratory responses immediately after activity. However, no evidence of an overall cardiovascular endurance performance test, the type of activity where vitamin E may be theorized to be beneficial, was indicated as one of the criterion tests.

Sharman (1971) utilized two groups of schoolboys, members of a swimming club, to study vitamin E. The athletes were maintained on a normal diet, at a boarding school, with the experimental group receiving 400 mg alpha-tocopherol acetate daily while the control group received a placebo. The subjects were matched on pretest performances, and undertook a six-week training period including swimming and other activities. Criterion tests at the conclusion of the experiment included vital capacity, body fat, resting EKG, heart rate response to a standardized step test, a one-mile run, a 400 meter swim, pull-ups, push-ups, two-minute sit-up test, and isotonic endurance with bench presses. Although some beneficial effects on performance were due to training, the statistical analysis revealed no significant effect of vitamin E on any parameters.

In a similar experiment, Shephard and his colleagues (1974) undertook a double blind investigation regarding the effect of vitamin E supplementation upon the performance of twenty varsity college swimmers, mainly middle distance swimmers. The athletes were matched on the basis of aerobic power, body weight and events, and assigned to either the experimental or placebo group. Criterion tests included maximal oxygen uptake, muscular strength, heart rate recovery and EKG analyses. The administration of the vitamin E, 1200 IU daily, was started in the experimental group at the initiation of the intense training season and ended eighty-five days later. It was a heavy dose, the amount recommended by those who advocate vitamin E as an ergogenic aid. Of the original twenty athletes, only fourteen completed the experiment, seven matched pairs. The training was heavy, averaging about 20,000 yards/week. The results illustrated no significant effect of vitamin E. Muscle strength tended to decline in both groups, but there was no significant difference between the groups. No differences in subjective reactions regarding the nature of training were noted. The authors indicated their experiment provided little support for the view that vitamin E improves either the performance of the well-trained athlete or his tolerance to a demanding training schedule.

Watt and others (1974) evaluated the effect of vitamin E upon oxygen consumption. In a double blind study, twenty active hockey players were matched according to their maximal oxygen uptake, and the experimental group (N = 10) received 1200 IU vitamin E daily for fifty days, while the control group received a placebo. All players were involved in the same training regimen. At the end of the training period both groups significantly increased their maximal oxygen uptake, but there were no significant differences between the two groups. The authors concluded that vitamin E had no beneficial effect upon the maximal oxygen uptake of active individuals.

In summary, Shephard and others (1974) noted that although some have reported highly significant effects of vitamin E upon athletic performance, the actual benefits are doubtful since many of the experiments had not been properly controlled. This review of the available literature supports that comment.

SUMMARY

Although the general implication of this review would be that vitamin supplementation is ineffective as an ergogenic aid and hence unnecessary in the diet of the athlete who is well-nourished, it is believed that more controlled experimentation is needed with the B complex vitamins, vitamin C and vitamin E. Although some studies have utilized rather large dosages, athletes have been reported to consume massive doses, for example, 10,000 mg vitamin C daily. Thus, there may be an analogy here between the field practices of athletes who consume copious amounts of anabolic steroids, and laboratory experimentation which utilize smaller amounts. The athletes attest to the value of the steroids, whereas many of the laboratory findings reveal no significant effects on performance. The difference may be in the dosages of anabolic steroids utilized, and the same may apply to vitamins. Can high dosages of certain vitamins elicit a pharmacodynamic effect on some body systems?

Shephard and his associates (1974) have noted that since vitamin E is relatively harmless, it is debatable whether further categoric disproof of its supposed ergogenic properties is either necessary or desirable. The same reasoning may also be applied to other vitamins. This author believes further research is both necessary and desirable to help further elucidate the role of supposed nutritional ergogenic aids as they relate to athletic performance. It should be substantiated that they are, or can be, beneficial, or proven that they are not. Only through controlled research may we eliminate false advertising claims for food supplements in athletics and the myths associated with nutrition and athletic performance.

CHAPTER SEVEN

THE ROLE OF MINERALS
IN PHYSICAL ACTIVITY

O F THE 103 KNOWN elements, eleven constitute the vast majority of living matter, with carbon, nitrogen, hydrogen and oxygen being major components. However, many of the remaining elements ranging from minute traces to major body constituents, may be detected in animals. Minerals, one form of elements, serve a variety of functions in the body. Some are utilized as building constituents, such as calcium and phosphorus in the bones and teeth. Others are important components of enzymes and hormones, such as iodine in thyroxine, zinc in insulin, cobalt in vitamin B_{12}, and iron in hemoglobin. Sulfur is a component of protein, the major building material of the soft body tissues. Minerals are also important in a number of regulatory functions in the body. Included among these functions are maintenance of normal pH through buffering action in the blood, regulation of muscular contraction processes, conduction of nerve impulses, clotting of the blood, maintenance of body fluid osmotic pressure, and regulation of normal heart rhythm.

According to the National Research Council (1974), mineral elements may be classified into two groups based upon body needs. The major minerals are those needed in the diet in levels greater than 100 mg/day; this group includes calcium (Ca), phosphorus (P), magnesium (Mg), sodium (Na), potassium (K) and chloride (Cl). The minor mineral elements, the trace elements, are those where only a few mg/day are needed. Biological functions in animals have only been demonstrated for seventeen trace elements. The National Research Council noted that while all these may eventually prove to be essential to man, at the present time only ten are. They include fluorine (F), chromium (Cr), manganese (Mn), cobalt (Co), copper (Cu), iron (Fe), zinc (Zn), selenium (Se), molybdenum (Mb), and iodine (I). Of both the major and minor elements, RDA have been determined for only six: calcium, phosphorus, iodine, iron, magnesium and zinc.

As is obvious from the functions of minerals in the body, they are important regulators of physiological processes involved in physical performance. The roles of sodium, potassium, calcium and magnesium are central to nerve impulse conduction and the resultant muscle contraction, and sodium in conjunction with the bicarbonate ion is an important buffer for lactic acid. Some of the trace elements may also be critical to physical performance, notably the role iron plays in oxidation processes. However, with the exception of sodium, chlorine, potassium and iron, there is little research available to ascertain any possible beneficial ergogenic effect of supplementation to the normal diet.

The first part of this chapter briefly covers the trace elements and several of the major elements and their possible roles in physical performance. No detailed coverage is offered. The basic nature and physiological role of sodium and potassium will be discussed in this chapter, but since they have been studied mainly in association with sweat losses incurred during exercise in hot environments, with the resultant water replacement, research relative to their role during exercise will be presented in the following chapter dealing with water. The main part of this chapter will center upon the role of iron in physical activity.

Calcium, Phosphorus, Magnesium and the Trace Elements

The vast majority, or 99 percent, of calcium is present in the skeleton, while 1 percent serves a number of physiological functions unrelated to bone structure. It is required as a component in a number of enzyme systems, particularly in muscle contraction in both the heart and skeletal muscle, nerve impulse transmission and blood clotting. Calcium metabolism is regulated by the parathyroid hormones, and there may be serious consequences of increased or decreased levels of circulating calcium. An increase may lead to respiratory or cardiac failure, whereas a decrease may cause muscle tetany. However, the normal individual on a sufficient diet will not suffer calcium deficiency. According to White (1974), a calcium deficiency of sufficient severity to affect the health of the nervous system has not been recorded. Although calcium is important for normal functioning of nerves, it does not necessarily follow that a person can have a healthier nervous system by increasing calcium intake. The same reason probably applies to the muscle system as well. No research has been uncovered which studied the role of supplemental calcium on aspects of physical performance. There appears to be no theoretical rationale or objective evidence to support that action.

Phosphorus, as phosphoric acid in its various combinations with organic substances, is highly involved in the metabolic energy processes in humans, is a main constituent of bone and other body structures, and is involved in other chemical reactions in the body. Many of the B vitamins are effective only when combined with phosphate in the body. Phosphate is present in nearly all foods, and dietary deficiency has not been reported in man (National Research Council, 1974). However, its role in conjunction with the B complex vitamins, which play a central role in the energy processes in the body, and its function as part of the high energy bond of ATP, have provided some theoretical evidence to support its use, as phosphates, as an ergogenic aid. The effect of the phosphates upon physical work capacity is discussed in Chapter Nine.

Magnesium is indispensable to man because it is intimately related to the activity of many enzymes, and may be involved in regulating body heat, muscle contractions and protein synthesis (White, 1974). Magnesium deficiency may lead to neuromuscular dysfunction, resulting in hyperexcitability and tetany. Although the National Research Council (1974) reported magnesium deficiency is rare because it is widely distributed in foods, Creff and Boursier (Unsigned, 1972c) indicated that all competitive athletes should receive 8 mg/kg body weight/day in their diets. They reported that it was essential to normal recovery after fatigue and the prevention of muscular cramps. Russian investigators (Unsigned, 1971a) reported a need for a 30 percent increase of magnesium in the diet of athletes in training. A recent report (Rose and others, 1970) has documented significantly reduced magnesium levels following a marathon race. The average RDA for an average American male is 5-6 mg/kg/day, apparently within range of the recommendation by Creff and Boursier. No research has been found that has studied the effect of magnesium supplementation upon athletic performance.

Some of the trace elements have functions related to the metabolic processes that are activated during exercise. However, these elements have not been studied as supplements to improve physical performance capacity. Zinc is an essential constituent of many enzymes, including carbonic anhydrase and lactate dehydrogenasé; these enzymes function in carbon dioxide disposition and the energy metabolism of the muscle, respectively. Copper is essential to prevent anemia, even in the presence of adequate supplies of iron; copper is also involved in energy metabolism as it is a constituent of cytochrome oxidase (Dowdy, 1969). Cobalt is a constituent of vitamin B_{12}, necessary for prevention of anemia. Chromium is required for maintaining normal glucose metabolism in experimental animals, and may have similar functions in man. Manganese appears to be essential for normal functioning of the central nervous system. Although all of these trace elements and others are important regulators of numerous physiological processes in the body, Mayer and Bullen (1959) noted that a pure or complete deficiency of trace elements in man is obviously unlikely.

SODIUM, POTASSIUM AND CHLORIDE

There is a high degree of interrelationship between the three elements, sodium, potassium and chloride. Sodium is the main cation (positive ion) of the extracellular fluid, and functions mainly for the maintenance of normal body fluid volume and osmotic equilibrium. It also serves a major role in nerve impulse conduction and muscular contraction. Potassium is the major cation of the intracellular fluid, and is primarily concerned with proper functioning of the cellular enzymes. According to Bajusz (1965) the physiological activities of sodium are almost directly antagonistic to potassium. Chloride is an anion (negative ion) and is closely allied with sodium in the maintenance of normal body fluid and electrolyte balance. Another role of chloride is the formation of hydrochloric acid in the stomach. Under normal circumstances found in athletes, the loss of chloride from the body parallels the loss of sodium. As these three elements are closely associated with body water losses during exercise in the heat, detailed consideration of their role in physical performance will be covered in the following chapter.

There is no RDA for sodium, but Mayer (1972b) has noted that the average American diet contains approximately 6,000 mg/day. Sodium is present in nearly all foods, not just table salt, although man has an intrinsic appetite for salt which helps assure sodium intake. The body possesses efficient homeostatic mechanisms to allow for a wide range of intake of sodium. Moderate levels of sodium intake are excreted rather quickly in the urine, a feedback mechanism controlled by decreased levels of the adrenal hormone, aldosterone. Conversely, if the dietary sodium intake becomes restricted, the adrenal gland secretes more aldosterone, which effectively facilitates reabsorption of sodium by the kidney. Too much sodium in the blood, hypernatremia, is associated with high body temperature. Too little sodium, hyponatremia, may lead to muscular cramps and weakness. Denton (1969) reported that extreme acute hyponatremia may cause a reduced blood pressure, resulting in reduced cardiac output and circulatory collapse.

Increased sodium intake has been associated with hypertension in animals, but the National Research Council (1974) has indicated there is little or no direct evidence to support the hypothesis that hypertension can be produced in an individual with normal blood pressure on the usual intakes of salt. On the other hand, hypertensive individuals may be able to reduce their blood pressure by decreasing the amount of salt in their diet. Nevertheless, Bajusz (1965) has cited international epidemiological surveys reporting significant relationships between incidence rates of hypertension and atherosclerosis in populations whose diet is high in sodium. Krehl (1966b) has indicated that salt usage is to be considered a bad habit in relation to preventive health for hypertension and other cardiovascular diseases.

As noted above, there may be potential dangers of too much or too little salt in the diet, and hence in the body. Although athletes need be concerned with both, most problems in athletics arise due to large losses of sodium and chloride through excessive sweating.

Sweat contains about 20-50 milliequivalents (mEq) sodium per liter. To convert milligrams to milliequivalents, simply divide 1000 mg by the atomic weight. Since the atomic weight of sodium is 23, 1000 mg is equal to 43.5 mEq. Thus, one liter of sweat may contain over one gram of sodium. Van Itallie and his colleagues (1960) have indicated that a slight sodium deficiency can impair athletic performance before any clinical signs of sodium deficiency are discernable; these clinical signs may include nausea, vomiting, headache, loss of appetite and muscular weakness which may develop into leg and abdominal cramps. Although the loss of one liter of sweat is not likely to elicit these effects, there are implications for sodium chloride restitution at higher levels of sweat loss. Discussion of the pertinent research follows in the next chapter.

Relative to its effect upon physical performance, chlorine will be considered with sodium, as sodium chloride. Although chlorine, as chloride in the body, has a variety of roles such as regulating acid base balance and osmotic equilibrium, most of the dietary intake of chlorine is in the form of sodium chloride. Therefore, it will be discussed in relation to salt losses and salt intake in the following chapter.

Potassium is one of the major cations of the body, and like sodium, the body possesses rather efficient homeostatic mechanisms to control normal levels in the body fluids. The ordinary intake is 50-150 mEq/day; the atomic weight of potassium is 39. Therefore, daily intake averages about 2-6 g. It is widely distributed in foods, and is especially abundant in oranges, grapefruit, bananas, beef and fish. Potassium deficiency is unlikely under normal circumstances. Bajusz (1965) has noted a variety of functions for potassium. It plays an important role in energy consuming reactions, helps in the synthesis of glucose and glycogen from lactate and pyruvate, and is important in the production of high energy compounds.

Hyperkalemia, or excess body potassium, is not too common, but may elicit EKG abnormalities. The renal control mechanism effectively controls hyperkalemia. On the other hand, hypokalemia may result from a number of conditions producing loss of potassium from the body, through vomiting, diarrhea, stress, poor dietary practices and dehydration. Krehl (1966a) noted that potassium depletion is a common event, which is associated with poor dietary practices. In athletes or others training at high levels over long periods of time in the heat, potassium may be lost through sweating. However, potassium is closely related to the storage of glycogen in the muscles; hence, when glycogen is metabolized during exercise, it may raise the level of potassium in the blood, possibly delaying the onset of hypokalemia and conferring another physiological advantage to the glycogen storage technique discussed in Chapter Three (Hultman, 1967a; Bergstrom and Hultman, 1966). On the other hand, the increased blood level of potassium may eventually elicit hypokalemia, as hyperkalemia is one means to increase renal excretion of potassium. White, Handler and Smith (1973) have noted that renal control is not as effective against hypokalemia as it is against hyperkalemia. Hypokalemia may lead directly to interference with muscle cell nutrition, and elicit muscular weakness which would be detrimental to physical performance capacity. Indeed, some have reported that potassium seems to serve as an antifatiguing agent (Klafs and Arnheim, 1973). Detailed coverage of the relevant research is presented in Chapter Eight.

IRON

Not so many years ago, a cantankerous little sailor named Popeye would perform superhuman feats immediately after consuming a can of spinach, a food noted for its high content of iron. Although spinach per se is not usually considered as a magical food by athletes today, which might be due to the fact that the form of iron in spinach is not readily absorbable (White, 1974), iron itself is construed to be some type of ergogenic aid. Zauner and Updyke (1973) reported that most endurance athletes take large daily dosages of iron hopefully to increase hemoglobin levels, and a world class distance runner, Jim Ryun, although advocating a rather routine diet, does consume iron tablets. Russian researchers (Unsigned, 1971a) have also indicated a 20 percent increased need for iron during athletic training. Buskirk and Haymes (1972) noted that there is a real need for insuring an adequate iron intake in the diet of women who participate regularly in strenuous physical activities. With the integral role that iron plays in the formation and physiological function of hemoglobin, myoglobin and the cytochromes, one can readily visualize its importance to oxygen transportation in energy metabolism of exercise. Thus, while the assurance of optimal supplies of iron in the diet is essential to the athlete as well as the nonathlete, the role of iron supplementation is controversial. Astrand and Rodahl (1970) have indicated, on the basis of the available evidence, that there appears to be no obvious justification for excessive iron intake in the athlete.

Iron Requirements and Metabolism

Iron is an essential nutrient to man, as it is a constituent of the oxygen transportation compounds, hemoglobin, myoglobin and a number of other enzymes. It is one of the few elements which may be deficient in the American diet, especially in females. There are wide differences in the physiological availability of iron compounds, the highest being when present as ferrous sulfate or the organice complexes such as ferrous ascorbate, ferrous fumarate and ferrous citrate. Among natural compounds, the heme iron of meat is a reliable source of available iron. There are many complex interactions and unknowns between the iron content of foods, the composition of the diet, and the absorption of the iron present in the diet.

In view of these complex interactions, and of the wide distribution of iron in food, a balanced diet is the best assurance that iron intake is adequate. Such diets contain approximately 6 mg/1000 calories, with an approximate 10 percent absorption rate (National Research Council, 1974). Good sources of iron include liver, heart, kidneys, lean meats, beans and egg yolk. The average adult male needs to retain approximately 1 mg/day iron in his body. Since the average diet supplies 6 mg iron/1000 calories, and the normal adult male diet is 3000 calories, the average daily intake would be 18 mg. With a 10 percent absorption rate, he would retain 1.8 mg, sufficient to meet his daily needs. The average developing male, age eleven to eighteen, and the female during the menstruating years, ages twelve to fifty, need approximately 18 mg/day in the diet, with retention of about 1.8 mg. However, since the average caloric intake of the female during these years may be only 2100-2400 calories, she may only retain 1.26-1.44 mg iron, and thus may possibly become iron deficient. A proposal to increase the iron enrichment of flour may help remedy this deficit, yet dietary education is essential. Women should be encouraged to eat more enriched cereals, meats and other iron-containing foods. The increased need for the female during the menstrual cycle is to replace the iron lost in the blood. White, Handler, and Smith (1973) noted that the average female loses .35 ml blood per period, and needs about 0.6 mg iron retention/day to replace this amount alone. The increased need for the growing and developing male is due to the iron requirement for formation of hemoglobin and other hemeproteins, since an extraordinary increase in total body hemoglobin occurs at puberty (White, Handler and Smith, 1973).

Figure 7-1 illustrates the metabolism of iron. Apoferritin combines with iron to form a compound called ferritin in the gastrointestinal tract, with the ferritin serving as a special carrier to regulate passage of the iron from the intestine to the plasma. The iron is transported through the blood bound to a serum globulin called transferrin. The normal plasma level for iron is 100 μg/100 ml. The liver plays a central role in the cycle of storing, transporting and utilizing iron in the body. The liver is a storage source of iron, containing approximately 700 mg present almost entirely as ferritin. Iron is also stored in the bone marrow and spleen. Iron in excess of the ferritin storing capacity accumulates in the liver as hemosiderin. Iron is transported by the blood via transferrin to other tissues for formation of hemoglobin in the RBCs, myoglobin in the muscle, and cytochromes in the muscle and other tissues. Iron is lost from the body via the intestinal tract as iron in bile, and also through the catamenic or gestational processes in the female, i.e. menstruation and fetal development of the child. (White, Handler and Smith, 1973).

Anemia and Physical Performance

In the adult, about 70 percent of the total body iron is essential

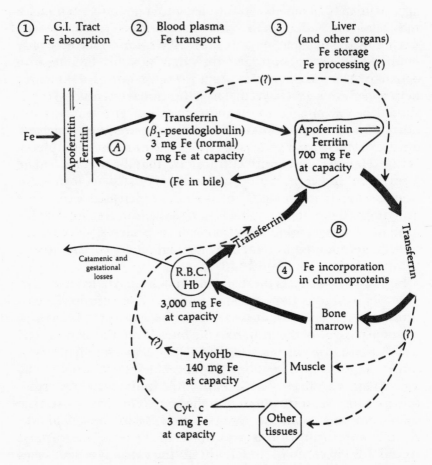

Figure 7-1 The metabolism of iron. The cyclic movement of iron is considered in two stages, A, the absorption, transport, storage and excretion cycle, and B, the storage, transport and utilization cycle. Note the central role of the liver in each cycle. From White, A., Handler, P., and Smith, E., PRINCIPLES OF BIOCHEMISTRY, 1973. Courtesy of McGraw-Hill Book Company, New York.

or functional, while the remaining 30 percent is nonessential or storage. Of the function iron, 80 percent is contained in the RBC in association with hemoglobin, whereas the remainder is in the myoglobin or intracellular iron containing enzymes (Committee on Iron Deficiency, 1968). According to Buskirk and Haymes (1972) only after the iron stores are depleted will the formation of hemoglobin be so depressed as to elicit iron deficiency anemia, a condition in which the RBC has decreased levels of bound iron. They noted, therefore, that iron deficiency anemia was extremely rare in males. The Committee on Iron Deficiency (1968) of the American Medical Association reported that in the normal individual, excluding pregnancy and infancy, iron deficiency anemia is generally due to blood loss. Nevertheless, the National Research Council (1974) reported a high incidence of iron deficiency in the United States. This may not be reflected by the development of anemia, since the iron stores may help deter the drop in hemoglobin iron content.

In contrast to the male, the female is more likely to suffer from iron deficiency anemia. Due to lower caloric intake she may have a dietary insufficiency in iron, and may also lose excess amounts during heavy menstrual flow. Hallberg and his colleagues (1966) reported a reduction in hemoglobin concentration and the mean corpuscular hemoglobin concentration in several subjects with a menstrual loss of 100 ml or more. Mayer and Bullen (1959) noted that the average female may lose up to 60 ml blood/period and not have signs of iron deficiency.

A number of reports have substantiated iron deficiency in American women. In a review of studies dealing with mineral nutrition in the United States from 1950-1968, Davis and others (1969) reported that iron intake in females was less adequate than in males. Two other reports (Alfin-Slater and Aftergood, 1973; Hutcheson and Hutcheson, 1972) indicated iron deficiency anemia was the most common deficiency disease in the United States today, especially in women and children under six years of age. The National Research Council noted that a recent ten-state nutritional survey revealed evidence of anemia in a considerable segment of the population, which was accompanied by the fact that iron intakes of many individuals were below the RDA.

Athletes, especially those in endurance activities which stress aerobic capacity, would appear to have their ability compromised if anemic. Several studies have been conducted with athletes to determine the levels of iron deficiency anemia, and the results do reflect some cases of iron deficiency and/or anemia. Stewart and his associates (1972) studied various blood parameters, notably their hemoglobin level, before and during the 1968 Mexico City Olympics. Although they noted suboptimal levels of hemoglobin in some endurance athletes, they did not attribute this to dietary deficiency as all the athletes exceeded the recommended daily intake of iron and protein.

A hematological study of Dutch athletes by deWijn and his colleagues (1971a; 1971b) revealed an occurrence of iron deficiency anemia in 2 percent of the male and 2.5 percent of the female athletes. In addition, another 3 percent of the athletes had mild anemia without signs of iron deficiency, while some athletes had iron deficiency without anemia. In total, they noted that 3.5 percent of the male athletes and 7.5 percent of the female athletes were iron depleted. The authors suggested this would be a detrimental condition for endurance athletes. They did implicate the diet as the cause of the low iron levels; however, the cause was not attributed to low levels of iron in the food, but to a high fat content in the diet which may inhibit iron absorption. Haymes (1972) studied plasma iron levels and total iron binding capacity and found 25 percent of the trained female field hockey players, 32 percent of the moderately active females, and 8 percent of the sedentary females were iron deficient. Overall it appears that some athletes, primarily females, may have iron deficiency anemia.

Some have contended that the early stages of training may produce a type of sports anemia, which has been related to inadequate intake of protein. The majority of the protein has been theorized to be used in the formation of muscle tissue, with a resultant shortage for hemoglobin formation. This may be related to the decreased plasma iron levels reported by Haymes (1975) in the initial seven weeks of training in women. She indicated that exercise increased the fragility of the red blood cell with subsequent release of hemoglobin and iron. On the other hand, Wirth and others (1975) found no significant changes in the serum iron levels of college age females who trained for a ten-week period.

Theoretically, anemia, with low hemoglobin levels, would pose a restriction to high level endurance capacity. Indeed, total body hemoglobin has been related to maximal oxygen uptake, and Haymes (1972) reported a linear relationship between maximal oxygen uptake and hemoglobin levels in both trained and untrained groups of subjects. A number of animal studies have been conducted to evaluate the effect of anemia upon endurance capacity, and one dealing specifically with iron deficiency anemia has been reported by Edgerton (1972). He found a decrease in performance when the animals were anemic. In humans, several pertinent studies have also revealed a debilitating effect of anemia upon endurance capacity and related physiological parameters. Sproule and his colleagues (1960) studied the response of nine anemic subjects to very severe exercise. The subjects had either sickle cell, iron deficiency or pernicious anemia. Age range was seventeen to sixty-five. Hemoglobin levels ranged from 5.2 to 9.3 g/100 ml blood. The exercise levels were individually geared to the patient. Although the anemic individual achieves maximal utilization of all hemodynamic adjustments, including cardiac output, during exercise, the oxygen supply is still limited due to the reduced supply of hemoglobin. A similar analogy would be endurance exercise at altitude.

A number of studies on blood donors has shown decreased endurance levels following the blood loss. Anderson and Barkue (1970) studied the relationships between variation in the blood hemoglobin concentration and the ability to carry out muscular exercise by measurement of quantitative changes in cardiovascular-respiratory functions. The subjects were blood donors and were classified as having iron deficiency anemia. Following exercise, the periods of time needed to restore functions to pre-exercise levels were prolonged under anemic conditions. Davies and others (1973) compared subjects with normal hemoglobin levels, 14.5 g/100 ml, to moderately anemic subjects, 9.2 g/100 ml, and severely anemic subjects 6.7 g/100 ml, and found decreased predicted maximal oxygen uptake for the anemic subjects as contrasted to the controls. It may justifiably be concluded that anemia will adversely affect the muscular endurance capacity of an individual in aerobic-type activities.

Iron Supplementation for Athletes

Iron supplementation has been used successfully on individuals with iron deficiency anemia. Hermansen (1973) reported that iron supplementation given to four selected subjects with iron deficiency anemia resulted in a pronounced increase in hemoglobin concentration and a slight increase in maximal oxygen uptake. Davies and Van Haaren (1973), although using submaximal exercise on a bicycle ergometer and the resultant heart rate as the criterion measure, reported a significant increase in predicted maximal oxygen uptake of an experimental group of anemic subjects who received 200 mg iron/day for three months. Anemic subjects with no supplementation did not experience this effect. Gardner and Edgerton (1972) conducted an experiment with twenty young females whose hemoglobin levels were below 12 g/100 ml blood. The criterion tests consisted of an anaerobic hand grip endurance task and a maximal oxygen uptake test on the treadmill. Several blood parameters were also evaluated. The experimental period was thirty days, and the subjects received a daily dietary supplement consisting of 150 mg ferrous fumarate. No specific training was used during the experimental period. Significant increases were noted in hemoglobin, packed cell volume, red blood cell count, and maximal oxygen uptake, indicating that iron supplementation to iron deficient females may have a beneficial effect upon physiological parameters associated with endurance capacity. However, in interpreting the results, one should note that no mention was made of a control group.

Although iron supplementation would be expected to benefit the iron-deficient anemic person, of what value might it be to the athlete? There has been relatively little controlled research done in this area, and yet, based on previous epidemiological studies dealing with iron deficiency, there may be apparent justification for recommending increased iron content in the diet or iron tablets for women athletes. Some authorities have recommended outright iron supplementation. deWijn and his colleagues (1971a; 1971b) suggested that prophylactic iron supplementation during training is indicated in many top athletes, while Mayer and Bullen (1959) recommended iron supplementation for women who lose over 60 ml blood during the menstrual cycle. White (1974) concurs with this latter recommendation. Many oral preparations of iron are available, and the simple ferrous salts such as sulfate and fumarate are the best absorbed and least expensive. Haymes (1973), after reviewing the literature, concluded that coaches should give serious consideration to the iron content in the diet of their female athletes. Buskirk and Haymes (1972), relating to the nutritional needs of the woman in sports, noted there may be a greater need for iron at the beginning of training, probably due to increased synthesis of myoglobin and the cytochromes.

Although the above recommendations may theoretically be valid, there appears to be no objective data to support the value of additional iron, in the form of iron supplement tablets, to the male or female athlete with normal hemoglobin levels. In a Swedish study, Ericsson (1970) reported significant increases in work capacity of elderly subjects, age ranging fifty-eight to seventy-one years, who received 120 mg iron daily for thirty days. A submaximal physical working capacity (PWC) test was used, and the males experienced a 4 percent increase while the females gained 12 percent. A single blind placebo experimental design was utilized. In spite of the fact that there was a significant increase in PWC in the iron supplement group, no correlations were found between the increase in PWC and the changes of hemoglobin levels. The authors hypothesized that the increase in PWC was due to factors other than total hemoglobin changes. In normal subjects, Davies and Van Haaren (1973) reported no significant effect of 200 mg iron daily for three months on predicted maximal oxygen uptake from submaximal exercise heart rate. Although not studying physical performance capacity, Weswig and Winkler (1974) evaluated the effect of iron supplementation upon hematological data of male competitive swimmers throughout an entire season. In a blind placebo design, seven swimmers received 325 mg supplement of ferrous sulfate six times/week, while seven others received a noniron placebo. A control group not in training was also used. At the end of the season, the authors reported no significant effect of the iron supplement upon RBC, hemoglobin, hematocrit, blood iron, plasma iron or plasma copper.

Although remote, there may be some danger from prolonged consumption of large amounts of iron. White, Handler and Smith (1973) noted that since there is no excretory pathway for excess iron, it tends to accumulate as hamosiderin in the liver in quantities sufficient to result in ultimate destruction of that organ. Hemochromotosis, characterized by pigmentation of the skin and hepatic cirrhosis, may result from excessive iron salt administration.

As an aside, the technique of blood doping, the infusion of blood into the athlete, may have therapeutic implications for the anemic athlete or those with subnormal levels of hemoglobin. A discussion of blood doping and the relevant research has been presented by Williams (1974).

In summary, it would appear prudent for the developing young male athlete, and the female athlete at all ages, to be conscious of the iron content in their diet. This concern is especially important to endurance athletes, but it would appear that the extra calories the endurance athlete consumes to meet his energy requirements would provide the necessary iron. Nevertheless, the athlete should be aware of iron-rich foods and include them in his daily diet. For the female athlete who experiences a heavy menstrual flow, iron supplementation by commercial preparations may be recommended. Hemoglobin and other hematological determinations may be made by a physician in order to determine the need for supplementation. Based on the available literature, which to be sure is extremely limited, there appears to be no value of iron supplementation in mature male athletes.

EIGHT____

THE ROLE OF WATER
AND MAJOR ELECTROLYTES
IN PHYSICAL ACTIVITY

WATER IS AN ESSENTIAL nutrient and a major component of the human body. In relation to some athletic events, such as long distance running in a hot environment, water may be considered to be an ergogenic aid as it may be needed to replace the four to six quarts of body fluid lost by the runner in attempts to maintain thermal homeostasis. In another athletic endeavor, mountain climbing, Sir Edmond Hillary, reviewing the records of the Swiss expedition to conquer Mt. Everest, concluded that the expedition failed due to inadequate hydration throughout the climb. Thus, the British team planned for adequate water supplies, and Sir Hillary attributed much of the success of their expedition to the fact that normal hydration was maintained during the last few days of the ascent (Unsigned, 1961).

Voluntary water restriction is a common practice in some sports, primarily amateur wrestling, but the practice is not universally approved. Zambraski and his colleagues (1974), using sixty finalists in the 1972 Iowa state high school wrestling championship as subjects, reported that many of the wrestlers were so dehydrated at the time of the weigh-in that they warranted closer medical supervision. They noted that the high urinary levels of potassium warranted concern for the possible existance of renal ischemia. In the past, water restriction during football practice, even in hot climates, has been used as a means to develop discipline and a Spartan attitude. Although this practice has been condemned for many years, the recent death of a collegiate football player was partly attributed to the absence of water on the practice field. Thus, based even on these few examples, it would appear important for coaches, trainers, and athletes to understand the role of water in various types of physical performance.

Water becomes increasingly important to the athlete as he exercises in the heat, for body temperature may be controlled through evaporation of sweat. Although sweat is primarily water, there are a number of electrolytes lost during active sweating which need to be replaced eventually. The major elements which are lost in sweat include sodium, chloride and potassium, with recent reports also indicating significant losses of magnesium. The function of these elements in the body was discussed in the preceding chapter, but since this chapter is concerned primarily with sweat losses during exercise in the heat, the role of electrolytes and electrolyte replacement solutions will be further considered.

FUNCTIONS OF WATER IN THE BODY

In the average man, the total amount of body water is approximately 57-60 percent of his total body weight. The water is compartmentalized in the body, although there is constant movement between the various compartments. Free water is more labile than bound water, which is attached more tenaciously to the colloids and hence not readily mobilized. About 55 percent of the body water is in the intracellular compartment. The remainder is in the extracellular compartments, consisting of the interstitial spaces, vascular system and miscellaneous spaces. The interstitial space is the area between the cells, whereas the vascular system includes the plasma water and cell water in the blood stream. Miscellaneous spaces include the cerebrospinal fluid, aqueous humor, vitreous humor and similar water compartments.

Water has a number of important functions in the body. It provides the essential building material for cell protoplasm, and it is a powerful ionizing agent, controlling the distribution of numerous solutes within and without the cells. The major and minor electrolytes are dissolved in water and function in an aqueous medium. Oxygen and carbon dioxide are dissolved in the body water to perform their physiological functions, as are the hydrogen ions which affect acidity changes and modify numerous physiological changes, especially during exercise. Water is the main transportation mechanism in the body, conveying to target tissues nutrients, waste metabolites and internal secretions such as hormones. In order for the taste and smelling mechanisms to function, the various substances are dissolved in water. Hearing waves are transmitted by water in the cochlea, whereas the aqueous and vitreous humor are essential to proper vision. Of prime importance for this discussion is the role water serves in temperature regulation. The cellular water absorbs the heat of oxidation in the cell, and through cardiovascular adjustments, transports it to the cutaneous circulation for dissipation to the environment. The excretion of sweat, mainly water, provides the material for evaporation and the resultant cooling effect on the body.

The requirement for body water depends upon the size of the individual. The average adult loses about 2000 ml, about two quarts, of water per day. Table 8-I represents the normal avenues for daily water loss and water intake. Urinary output is the main avenue for water loss. Insensible perspiration, which is not visible, is almost pure water and ranges between 600-700 ml/day. Water in the feces and exhaled air account for minor losses. These values would change during exercise in a hot environment, with skin perspiration losses increasing markedly. Fluid intake is the main means to replenish body water losses, and assumes an even greater role during heat stress. However, food itself contributes to body water stores in two ways. Food contains water in varying amounts, with lettuce, celery and other such vegetables being over 90 percent water. Many foods are more than 60 percent water, and even bread contains 36 percent. The metabolism of foods for energy also produces water. Wilson and his colleagues (1967) have reported the following amounts of water, in grams, are produced during the metabolism of the three main foodstuffs: 0.6/g carbohydrate; 1.07/g fat; 0.41/g protein. In addition, glycogen also has over 2 g water bound to it, which is also released during its metabolism in exercise.

Body water is maintained at a normal level through kidney function. Normal body water level is called normohydration,

TABLE 8-1

DAILY WATER LOSS AND INTAKE FOR WATER BALANCE

Water Loss

Urine Output	1100 ml
Fecal Water	100 ml
Lungs - expired air	200 ml
Skin - insensible perspiration	600 ml
TOTAL	2000 ml

Water Intake

Fluids	1000 ml
Water in Food	700 ml
Metabolic Water	300 ml
TOTAL	2000 ml

whereas loss of body fluid by dehydration results in a state of hypohydration. Hyperhydration represents a state of increased body water supply. Normal kidneys function by eliminating excess water during hyperhydration, and conserving water during hypohydration. Kidney function is complex, but one of its main roles is to regulate body water. This function is controlled by a hormone, the antidiuretic hormone (ADH), which is released by the pituitary gland dependent upon the osmotic equilibrium of the blood. There are specialized cells called osmoreceptors located in the hypothalamus which detect changes in the osmolarity of the blood, the osmolarity depending upon the concentration of substances in the blood per unit of total volume. When the osmoreceptors are affected, the hypothalamus controls the secretion of ADH by the pituitary. The ADH directs the kidney to reabsorb more of the water passing through its tubules. For example, during water deprivation, as the individual loses water from the body the blood volume will shrink and there will be more solute per unit of blood. This will influence the osmoreceptors in the hypothalamus to direct the pituitary to release more ADH. The ADH will enhance kidney reabsorption, and body water will be conserved. The reverse occurs during hyperhydration. The sensation of thirst is usually a good guide to body water needs, and is partly controlled by the hypothalamic osmoreceptors. However, as will be noted later, there may be times when thirst is not an adequate indicator of needed water replacement.

As related to athletic performance, the most important practical function of water is to serve as a means of controlling body temperatures through evaporative processes. Although this is even important during cool, or even cold weather if one exercises severely enough, it becomes increasingly important as the temperature and humidity levels climb. One of the major research topics in sports medicine involves the effects of dehydration and subsequent rehydration upon physical performance, especially in the heat. Thus, before considering the effects of hypohydration and hyperhydration on performance, a brief review of temperature regulation in man will be presented.

Temperature Regulation in Man

Of the various environmental factors that may influence work performance — such as altitude, wind, solar radiation, air pollution and humidity — the most common condition which affects performance capacity in trained athletes, as well as the normal individual who exercises regularly, is the temperature. Anyone who jogs or runs for exercise is probably aware of the effect that temperature changes may have on their ability to perform. Unless the environmental temperature is extremely low, cold does not pose much of a problem to the individual who is exercising. However, as the temperature begins to rise, the combination of the environmental heat stress and the increased metabolic heat produced during exercise may elicit physiological adjustments which at the least may prove detrimental to endurance capacity, and at the extreme may be fatal.

Ribisl and Zuti (1972) and Consolazio and his associates (1963) have noted that the energy cost of exercise in the heat is greater than comparable work in cold or temperate environments. It is a known fact that marathon runners and other endurance athletes do not particularly appreciate high environmental temperatures on the day of competition. More serious consequences may result from unsound exercise practices in the heat, as Fox and his colleagues (1966) reported a total of twelve deaths due to heat stroke over a three-year period in college and high school football players. Thus, it is imperative that all coaches, trainers, athletes and every other individual who exercises regularly be cognizant of current knowledge and potential problems associated with exercise in a hot environment.

The body temperature in cold-blooded animals such as snakes varies directly with the environmental temperature, whereas warm-blooded man is able to maintain a constant body temperature under varying environmental temperatures. In man, body temperature regulation is effective in the environmental temperature range of 68 to 92° F. The normal body temperature of 98.6° F (37°C) remains relatively constant and represents the core temperature, which consists of the cranial, thoracic, abdominal, pelvic and deeper muscle masses. Actually normal body temperatures may range from 97 to 99° F. On the other hand, the shell temperature, which represents the temperature of the skin, subcutaneous tissues and superficial aspects of the musculature, varies considerably dependent upon the surrounding environmental temperature.

In order to maintain the normal core temperature, there is a constant interplay of factors which contribute to heat production and heat loss in the body. Resting or basal heat production is provided through normal oxidative processes of the three basic foodstuffs: carbohydrate, fat and protein. Disease, a higher basal rate, the specific dynamic action of food, shivering, unconscious muscular contraction, and exercise are several factors which may increase heat production.

Heat loss is governed by four physical means: conduction, convection, radiation and evaporation. In normal environmental temperatures, body heat is transported from the core to the shell by way of conduction and convection, the blood being the prime carrier of the heat. Then the vast majority of heat radiates from the body, with a smaller amount being carried away via evaporation of insensible perspiration. A cooler environment, increased air movement, increased skin circulation, or increased radiation surface would facilitate heat loss, whereas an increased environmental temperature above 92° F would possibly reverse the radiation process, with heat radiating to the body rather than away from it. If any of the factors governing heat production or heat loss increase and are not counterbalanced by an antagonistic adjustment, then the body temperature will deviate from its normal value.

During exercise, man may increase his energy expenditure twenty-fold or greater. From a resting oxygen consumption level of 250 ml/minute, a well-conditioned athlete may increase his oxygen uptake to 5 liters/minute or more. This represents an increase in caloric expenditure from 1.25/minute to 25/minute. Measures of oxygen consumption represent energy expenditure and heat production in the body, and the three factors are directly proportional to intensity of work done by the individual. The increased heat production during prolonged exercise must be dissipated or the body temperature may be elevated to a dangerous level. The body temperature may be elevated to 102 to 104° F during hard exercise as total heat loss may not balance total heat production, but if it exceeds 106° F, temperature regulation may become seriously impaired. Thus, since the amount of heat lost through conduction, convection and radiation does not change appreciably during exercise, evaporative heat loss becomes the main means of eliminating the excess metabolic heat.

Although the mechanisms underlying regulation of body temperature during exercise are not precisely known, the hypothalamus has been identified as the central control for physiological adjustments to counteract temperature changes. Afferent impulses from temperature receptors in the skin, as well as temperature changes in the blood, are received by the hypothalamus, which then may help govern the blood flow to the cutaneous circulation and also may control the secretory nerve fibers to the sweat glands. Thus, as man exercises, the blood passing through the active musculature will pick up the heat generated by the increased level of oxidative processes during exercise and circulate it to the hypothalamus. The hypothalamus, functioning similarly to a thermostat, detects the increased temperature, and initiates, through sympathetic neural control, a release of normal vasoconstrictor tone in the cutaneous circulation. This causes a vasodilation in the circulation of the skin, thus placing the warm blood (core) closer to the body surface (shell). At the same time, increased activity of the sweat glands produces more perspiration, which when evaporated will conduct the heat away from the body. This explanation of course has been extremely simplified; for a more detailed explanation of the physiology of temperature regulation during exercise, the reader is referred to Astrand and Rodahl (1970) and Snellen (1969).

As indicated previously, evaporation of sweat is the major means of dissipating body heat while exercising in a hot environment. If a normal size individual (70 kg body weight) were to perform an aerobic task, such as jogging for an hour, he might conceivably be performing at an oxygen uptake level of 3 liters oxygen/minute. If each liter of oxygen equalled 5 calories, then he would be expending 15 calories/minute, or 900 calories/hour. Assuming a mechanical efficiency rate of 25 percent, then 75 percent, or 675 calories would need to be dissipated if the core temperature were to remain the same. Since the specific heat of the body is .83 (.83 calories will raise 1 kg of the body 1° C), then 58 calories (70 kg X .83) would raise the body temperature 1° C in the normal man. Thus, unless body heat was dissipated, the body temperature would increase over 11° C (675/58) in the above example.

When evaporation occurs, 0.58 calories are lost for each gram of water evaporated. Thus 580 calories are dissipated through the evaporation of one liter of sweat. In this example, the individual would lose over a liter of sweat if perfect evaporation occurred. As the evaporation of sweat is not perfect, i.e. sweat that drips off the body does not conduct away body heat, the subject will probably lose even more body water. Assuming a total water loss of approximately 1.5 liters in the above example the subject would lose approximately 3 pounds body weight, as a pint of water equals one pound. Indeed, some individuals may lose as much as 4 liters of sweat/hour, or 8 pounds of body weight. In contrast to a hot, dry environment, loss of body water is increased in a hot, humid environment as the increased humidity decreases the ability of the body sweat to evaporate. Consequently, high humidity in conjunction with a hot temperature combines to increase the heat stress placed upon the exercising individual. Although electrolytes are also lost during exercise in the heat, the main problem is the loss of body water. The following section discusses the physiological effects of dehydration and resultant hypohydration.

DEHYDRATION AND PHYSICAL PERFORMANCE

Dehydration and the resultant effects of hypohydration upon physical performance are, for several reasons, of interest to those associated with sports and sports medicine. The distance runner may experience severe dehydration. Buskirk and Beetham (1960) reported an average weight loss of 6 percent of the starting body weight following completion of the Boston Marathon, even though no effort was made to curtail drinking during the race. Magazanik and his colleagues (1974) reported an average loss of 3.7 percent of the body weight, with a range of 1.7 to 6.2 percent, even with replacement along the route. The climate was about 68 to 77° F. Snellen (1969) suggested that dehydration during marathon running may produce a "thirst fever" augmenting the internal body temperature independent of the metabolic rate effects. Many athletes also use dehydration techniques in attempts to reduce weight for certain sports where a lower weight classification may serve as an advantage. Examples include wrestling, judo, boxing, light weight crew, and 150-pound football. Even though dehydration to make weight in sports has received severe criticism from sports medicine groups, the procedure is still utilized by many coaches and athletes in attempts to secure some theoretical advantage in strength.

Zambraski and his associates (1974), although they reported

some severe cases of dehydration in wrestlers prior to a state tournament, noted that the acute or chronic effects of dehydration in wrestlers have not been extensively investigated or documented. There have been a number of studies undertaken to assess the effect of dehydration upon physiological performance during exercise, but this does not provide evidence that dehydration will adversely affect the wrestler's actual performance. As Costill (1972b) has implied, the results of research are difficult to extrapolate to the sport of wrestling, for although strength and endurance are important contributors to success, so also are skills and the advantage one has at wrestling in a lower weight class in relation to strength, leverage and maturity. Additional research is definitely needed in this area.

Dehydration may be accomplished either by a thermal stress, a metabolic stress or a combination of the two. Kozlowski and Saltin (1964) studied the effect of different types of heat stress upon the body fluids and loss of electrolytes. The three experimental conditions were (1) thermal — a sauna at 176° F, (2) metabolic — hard muscular work at 65° F, and (3) combination — medium exercise at 98° F. The average weight loss under each condition was 3.1 kg. There was no significant difference in the loss of electrolytes between the three conditions. However, hard muscular exercise in a cool environment did not appear to decrease extracellular fluid and plasma as much as thermal stress. They noted that the metabolic water loss from combustion of carbohydrates and fat, plus the water stored with glycogen, would account for increased losses of intracellular water during exercise. Greenleaf (1967), after a review of the literature, noted that hypohydration by thermal means decreased plasma volume and extracellular water ten times more than if the same degree of body weight loss was induced by exercise hypohydration. Heat affects the extracellular fluid whereas exercise affects the intracellular fluid.

Effect of Dehydration on Strength

Bosco and others (1968) studied nine subjects over a three-week period who were subjected to three different schedules of water intake. During the first week daily intake was 1500 ml. The second week intake was ad libitum, and the third week was 900 ml/day. Isometric strength was measured in six different muscle groups, but decreased significantly only in the elbow flexors although a general decrease was noted in the other groups. The level of dehydration was 3.1 percent of the body weight. The absence of a significant decline in five of the six measures would lend support to the contention that dehydration does not appreciably affect strength. Ahlman and Karvonen (1962) studied dynamometer strength levels of thirty-two wrestlers following both a thermal and metabolic dehydration of 2 kg body weight. They found a slight increase in the strength level following dehydration, and attributed it to a learning or warm-up factor. Costill (1972b), after a review of the literature, concluded that in events of a brief nature with intense muscular effort such as weight-lifting, dehydration has no effect.

Effect of Dehydration Upon
Submaximal Work Performance

The majority of research indicates that physiological responses to submaximal work deteriorate following dehydration. In most of these cases, dehydration will reduce the blood volume and hence the cardiovascular adjustments to exercise will result in a decreased stroke volume and an increased heart rate. If the heart rate is the criterion measure of physical working capacity, which it is in many submaximal PWC tests, then performance will be regarded as lower since the heart rate response is higher. Ahlman and Karvonen (1962) reported a high resting and exercise heart rate in thirty-two wrestlers following dehydration. The exercise was submaximal, as recorded heart rates were about 140. Saltin (1964b) noted no change in oxygen consumption at submaximal workloads, but the heart rate was higher. Herbert and Ribisl (1972a) noted a significant decrease in a modified PWC_{170} test following a 4.8 percent dehydrated weight reduction. A previous report by Herbert (1969) produced similar results. Saltin (1964a), testing three subjects after a 5.2 percent body weight loss via thermal dehydration, reported no significant change in cardiac output as compared to the same submaximal test in a normohydration state; however, the stroke volume decreased with a compensating increase in the heart rate. In summary, while submaximal exercise cardiac output and oxygen consumption do not change following dehydration, heart rate increases do occur to compensate for the reduced stroke volume resulting from decreased blood volume.

Effect of Dehydration Upon
Maximal Work Performance

Although submaximal tests are useful in evaluating physiological responses to exercise under different conditions, they do not have exact predictability relative to physiological adjustments to maximal exercise. The main tests for assessing maximal physical working capacity are the maximal oxygen uptake test and the exhaustive work test.

Several reports have indicated a significant decrease in maximal oxygen uptake following dehydration. Buskirk and others (1958) dehydrated fifteen subjects 5.5 percent of their body weight and reported a detrimental effect upon maximal oxygen uptake. Craig and Cummings (1966) reported a 27 percent drop in maximal oxygen uptake in nine men who were dehydrated 4.3 percent of their body weight. Even when rehydrated to within 1.9 percent of their weight, the maximal oxygen uptake was still 10 percent lower.

On the other hand, the majority of the literature indicates there is no gross impairment in maximal physiological functioning, even to a level of 4 to 5 percent dehydration in trained athletes. However, even though the measured physiological processes appear not to be adversely affected, maximal work time to exhaustion is severely curtailed. Blyth and Burt (1961) reported a significant decrease in treadmill run to exhaustion following dehydration. However, the run was performed in an extremely hot condition, an ambient temperature of 120° F. Saltin (1964a) noted that a 5.2 percent dehydration produced no significant change in maximal oxygen uptake, cardiac output or stroke volume, but did decrease maximal work time. In a subsequent study

(Saltin, 1964b), similar findings were reported. Kozlowski (1966) also reported that exercise dehydration on the level of 5.2 to 8.0 percent of the body weight elicited a significant decrease in maximal work performance, but not in maximal oxygen uptake. Bock and others (1967) placed ten subjects on total abstinence from water for forty hours. Test results indicated no significant effect upon maximal oxygen uptake, even with weight losses up to six pounds. Although the decrease in maximal oxygen uptake was not significant, seven of the ten subjects did have lower values.

Astrand and Rodahl (1970) effectively summarized the current viewpoint relative to the effects of dehydration upon maximal performance. They noted that following a 5 percent loss of body weight from dehydration, maximal oxygen uptake, cardiac output and stroke volume are not modified. However, the work time to exhaustion is definitely reduced after dehydration. They hypothesized that the explanation must be at the cellular level, since the aerobic power was not impaired. Change in the intracellular compartment due to dehydration may disturb the electrolyte balance and thus adversely affect muscular contraction and its susceptibility to metabolites.

From a practical viewpoint, Costill (1972b) noted that under conditions of heat stress and prolonged exertion, such as soccer, football and long distance running, water losses as little as 2 percent of the body weight may impair circulatory and thermoregulatory functions. He noted that under these conditions, adequate fluids should be made available to the athlete in order to prevent the debilitating effects of dehydration.

REHYDRATION AND HYPERHYDRATION

Since dehydration causes a reduction in work capacity in the heat, the natural reaction of the athlete is to attempt to maintain normohydration. The nature of the athletic event may partially determine the technique to be used to achieve normohydration. Although the wrestler rarely performs in a hot environment, he may replenish his dehydrated weight losses by rehydrating from the time of the weigh-in to the match time. Collegiate rules allow for a five-hour period between weigh-in and the match, hence the wrestler has sufficient time to regain a good percentage of his lost water weight. The football or soccer player may replenish fluids during frequent breaks of action. The long distance runner may carry or receive fluids for ingestion during the race, and he may also take advantage of the technique of hyperhydration, often called superhydration.

As the effects of dehydration have been studied in relation to submaximal and maximal performance parameters, so too has rehydration. The following paragraphs will discuss rehydration in that light. Later sections will cover the electrolyte solutions and fluid replacement schedules.

Since college wrestlers may undergo considerable dehydration in order to make a particular weight class, several investigations have studied the effect of rehydration upon their physical working capacity. Herbert and Ribisl (1972a), using a submaximal PWC_{170} test, noted a significant decrease in performance following 4.8 percent dehydration of body weight. PWC_{170} was still below normal just prior to competition, even though the nine wrestlers had undertaken voluntary partial rehydration. They were still 2.2 percent below normal weight. However, the rehydration did increase PWC_{170} above performance in the dehydrated state. Ahlman and Karvonen (1962) studied 32 wrestlers before dehydration, after an average dehydration of 2 kg, and about three hours following rehydration and a light meal. The criterion test was heart rate response to a 1200 kpm work load on a bicycle ergometer. They reported that losing 1 to 3 kg of water before competition adversely affects the cardiovascular system and the effect does not pass within three hours even though food and water are ingested. Vaccaro and his colleagues (1975), studying college wrestlers, noted that under competitive conditions, wrestlers cannot regain in five hours all of the fluid which was lost in order to make weight. Zambraski and others (1975) suggested the rule governing the time allocated for rehydration should be re-examined. On the other hand, Palmer (1968), using seven trained men as subjects, indicated that rehydration over a five-hour period would return physiological processes to normalcy. He studied exercise and recovery heart rates for a submaximal task under normal, dehydrated and rehydrated conditions. The subjects lost

4.75 percent of their weight via dehydration, and replenished it during the five-hour rehydration period. Heart rate responses returned to normal following rehydration. These four studies involved the effects of rehydration on submaximal exercise parameters, and are not very valid predictors of maximal capacity. This viewpoint was noted by Herbert and Ribisl in their report. No reports were uncovered which studied a rehydration effect, following a dehydration period and prior to performance, upon maximal capacity.

Water replacement during exercise is practical in several athletic activities which are conducted over prolonged periods of time. Costill (1972b) has done considerable research in the area of fluid replacement during exercise in a hot environment, primarily marathon running. He noted that while the literature supports water replacement during marathon running as effective in maintaining a steady rectal temperature and cardiovascular responses, several factors work against its effectiveness, including the rapid loss of fluid by sweating, the lower rate of gastric emptying, and inadequate thirst sensation. Costill's work in recent years has centered upon the various glucose-electrolyte solutions, which are covered in a later section.

Noting that a number of deaths in football have been attributed to heat stress, several investigations were undertaken to evaluate the relative merit of various water replacement schedules. Burt and his associates (1962), studying endurance performance during a treadmill run in the heat, found that water ingested every sixteen minutes produced the longest time to exhaustion in contrast to two other water replacement schedules, i.e. before the trial and at thirty-two minute schedules. However, Burt did note that one complicating factor in the experiment was the fact that more water was administered during the sixteen and thirty-two minute schedules.

Updyke and his associates (1966) evaluated the effectiveness of different water replacement schedules upon various physiological responses during seventy-five minutes of intermittent treadmill running. The subjects undertook the treadmill task in the heat with five conditions, which were ranked according to their effectiveness in helping to combat the adverse effects of the heat.

From best to worst, the conditions were (1) 1 liter of cold water ten minutes before and 1 liter at thirty-five minutes into the work session; (2) 1 liter of cold water prior to the start; (3) .5 liter at twenty-one and sixty-one minutes into the work; (4) .25 liter at twenty-one, thirty-five, sixty-one and seventy-five minutes into the work; and, (5) no water replacement. The results of this experiment may have implications for hyperhydration.

Londeree and others (1969) conducted a similar experiment which also suggested hyperhydration may be beneficial. They studied ten well-trained male students during a treadmill exercise at a constant temperature of 90° F and relative humidity of 70 percent. Criterion measures were heart rate, rectal temperature, blood pressure, sweat loss and specific gravity of the whole blood and plasma, which were measured before and after the one hour run. The subjects were attired in full football gear, and each undertook the test under five conditions: (1) 1 liter ten minutes before the test; (2) 1 liter thirty-five minutes into the test; (3) .5 liter ten minutes before and twenty-one minutes into the test; (4) .5 liter at twenty-one and thirty-five minutes into the test; and (5) no water. The water was cold at about 45° F. The results indicated that the early administration of cold water was more effective than late administration in helping to combat the effects of heat during exercise; this hypothesis was supported by heart rate and rectal temperature data. However, this beneficial effect was more prevalent during the early part of the work task, and this advantage was reduced during the later stages. No conclusion was reached relative to the whole versus the part technique; if anything, they noted no difference whether the liter of water was given all at one time, or in two parts in the early stages.

Hyperhydration, synonymous with superhydration or overhydration, may be effectively applied to endurance performance in the heat. Especially in marathon running, where the rules prohibit watering stations during the early stages of the race, hyperhydration may be especially important. In one of the earlier reports, Blyth and Burt (1961) noted that the performance of eleven athletes in a superhydrated state, while doing an exhaustive treadmill run at a temperature of 120° F, was significantly superior to their performance under the condition of normal water balance. Using soldiers as subjects, Moroff and Bass (1965) studied the effect of overhydration upon physiological responses to a 1.5 hour walk at 3.5 MPH in a climatic condition of 120/80° F dry bulb/wet bulb. On one day each man drank 2 liters of water before the walk, and none on the control day. During the exercise, 1200 ml was ingested. The overhydration resulted in significantly lower heart rate and rectal temperature, and a significantly higher sweat rate than the control condition. Discussing a related study, the authors indicated that overhydration was also successful in eliciting the same effects in acclimatized men. Greenleaf (1967) also reported a significantly lower heart rate and rectal temperature following overhydration as compared to normohydration, in men walking at about 3.4 mph in a temperature of 120° F. Similar findings were reported in a subsequent study (Greenleaf and Castle, 1971). On the other hand, Soule (1974) reported no effect of hyperhydration upon submaximal exercise oxygen uptake. Overall, it appears that hyperhydration with cold water prior to exercise in the heat may effectively reduce hyperthermia and the stress upon the cardiovascular system. Not only should cold water be ingested before performance, it should also be administered during the race, preferably as an electrolyte-glucose solution.

One of the myths which circulated some years ago concerned the inadvisability of ingesting water prior to performance, the assumption being that the water would distend the stomach and restrict the descent of the diaphragm, thus handicapping respiration. Several studies have investigated the effect of acute water ingestion upon selected athletic events. Little and others (1949) gave 1 liter of water to four trained men just prior to a strenuous treadmill run, and in later tests, just prior to 50-and 200-yard swims and a 220-yard dash. The general results revealed no adverse effect upon performance. Blank (1959) used thirty-three collegiate runners, testing each on a 220 yard dash twenty-seven times over a track season. Each subject performed nine times under each of three conditions: no liquid, one pint of water five minutes prior to the test, and free consumption of water five minutes prior to the test. There was no significant difference in performance. Foley (1971) reported that the ingestion of a large volume of water, 1-1.5 liters, ingested immediately prior to swimming a 200-yard individual medley, resulted in a significantly slower time. A smaller volume, .5 liter, was not significantly different than a control condition. He concluded distention of the stomach handicapped performance, not the water itself.

It is highly unlikely that an athlete would voluntarily consume a large quantity of fluid immediately prior to performance, especially in a short event where it has no possible beneficial effect. In long endurance events however, large quantities may be consumed during the hour prior to competition, and if taken immediately prior to the start, .5 liter should not pose any problem.

ELECTROLYTE REPLACEMENT

During exercise in the heat, man loses increasing amounts of body water via evaporation of sweat. In some cases, the amount may be 2 to 3 gallons over a period of several hours. Along with the sweat, a number of body electrolytes, principally sodium, potassium, chloride and magnesium, are lost. However, since the sweat is hypotonic in comparison to the body fluids, there is an elevation in serum electrolytes. Nevertheless, the loss of large amounts of electrolytes will disturb normal ionic balance in the body and may interfere with the efficient functioning of the nervous and muscular systems. Greenleaf (1967) reported that muscle cramps appear if the body salts become too diluted; as a more serious consequence, Mathews and Fox (1971) have indicated that excessive losses of sweat may increase the electrolyte concentration in the body, possibly leading to ventricular fibrillation and resultant death.

The main concern for the athlete, such as the marathoner, during competition is the attempt to maintain water balance as normal as possible due to rationale previously stated. Although athletes may experience a considerable reduction in electrolytes after two hours of running in the heat, Costill (1974) did not find these changes were responsible for fatigue. However, Costill emphasized the point that runners in training who do not replenish their salt losses may accumulate an electrolyte deficit over a few days of hard training, especially in hot environmental conditions where fluid loss will tend to be high.

Cade (1971) studied the changes in body fluid composition of ten men who underwent two hours of vigorous exercise in a warm environment. The concentration of sodium in the sweat ranged from 37-114 mEq/liter, while that of potassium was 10-65 mEq/liter. He calculated the mean sodium loss at 177 mEq; however, the serum concentration increased since sweat was always hypotonic to plasma. Rose and others (1970) measured serum electrolyte level before and immediately upon completion of the Boston marathon. They also reported a significant increase in serum sodium and potassium. A significant decrease in serum magnesium was noted, with no change in chloride levels. Kozlowski and Saltin (1964) contrasted thermal and metabolic dehydration techniques, and indicated no significant difference between the two methods upon electrolyte loss, except that potassium losses were greater during the exercise dehydration as contrasted to thermal dehydration in a sauna.

Since it is a well-established fact that electrolyte losses can be considerable following exercise in a warm climate, man has experimented with various forms of replacement in order to maintain or increase physical performance capacity. Thus, while salt tablets were the main means to replenish electrolyte losses in the past, there is an increasing popularity of a number of sport drinks, such as Gatorade®, Energade®, Olympade®, Instant Replay® and Take-Five®, all designed to help restore normal electrolyte levels and provide a little glucose. Research and opinions concerned with salt replacement and the sport drinks are considered below.

Salt Tablets

One of the most common practices in the past, and still prevalent in some high schools and colleges today, was to have available a dispenser of salt tablets in the dressing room of the athletes. Athletes who exercised several hours in the heat were advised to take several tablets daily. However, to the thinking of many young athletes, if two tablets were good, then eight to ten must be better. In a recent scholastic athletic journal, the practice of ingesting large quantities of salt tablets was recommended by a physician. Depinto and others (1971) recommended that an athlete losing 15 pounds in a football game may need a dozen or so salt tablets daily, whereas others such as tennis players who lose 5 pounds in a match need ten to twelve daily. They further indicated that it is impossible to get adequate amounts of salt with your food, and that low salt intake may cause fatigue, muscle cramps, low blood pressure, improper functioning of the adrenal and thyroid glands, and the individual will suffer from "natural laziness." They stressed the point that a little excess salt is harmless, as it readily passes out of the skin, kidneys and bowels. Although the body does have an effective homeostatic control mechanism for sodium balance via the effects of aldosterone upon the kidney, and excess salt usually is excreted, the advice by Depinto and his associates applies primarily to the nonacclimated athlete during the early stages of training before he becomes acclimated. Otherwise, the advice is contrary to general recommendations for the acclimatized athlete.

For example, Cade (1971) noted that the uniform increase in plasma sodium concentration during exercise and thermal induced sweating, together with the demonstration that sweat is a hypotonic solution, casts doubt on the wisdom of salt ingestion without adequate water intake by athletes who exercise in hot environments. Indeed, ingestion of salt without water during exercise would aggravate the basic physiological disturbance. Astrand and Rodahl (1970) have supported this viewpoint, and indicated that extra salt intake is contraindicated under these conditions.

Nevertheless, salt replacement is important, and salt tablets may be useful when sweat losses are high. In an extremely pertinent study conducted over thirty years ago, Taylor and his associates (1943) studied dietary levels of sodium chloride under various conditions while exercising on a treadmill. They evaluated the effects of a low (6 g), moderate (15 g) and high (30 g) level of sodium chloride in the diet upon performance in both a normal and hot environmental condition. They evaluated rectal temperature, exercise heart rate and sweat rate while walking intermittently on a treadmill for a half day. The men on the low salt diet suffered more heat exhaustion and had higher heart rates and rectal temperature during work. No differences were noted between the moderate and high conditions. It was concluded that the sodium chloride requirements of acclimatized men who are sweating 5-8 liters/day is not greater than 13-17 g/day. An increase in salt above this level results in increased loss of salt and water in the urine with no apparent advantage.

Salt tablets may not be necessary to restore lost electrolytes. In their excellent publication, *Nutrition for Athletes*, the American Alliance for Health Physical Education and Recreation (1971) noted that salting of the normal daily food intake will take care of sodium lost during exercise perspiration. According to their figures, the untrained individual may lose up to 1.8 g of sodium/ quart of sweat; the acclimatized athlete loses only 1.1 g sodium/ quart. Thus, if an athlete lost 12 pounds during a practice or a run, he would lose approximately 6 quarts of sweat, since a pint of water is equal to 1 pound. Six quarts of sweat would contain, at the most, 10.8 g sodium in the unacclimatized man. Since the average meal contains 3-4 g sodium if well salted, three meals per day would offer 9-12 g sodium, about enough to just cover the losses incurred in the sweat. However, sodium is lost through other processes in the body, and hence the recommendation of Taylor and his associates for 13-17 g day is reasonable. The athlete may increase his sodium intake by more liberal salting of his food, which may be adequate. One-half teaspoon of salt approximates 1 g sodium.

If salt tablets are necessary, they should be taken only with liberal amounts of water or similar fluids. In general, 1 pint of water should be consumed with each 7-grain tablet. Each 7-grain tablet is approximately .5 gram, since 15.4 grains equal 1 g. Mathews and Fox (1971) noted that no salt tablets needed to be taken unless the weight loss exceeded 6 pounds/day. In addition, acclimatized men need less salt than unacclimatized individuals since their sweat contains less salt. In general, for the nonacclimatized individual, Mathews and Fox recommend one salt tablet per pound weight loss over 6 pounds. Thus, if a subject lost 9 pounds of weight during practice, he may use three tablets. The acclimated athlete is advised to take one tablet for each pound of weight loss above 7 pounds. A recent article (Unsigned, 1975a) recommended salt tablets during the first three weeks of football practice until the players became acclimatized to practice in the heat. Dosages should be given according to the weight of the player, in amounts of 3 g daily for those under 145 pounds, 5 g for those between 145 to 180, and 8 g for those over 180.

Individual preferences should be established for athletes, since they may be able to achieve adequate salt replacement through the diet alone if salting is adequate. However, due to the link between excessive salt intake and hypertension, it may be advisable to recommend against excess salting of the meal. If the athlete acquires a taste for heavily salted food, this may persist later in life when he may no longer need electrolyte replacement. Thus, under heavy sweat losses, controlled salt tablet intake may be advisable. In sports where excessive dehydration is common, the coach should record and observe weight losses, and attempt to replenish water loss at the rate of 1 pint per pound loss, and should only be concerned with electrolyte replacement when the weight loss is over 5 to 6 pounds a day. Of course, body size should be considered, as the loss of 8 pounds in the 130 pound athlete is not comparable to the same loss in a 200 pounder. Salt replacement may be most important during the period of acclimatization, or during the first seven to fourteen days of training.

Some salt tablets may not be tolerated too well by the athlete and may lead to nausea and gastric distress. A timed release tablet called Slow Sodium® reportedly was used successfully by English soccer players competing in hot environments. Darden (1975) reported that Slow Sodium goes well with fluids, and that the ingestion of the tablets before the onset of acute sweat loss makes it possible to at least partially replace the salt loss as it is occurring.

Potassium Depletion

While much concern in the past was directed towards the possible debilitating effects of sodium chloride loss, some recent reports indicate an increasing concern for potassium loss. Rose (1975) reported that progressive hypokalemia is a slow, insidious process. He noted that unless the potassium level is quite low it is often unrecognized, but an unusual degree of muscular weakness and fatigue in the presence of a good state of aerobic fitness could be an indication of potassium insufficiency in the diet. Rose produced evidence indicating that prolonged aerobic training could elicit progressive hypokalemia. Schamadam and Snively (1967) noted that a relationship exists between potassium depletion and heat stress disease among otherwise healthy individuals when exposed to basic military training or preseason football training. They decried the indiscriminate use of salt tablets.

Knochel and Vertel (1967) also reported that the widespread practice of vigorous salt supplementation during athletic and military training may induce significant potassium losses. They hypothesized that potassium depletion may be an important factor leading to heat injury during exercise in a hot environment. The authors do not belittle the use of salt supplementation, but suggest that it be done a little less vigorously. Also, potassium should be supplemented in those individuals losing copious amounts of body fluids during sweating. Costill (1972b) also noted that the indiscriminate administration of salts should be prohibited in order to prevent excess potassium losses and possible subsequent heat injuries. He stated that the ingestion of salt prior to activity may reduce sweating and possibly induce excessive potassium losses.

Macaraeg (1974b) indicated that during exercise in the heat, the body loses potassium in two ways. The first is in the sweat itself, and the second is via increased excretion by the kidney. As more sodium than potassium is lost in the sweat, the adrenal gland responds to a low plasma sodium level and increases the absorption rate of sodium by the tubules in the kidney. As aldosterone stimulates the active reabsorption of sodium, a concomitant excretion of potassium occurs as the potassium ions are exchanged for the sodium ions.

According to the several investigators cited above, the intake of sodium chloride tablets may increase potassium losses. The physiology underlying this increased potassium depletion is not clear. The regulation of potassium ion concentration is controlled in at least two different ways, either by an aldosterone feedback mechanism that functions directly opposite to that for sodium regulation, or by high extracellular fluid potassium levels (Guyton, 1971). The salt tablets would tend to increase the plasma sodium level, hence decreasing aldosterone secretion and thus favoring retention of potassium. High extracellular fluid potassium may occur during exercise independent of sodium chloride intake, since it may be released when glycogen is metabolized. Indeed Rose (1975) has documented the fact that vigorous exercise produces hyperkalemia, or high blood potassium levels, and thus renal excretion of potassium would occur.

Potassium may be lost during exercise in sufficient amounts to adversely affect muscular performance. Macaraeg (1974b) cited several possible ways. First, it may be possible that potassium depletion will disturb utilization of carbohydrates, and the energy production in man from carbohydrates may be slightly compromised. Secondly, potassium deficiency may interfere with the release of potassium ions from the contracting muscle cells, and possibly arteriolar dilatation would be hindered, thus creating local muscular ischemia due to impeded blood flow. Low potassium concentration may also cause hyperpolarization of the nerve and muscle fibers, which may inhibit transmission of action potentials with a resultant inhibitory state.

With these thoughts in mind, increased potassium in the diet or fluids has been recommended for athletes who exercise in the heat. Potassium is a constituent of most of the major sport drinks available commercially. Schamadam and his colleagues (1968), through questionnaire analysis of athletes at Arizona State University, reported some success in the prevention of heat stress with effervescent tablets containing potassium. They suggested the use of one to two potassium bicarbonate tablets (2.5 g; 25 mEq potassium) or other multiple mineral tablets. Rose (1975) recommended particular attention to the diet, citing citrus fruits and bananas as two of the many foods high in potassium.

Electrolyte Solutions

As discussed throughout this chapter and in Chapter Three, electrolyte and glucose depletion may occur during prolonged exercise. Although the majority of the research has centered around long-distance runners, other athletes who exercise for long periods of time may also deplete energy and electrolyte stores. For example, Bolliger (1974) noted considerable fluid losses in tennis players in the heat. He found that they only replaced 17 to 56 percent of the fluid during a match, and thus recommended systematic replenishment of 150 ml sugar water at each change, or approximately every five to ten minutes. In the past decade, a number of commercial preparations have been produced with the advertised value of replacing sweat losses with fluids of similar electrolyte composition; glucose is also a major constituent to help partially replenish sugar losses. The best known thirst-quencher is Gatorade, an orange or lime flavored solution containing the following ingredients per liter: sodium (21.0 mEq), potassium (2.5 mEq), chloride (17.0 mEq), phosphorus (6.8 mEq), and 5 percent glucose. One quart of the thirst quenchers contains about 1 g of salt. The caloric content is approximately 5/ounce. It is devoid of fat and protein, and is isotonic and isosmotic with body fluids. Rose and his associates (1970), noting significant decreases in magnesium during marathon running, suggested that it be included as one of the electrolytes in the solution. Macareag (1974b) reported on the possible uses of such a solution at the 1970 Asian games in Bangkok, Thailand. The solution was Sustagen®, containing electrolytes similar to those in Gatorade, but also including magnesium (2 mEq/liter).

Plain water is one of the best thirst quenchers available. According to the manufacturers of the various sport drinks, water will ultimately satisfy both the physiological and psychological thirst of the athlete, but is not ordinarily absorbed from the digestive tract until it reaches osmotic equilibrium with the fluids in the body. Thus, the sport drinks will theoretically be more effective than plain water in rapidly replenishing body water, as they are already isotonic and isosmotic with body fluids. However, Rose (1975) indicated that money spent on electrolyte supplements is lost unless the ionic concentrations are right. Moreover, in moderate repeated dehydration over several days, glucose-electrolyte solutions appear to be no more effective than plain water in restoring electrolyte levels. Costill and his associates (1975) studied the value of replacing sweat losses with either glucose electrolyte solution or water in twelve subjects who were subjected to a 3 percent exercise dehydration on five consecutive days. The fluid ingested replaced the sweat losses. They concluded that the addition of electrolytes to drinking water is of minimal value under these conditions of moderate dehydration when subjects are allowed to ingest food and drink ad libitum.

A number of studies have evaluated the effect of these various glucose and electrolyte solutions as they relate to physical performance. Several reports have studied the absorption rate of the various substances in solution. Fordtran and Saltin (1967) studied the effect of prolonged severe exercise on active and passive absorptive processes in the small intestine, and on gastric emptying in four male and one female normal subjects. Subjects worked for one hour at about 71 percent maximal oxygen uptake. The subjects consumed 750 ml of a different solution during each trial; the solutions varied from water to saline solutions, with glucose also added. Their results indicated that isotonic saline solutions are emptied from the gastrointestinal tract more rapidly than water. However, the addition of glucose to the test solutions retarded the rate of water and sodium emptying, and hence deprives the body of the benefits of these solutions following oral replacement. On the other hand, judging the evidence from the literature and their own experiments, they noted that gastric emptying and intestinal absorption of saline solutions would be rapid enough to replace the sweat losses incurred during exercise, even in a hot environment. Costill and his colleagues (1970) challenged this statement, noting that Fordtran and Saltin recovered 500 ml of the 750 ml ingested, suggesting only 250 ml was absorbed.

Costill and his associates (1970) evaluated physiological responses with and without fluid intake during a two-hour run. Four runners each performed 3 treadmill runs at about 70 percent maximal oxygen uptake. One condition involved no fluids, a second was water only, and a glucose-electrolyte solution similar to the sport drinks was administered during the third trial; the temperature of the fluids was about 50 to 55° F. The fluids were administered at a rate of 100 ml every five minutes for 100 minutes, a total of 2000 ml. The results indicated both fluids exerted a lowering effect upon rectal temperature after about forty-five minutes of exercise. The serum electrolyte solution maintained the serum electrolyte level near the pre-exercise level, elevated the blood glucose, and maintained carbohydrate metabolism during the final sixty minutes of running. They also indicated that the fluid replacement in their study was greater than the rate of gastric emptying, and that it is highly unlikely that fluid replacement could keep pace with fluid loss. Although the effectiveness is lessened through limited gastric emptying, rapid water loss through sweating, and rules against fluid ingestion, it is still of considerable value to ingest fluids during distance races.

In a later report, Costill and others (1973c) studied the factors that limit gastric emptying time, since it posed the major problem to fluid restoration. A series of experiments was undertaken to determine the effects of various solution volumes, solution temperature, osmolarity of the solution, and sodium chloride content. Additional testing included the interaction of different levels of work intensity and duration. The results indicated little effect of sodium chloride on gastric emptying, but even the addition of a small amount of glucose (2.5 g/100 ml) elicited a marked reduction in gastric emptying. The cold solution at 41° F was evacuated from the stomach more readily than the 95° F solution. Also, high intensity workloads above 70 percent maximal oxygen uptake slowed the rate of gastric emptying. The investigators concluded that feedings during distance running or prolonged events should minimize glucose feeding in order to replenish fluid losses. Less than 2.5 g/100 ml fluid should be utilized, and consumed in quantities of 200-300 ml every fifteen minutes. The fluid should be chilled. Since some of the commercial preparation may contain about 5 g glucose/100 ml, they may deter the effective replacement of fluid lost during exercise in the heat.

Ergogenic Aspects of Glucose-Electrolyte Solutions

In an early study, Pitts and his colleagues (1944) investigated the effects of water, salt and glucose upon work in the heat, with the main aim of maximizing performance. Six acclimated young men undertook a prolonged walking workload on a treadmill in either a hot dry or hot wet environment. The criteria measured were heart rate, rectal temperature and sweat rate. The best results were obtained when the fully acclimated young men replaced the sweat they lost by water on an hour-to-hour basis. Replacement of salt via an aqueous saline solution, equal in volume to the sweat, produced essentially the same results as the water replacement. There was a slight tendency for the saline solution to better maintain sweating. Large doses of glucose induced nausea in the subjects, whereas small doses in water equal to the sweat lost elicited no significant advantage. Ladell (1955) reported lower sweating rates in man after drinking saline solution than after drinking water. The exercise consisted of a bench-stepping task in a hot, humid environment.

Costill (1972a) investigated the effect of various types of fluid replacement upon plasma and blood volume following a 4 percent reduction of body weight by thermal means. Three different solutions were utilized to rehydrate the eight male subjects. The composition was similar to the commercial sport drinks for two of the drinks, the only difference was that one was carbonated and the other was not; the third solution was water, while a fourth condition involved no replacement. The solutions were ingested over a three-hour period. Since the electrolyte solutions were relatively more effective in restoring the blood volume, Costill suggested consideration should be given to the electrolyte composition of the ingested fluid when replenishing dehydrated water losses. He noted that the five-hour time period between weigh-in and competition is sufficient for the dehydrated wrestler to replenish his vascular fluid losses. Herbert and Ribisl (1972b) utilized Gatorade during a forced rehydration study. They measured metabolic responses to a standardized treadmill task, and subjected the subjects to four trials; body weight remained constant in the control trial, and was decreased 3, 5 and 7 percent, respectively, in the other three trials. The authors concluded that wrestlers who rapidly reduce their weight beyond 3 percent will experience slight impairments in metabolic efficiency; however, if concerted efforts are made to replace all fluid losses with a physiologic solution, complete performance recovery can occur. Only carbonated Gatorade was used in the study and no comparison was made with water replacement.

Several studies compared water with the glucose-electrolyte solutions relative to their effect upon physiological parameters during exercise. Costill and Sparks (1973) studied the effect of rapid fluid replacement upon heart rate response to a level treadmill run at a speed of about 5.8 m.p.h. The subjects underwent thermal dehydration of 4 percent of the body weight on three separate occasions, and were then exposed to one of three experimental trials. The trials involved fluid replenishment with either demineralized water or a glucose-electrolyte solution, and a third control condition without rehydration. The replacements were administered over a three-hour period. The results indicated the exercise heart rate returned to normal when the subjects reached approximately 62 percent rehydration, and the glucose-electrolyte solution was apparently not significantly differentiated from the water treatment in this regard.

In another report, Costill (1972b) studied the effects of rehydration with different osmotic solutions upon heart rate responses to a standardized treadmill run. Thermal dehydration was set at 4 percent of the body weight and fluid replacement was accomplished by two hypertonic solutions, one isotonic solution, and water only. A no rehydration trial was also used. Although the heart rate responses were lower following all rehydrated conditions, no one condition was significantly better than the other.

Witten (1972) studied the effect of fluid replacement by either Gatorade, Coca-Cola® or water, against a control period of no rehydration, upon heart rate response to exercise following a 2 percent dehydration loss of body weight. Six subjects undertook all four trials. The subjects were dehydrated for seventy minutes, rehydrated in fifteen minutes the fluid lost, and rested another seventy-five minutes before taking the Balke treadmill test. The test was terminated at a heart rate of 180. No significant differences were noted between the treatments. It would appear, based on the available evidence, that the sport drink solutions do not confer any advantage as a replacement fluid in dehydrated conditions, relative to heart rate responses to exercise.

Whether or not the glucose-electrolyte solutions confer an ergogenic effect and hence increase performance capacity is a question of interest to many athletes and coaches. The following reports have in general revealed no significant beneficial effects in comparison to other fluids, including water. Eaves (1968) studied the effect of four different liquids upon the endurance of college wrestlers. Five wrestlers dehydrated 6 percent of their body weight on four occasions and then rehydrated 2 percent of their body weight by consuming either Take-Five, Gatorade, Coca-Cola or water. No statistically significant differences were noted between the treatments. O'Conner (1967), using a repeated measures design, compared the acute effects of Gatorade, as compared to a placebo and control condition, upon performance in a 1-mile run. There were no significant differences between the treatments.

Mathews and others (1969) investigated the effects of Gatorade, Coca-Cola and water upon exhaustive endurance capacity and several other variables. A no rehydration control condition was also used. Six subjects were dehydrated 2 percent of their body weight on four different occasions, and each subject undertook each treatment. There was no significant difference between the four conditions on endurance time, core temperature, heart rate or maximal oxygen uptake during the Balke treadmill test. The results appear contradictory to prior evidence when comparing the rehydration conditions with the no rehydration condition. However, the 2 percent dehydration may not have been severe enough to affect performance.

Patton and Randolph (1972) compared a dextrose solution, Gatorade, Take-Five, and a non-nutritive placebo on the endurance capacity of twenty subjects on a treadmill test. The exercise test to exhaustion was performed under a heat stress condition in high temperature and humidity. There were no significant differences between the treatments. In a double blind experiment, Cade and his colleagues (1972) evaluated the effect of a glucose-electrolyte solution versus a water replacement and no replacement condition upon several parameters. The work task consisted of a seven-mile run-walk, and the criterion measures of performance were the overall time plus the maximal ability to run the last 880 yards of each mile. The task involved a sequence consisting of: walk 220 yards, run 440 yards, walk 220, run 880. This procedure was undertaken for the last six miles. In a second experiment, a run to exhaustion was used. The authors noted that the performance of the athletes in both sets of experiments was better when a glucose-electrolyte solution was used. The authors did not speculate as to whether the increased performance was due to a decreased heat stress or maintenance of blood sugars.

In summary, there appears to be no conclusive evidence of an ergogenic advantage which may be attributed to the glucose-electrolyte preparations. While the commercial preparations do offer a scientifically sound means of replenishing body fluids lost through exercise in the heat, they do not appear to help increase performance capacity. Nor are they any more effective than extra salt and water in replacing lost body fluids and electrolytes over a day's period. Their increased potassium content may be helpful, but their main appeal may be their convenience. A homemade solution may be made from water, flavoring, some salt, and a simple sugar or glucose syrup.

HEAT ILLNESSES

Heat injuries can prove to be fatal, and a number of athletes who exercise for prolonged periods of time in the heat have suffered the extreme consequences of heat stroke. Many athletic governing bodies have established rules relative to athletic training in hot environments, primarily in American football. Certain precautions are usually mandatory during early season practice. The American College of Sports Medicine recently issued a position statement on prevention of heat injuries in distance running, noting that distance runners may incur a 6 to 10 percent body water deficit. They noted that dehydration of these proportions severely limits subsequent sweating and exposes the runner to the various health hazards of hyperthermia.

Figure 8-1 represents a flow chart of heat regulation and heat disorders. When a heat stress is imposed on the body, the chief physiological adjustments to control body temperature are sweating and vasodilation. Thus, the blood conveys the body heat from the interior to the cutaneous circulation and the evaporation of sweat facilitates cooling. As the heat stress, such as exercising in a hot environment continues, vasodilation and sweating may

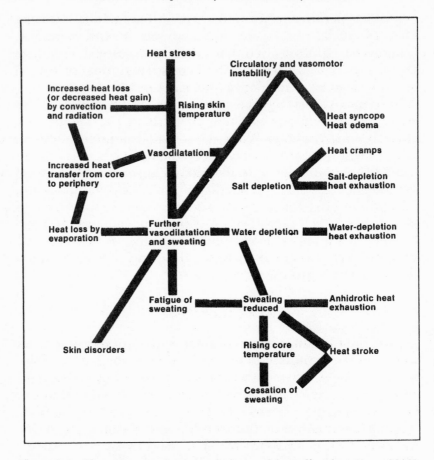

Figure 8-1   Flow chart on heat regulation and heat disorders. From MAN, SWEAT AND PERFORMANCE, 1969. Courtesy of Becton, Dickinson and Company, Rutherford, New Jersey.

continue, with possible circulatory instability. Due to decreased relative blood volume, heat syncope or fainting may occur. This is one of the milder forms of heat illnesses and may be treated by rest in a cool area with the administration of cold fluids. If the individual continues to be exposed to a heat stress, salt and water depletion may occur. Heat cramps appear to be caused by excessive loss of body salt through profuse sweating. They usually appear late in the day following ingestion of large amounts of unsalted water, and result in severe muscular cramps in the calf of the leg and/or the abdomen. Appropriate therapy would consist of rest and adequate salt intake; however, as previously noted, salt should be replaced only in conjunction with adequate fluid intake. The use of glucose-electrolyte solutions may possibly be effective during activity in preventing heat cramps as these solutions may rapidly replace lost electrolytes to the plasma and tissues. Salt depletion heat exhaustion occurs most frequently in individuals who are not acclimated to work in the heat, and is also caused by inadequate replacement of salt. The treatment is similar to that for heat cramps.

Excessive water depletion poses the most serious problem. Water depletion heat exhaustion resembles fainting, and is caused by inadequate circulation to the brain; the blood volume is distributed primarily to the skin in an effort to cool the body, and hence the brain circulation is not adequately maintained. The skin usually becomes pale, cool, clammy and is profuse with sweat. Heat exhaustion may incapacitate the individual for a few hours, but is usually responsive to treatment consisting primarily of cooling the individual in a reclining position. Mild stimulants, such as iced coffee or tea may also be used. The individual should rest and be observed for several hours in order to prevent a relapse.

A highly motivated individual may push himself beyond the early warning stages of more serious heat injury. As he continues to exercise, the sweating mechanism may become ineffective in maintaining the body temperature. Sweating may actually cease and the core temperature will elevate rapidly as the individual continues to exercise, resulting in heat stroke. Heat stroke is the most dangerous condition resulting from exposure to high temperature, since it may lead to death. Although it may be caused by simple exposure to combined conditions of high temperature and humidity, it is usually associated with exercise in the same conditions. The combination of the environmental and metabolic heat of exercise with the decreased evaporative heat ability in a hot, humid environment elevates the body temperature. As the body temperature rises, the hypothalamus becomes overheated, its heat-regulating ability may then become diminished, and sweating will diminish or cease. As the body temperature rises to 106° F or greater, the essential elements in the cell, the parenchyma, may be damaged. Death may result if critical areas of the brain are irreparably damaged (Guyton, 1971). During heat stroke the temperature may reach 110° F, and the skin will be hot and dry as contrasted to the cool and wet conditions of heat exhaustion. When heat stroke is detected, the individual should be cooled as rapidly as possible, by placing him in a tub of ice water or by other means. Immediate medical attention is imperative. It should be stressed that even though the normal young, unacclimatized, thin male may suffer the consequences of excessive exercise in the heat, other groups of individuals may be even more susceptible. Aged, female or obese persons are less able to cope with strenuous exercise in the heat, and hence may more easily fall victim to the various heat disorders. According to Henschel (1971), age per se is not a limiting factor in mild or moderate thermal stress, but at high levels of thermal stress, which would occur during exercise in the heat, tolerance to the heat is decreased in older individuals. Henschel has also noted a lower tolerance time to severe heat by women, which may be due both to their extra amount of body fat which serves as an insulation against the dissipation of body heat, and the lower and slower rate of sweat production as compared to the male. He noted that the skin temperature at the onset of sweating was 4° F higher in females than in male subjects, even though the total number of sweat glands, as well as the number per unit of skin surface, were both greater in the females. The obese individual, due to his larger amount of subcutaneous fat and greater energy production during exercise, is more susceptible to heat stroke. The increased heat production and inability to dissipate the heat due to the insulating properties of body fat combine to deteriorate performance and predispose to heat disorders.

Prevention of Heat Illness

The athletic coach and trainer, as well as the athlete, should be aware of the potential dangers of hot environments. A temperature reading from a dry bulb thermometer, although helpful, is not fully adequate to assess the heat stress which may be imposed upon an athlete. Even if the dry bulb temperature is only 70 to 75° F, a high relative humidity may increase the risk of overheating.

There are several means to assess the index of heat stress. The ordinary dry bulb (DB) thermometer measures the air temperature, and usually is located in the shade. The natural wet bulb (WB) thermometer is an ordinary thermometer with a moist wick surrounding the bulb. A sling psychrometer consists of a dry bulb and wet bulb thermometer. Since evaporation cools the wet bulb thermometer, it presents a lower reading than the dry bulb. The difference between the two readings is a measure of dryness of the surrounding air. The larger the difference, the greater the dryness. When the two temperatures are the same, there is 100 percent humidity. Since the wet bulb thermometer reflects humidity, some guides to athletic practice have been based upon wet bulb readings. Murphy and Ashe (1965) presented the guide in Table 8-II for football practice.

TABLE 8-II

WET BULB TEMPERATURE GUIDELINES FOR

FOOTBALL PRACTICE

Wet Bulb Temperature	Recommendation
Under 60°F	No precautions necessary
61-65°F	Alert observation of all squad members, particularly those who lose considerable weight
66-70°F	Insist on water and salt intake on the field
71-75°F	Alter practice schedule; provide frequent rest periods, water and salt replacement
Above 76°F	Postpone practice or conduct it in shorts

Although use of the sling psychrometer is better than the dry bulb, Minard (1961) contended that in cases of high solar radiation and low humidity, the wet bulb thermometer alone is a relatively poor guide or index to heat stress. He suggests the use of a Wet Bulb Globe Thermometer Index (WBGT). The globe (G) thermometer is a hollow copper sphere painted black on the outside, with an ordinary thermometer inside with the gauge exposed for reading. The black surface absorbs solar and local radiation. In an unshaded outdoor position, the globe thermometer is usually higher than the DB. The WBGT takes into account the four physical variables determining the heat stress: radiation, air temperature, humidity and air movement. The WBGT Index is computed as: .7 WB + .2G + .1 DB. A recommended guide is presented in Table 8-III. Sling psychrometers are available at reasonable prices, as are devices such as the Physiodyne®, a compact battery-operated instrument that instantaneously detects and correlates relative humidity, thermal radiation and air temperature. Spickard (1968) offered a diagram for the individual who wished to construct his own WBGT.

TABLE 8-III

WET BULB GLOBE THERMOMETER (WBGT) RECOMMENDATIONS

FOR FOOTBALL PRACTICE

WBGT Temperature	Recommendation
82-84.9°F	Alert
85-87.9°F	Active practice curtailed in unacclimated men
88-89.9°F	Active practice curtailed in all men except those most acclimated
90°F	All active training stopped

*Courtesy of Becton, Dickinson Company.

The most common form of heat illness results from a large loss of body water. Even after mild exercise dehydration, the body temperature may be elevated due to reduced sweating (Ekblom, 1970). Thus, it is imperative that body water be replenished during exercise in the heat. Although water restriction to athletes was a common practice in the past, the Committee on Nutritional Misinformation of the National Research Council (1974) has reported that there is no evidence to indicate man can adapt, or be physically trained, to tolerate water intake lower than his daily losses. There is no basis for restricting water intake to athletes, and it is essential that they have free access to fluids whenever sweat losses are likely to be high. Body water levels are maintained relatively constant, and the sensation of thirst over a twenty-four-hour period of time normally will govern the replenishment of body water lost through thermal or exercise dehydration. However, in athletes who are continually subjected to high losses of body water, and may experience several such dehydrations daily, the sensation of thirst may not adequately replenish lost body fluids. In these cases, according to Westerman (1970) the best rule for fluid replacement is on a weight-to-weight ratio. One pint (16 fluid ounces) should be ingested for each pound of weight loss.

Acclimatization

It is a well-established fact that acclimatization to the heat will help increase performance in comparison to an unacclimatized state. Physical conditioning alone also confers some advantage to exercising in the heat (Buskirk and others, 1958; Kral and Hais, 1963). Simply living in a hot environment confers a certain measure of acclimazation to heat (Wyndham and others, 1964). However, this passive acclimatization is not sufficient to deter potential problems associated with exercise in the heat. Thus, before an individual is subjected to strenuous exercise in a hot environment, he should undergo a period of active acclimatization. By participating in moderate exercise in the heat, the individual will undergo several physiological adjustments which will render him less susceptible to the ills of excessive heat stress. In many states, a period of acclimatization, without full gear during the latter part of summer, is mandatory prior to football practice. During acclimatization, the circulatory system and sweating mechanisms undergo several important changes to help the individual function more effectively while exercising in the heat. According to Astrand and Rodahl (1970), most of the changes are accomplished in four to seven days, and acclimatization is complete in approximately two weeks. Regarding the circulatory system, acclimatization increases the total blood volume, increases the skin blood flow, and decreases the time needed to shunt the blood to the skin. Before acclimatization, the blood flow to the skin increases at the expense of blood flow to other tissues, including the active musculature. This decreased blood flow to the muscles would hamper performance capacity. Following acclimatization, the increased blood volume helps restore normal circulation, thus helping to restore normal physical working capacity. According to Guyton (1971), the maximal rate of sweating is approximately 1.5 liters/hour in the unacclimatized individual, but is nearly 4 liters/hour in the person maximally acclimatized to heat. Thus as man becomes acclimatized, the onset of sweating becomes quicker and the sweat rate increases, facilitating greater evaporative heat loss. In addition, the amount of salt lost in sweat is decreased, preventing excessive loss of electrolytes.

Following a period of acclimatization, man is better able to tolerate exercise in the heat due to alterations in the cardiovascular system and sweating mechanism.

Guidelines for Exercise in the Heat

In summary, the following guidelines may be applicable to all individuals, athletes and otherwise, who may perform strenuous exercise in hot environments.

1. Be conscious of temperature and humidity conditions. If you live in a temperate zone where the temperature may fluctuate rapidly within a week, be cautious of exercising your usual amount on a hot day, especially when the humidity is high.

2. When the hot weather begins, moderate your activity until acclimatized. If initiating a strenuous exercise program in hot weather, allow one to two weeks for acclimatization; exercise at lower levels.

3. Exercise in the cool of the morning or evening in order to avoid the heat of the day.

4. Exercise in the shade, if possible, as the solar radiation poses

an additional heat stress.

5. Wear loose, white porous clothing when exercising. The whiteness will reflect radiant heat, and the porous clothing will permit evaporation to occur.

6. Keep a record of weight losses. Replenish fluids based on the guidelines in this chapter. A pint of fluid for each pound lost is a sound guide.

7. Replenish lost electrolytes (salt) if excessive loss of body water occurs. Salt foods excessively, as this will normally account for normal electrolyte losses. Eat foods that are high in potassium content.

8. If you are performing strenuous exercise over a prolonged period in the heat, hyperhydration or the ingestion of extra amounts of fluid prior to exercise may be beneficial. Intake of commercial thirst-quenchers or other fluids during exercise may help deter dehydration and loss of performance capacity. Do not consume solutions with large glucose concentrations, as they may deter fluid absorption.

9. Avoid excessive intake of protein, as the specific dynamic action of protein is greater than that of carbohydrates or fat and may contribute to the heat stress.

10. If you are either aged, female or obese, you are less likely to tolerate exercise in the heat and should therefore use extra caution.

11. Be aware of the signs and symptoms of heat exhaustion and heat stroke, as well as the treatment for each. Muscle cramps, dizziness, extreme fatigue and coordination problems may signify oncoming illness.

12. Do not avoid exercise in the heat completely, but be cognizant of the problems related to prolonged exposure. Coaches, trainers and administrators should have an emergency procedure available in case of heat illness. For those individuals responsible for the conduct and administration of competitive distance races, it is advisable for them to be familiar with the position statement advanced by the American College of Sports Medicine, found in Appendix G.

CHAPTER **NINE** _____

ERGOGENIC FOODS

THROUGHOUT THE YEARS a number of different foods or compounds have been utilized in attempts to increase athletic performance because they theoretically possessed some ergogenic effect. The popularity of many of these foods, such as gelatin and lecithin, has faded somewhat; however, multivitamins, protein tablets and wheat germ oil, among others, are still extolled as ergogenic foods, and advertised with this implication in leading coaching magazines. Fleming (1968), in a recent book entitled *Super Food for Super Athletes,* discussed a number of super foods, foods that have been invested of their dynamic energy by the sun and mineralized by the earth. At one time, the intake of such compounds was considered by some athletic governing bodies to be a form of doping or drug use. However, the Medical Commission of the International Olympic Committee (1972) stated that the simple replacement of missing or expended body matter, such as glucose, calcium, lecithin, phosphate, protein compounds and vitamins, is no longer regarded as doping, even when administered by injection before competition.

While the ergogenic drugs have been banned from use in athletics and may be more difficult to secure the athlete may increasingly begin to use the so-called ergogenic foods as the magic potion. The role of several alleged aids have been discussed previously. Protein supplements were covered in Chapter Five, while the vitamins and minerals were explored in their respective chapters. The role of glucose was reported in Chapter Three, but several other comments are made below, followed by a brief discussion of honey, another form of sugar. The remaining alleged ergogenic aids that are discussed include gelatin, lecithin, phosphates, multiple supplements, wheat germ oil, alkaline salts, aspartates, alcohol and caffeine.

208

GLUCOSE AND DEXTROSE

Karpovich and Sinning (1971) noted that some coaches, knowing that sugar is the fuel for muscular contraction, have attempted to give up to one-half pound daily to their athletes. The results were gastric disturbances. As reported previously in Chapters Three and Eight, the intake of glucose during prolonged work may be helpful in alleviating the symptoms of fatigue, probably by helping to maintain the blood glucose level and optimal functioning of the central nervous system. However, the intake of sugar just before performance will have no significant effect, particularly upon events of short duration.

In early research, Vogeler and Ferguson (1932) gave 4.8 g dextrose to eight subjects prior to performance in a 40-yard dash and several strength tests. A calcium carbonate tablet flavored with cinnamon was used as the placebo. The tablets were ingested five minutes prior to testing. Based upon percentage changes, the authors indicated that sugar conveys a small but beneficial effect upon performance in both speed and strength. However, the statistical interpretation would be open to question. In the same year, Pampe (1932) noted no beneficial effect of 50 to 100 g sugar upon muscular work. Wrightington (1942) studied the effect of 50 g sucrose or an equicaloric amount of glucose upon mechanical efficiency on a bicycle ergometer. The sucrose increased the respiratory quotient from .84 to .92, but the author concluded that neither glucose nor sucrose elicited a significant increase in mechanical efficiency. Karpovich (Karpovich and Sinning, 1971), in numerous early studies, also found no beneficial effect of glucose or cane sugar on events of intense muscular effort for short duration.

In a more recent report, Scherrer (1971), using thirty highly-fit freshmen college students, studied the effect of 100 g dextrose upon strenuous sprint ability on a bicycle ergometer. Each subject undertook the test three separate times: experimental condition, placebo, and control. Performance was significantly greater during the initial sprint when dextrose was ingested, as compared to the control when nothing was ingested. Since no significant difference existed between the placebo and dextrose trials, it must be concluded that the dextrose did not exert an ergogenic effect on these anaerobic work tasks. Orava and his colleagues (1974) investigated the effects of a carbohydrate-rich solution, Sportti-C®, in amounts of 1 g glucose/kg body weight, on various blood parameters and cardiovascular responses to submaximal exercises while on a bicycle ergometer and while running. The placebo condition involved the use of Coca-Cola. The general results indicated no significant changes in cardiovascular parameters, or in subjective and objective performance abilities.

Even after the generally negative reports relative to the effect of glucose intake upon physical performance, Arnold (1971) noted that it is still a good idea to eat one or two tablets of glucose about thirty minutes before the shorter races for a neurophysiological effect. He also indicated that for races of a mile or so, an ounce or two of glucose may be helpful. He presented no data to support these contentions.

The intake of large amounts of sugar would produce a rapid rise in the blood sugar level (hyperglycemia), which would trigger the release of insulin from the pancreas. The insulin would rapidly store the blood sugar in the muscles and liver, and possibly cause a low blood sugar level (hypoglycemia), which might give the athlete a feeling of weakness several hours after ingestion. The reduced blood sugar would affect the central nervous system to elicit these symptoms. However, with the onset of exercise, the release of epinephrine would stimulate glucose release from the liver, hence elevating the blood glucose level.

The general conclusion is that the ingestion of sugar immediately prior to performance will exert no significant bearing upon the outcome of the event. It may even be detrimental in long-distance events since it may draw water into the gastrointestinal tract, thus causing minor gastrointestinal disturbances or possibly restricting water for perspiration during endurance races in a hot environment.

HONEY

One of the main foods of athletes over the years has been, and still is, honey. Even for the general public, Jarvis (1958), in his best seller *Folk Medicine,* suggested that honey gives quick energy release, enables athletes and others who expend energy heavily to recuperate rapidly from exertion, and relieves pain in arthritis. He claimed that it is an excellent source of potassium, iron, calcium, phosphorus, magnesium and is high in riboflavin and nicotinic acid. However, a perusal of nutrition tables reveals that many of these substances are found in small or trace amounts in a tablespoon of honey, and White (1974) indicated that honey is a poor source of nutrients.

Forty percent of the sugar in honey is fructose. Arnold (1971) indicated that in cases where swimmers may have to perform in meets on consecutive days, and thus may deplete glycogen stores, fructose would be better to take than glucose, as fructose is converted rapidly into glycogen. He noted that it cannot be used immediately for energy in the muscle, as glucose can, but must be converted to glycogen first. Thus, Arnold suggests eating fructose, which may be obtained in honey, as a rapid means of restoring glycogen in the body. However, Arnold provided no experimental evidence relative to the superiority of fructose over glucose in replenishing muscle glycogen supplies in athletes undergoing glycogen repletion techniques, much less any evidence to support the superiority of fructose relative to increases in performance capacity in comparison to a normal diet.

One of the main protagonists for honey as an ergogenic aid is Percival (1955), who published his experiences with honey relative to athletic nutrition in the periodical, the *American Bee Journal.* The reader may perceive the implications. His experiences are also cited at length in *Folk Medicine* (Jarvis, 1958). Percival, representing the Sports College of Canada, cited his research in an attempt to find the ideal preactivity meal and postactivity recovery aid. He noted that honey supplies the necessary energy requirements, has high caloric content, is popular with the athletes due to its taste appeal, is versatile in combination with other foods, and is a pure food. Without reporting any experimental design or quantified results, Percival noted that athletes participating in endurance tests, such as distance running and repeated 50-yard sprints and 100 yard swims, performed better when fed two tablespoons of honey thirty minutes prior to testing, and a definite drop in performance when the honey was withdrawn. Other advantages attributed to honey were facilitated recovery from fatigue; maintenance of sustained effort during hockey, football and basketball; and the prevention of weight loss during training. He concluded, without reservation, that honey is an ideal energy and fatigue recovery fuel.

The absence of any experimental data makes it difficult to digest his conclusion, and the role of honey must be similar to that of glucose, i.e., it may be of limited use during events characterized by prolonged effort. It may be that Percival's data was biased by the placebo effect, as no mention was made of placebos in his discussion.

GELATIN

Gelatin is derived from collagen, a protein substance in the connective tissue. Since gelatin is composed of approximately 25 percent glycine, an amino acid, it has been considered by some athletes to be a good source of protein. Glycine is also known as aminoacetic acid or glycocoll. However, McCollum (1957) has noted that gelatin is poorly constituted to meet the body needs for tissue protein synthesis, as it does not contain all the essential amino acids. Plain dry gelatin, not the dessert type, is almost pure protein with some water. A cup of the dessert gelatin, prepared with water, contains about 4 g protein and 34 g carbohydrate. However, the rationale most commonly noted concerning the ergogenic effect of gelatin is its relationship to creatine formation; since glycine, a constituent of gelatin, is considered a precursor for the formation of creatine, some have contended that gelatin may help form phosphocreatine in the muscle (Kaczmarek, 1940).

The results of early research are controversial, with some finding a beneficial effect and others reporting no effect of gelatin upon physical performance. Several reports from the Mayo Clinic may have triggered research in this area; they revealed that glycine decreased fatigability in normal men. Thus, Ray and others (1939) reported that 60 g gelatin a day elicited tremendous increases in the work capacity of six men on a bicycle ergometer, whereas four women experienced no such effect. The workload was submaximal, representing about 270 to 360 kpm. The results were also very variable among subjects. Kaczmarek (1940) also reported fantastic increases following gelatin supplementation. He studied the effects upon a number of male athletes and non-athletes, as well as some fifteen to seventeen-year-old-females. The dietary supplement consisted of 1.5 ounces of gelatin daily for six weeks to the athletes, and for three weeks to the nonathletes. The subjects also undertook three to four weeks preliminary training. During the entire experiment, all subjects undertook an exhaustive bicycle ergometer test sixty times/week. Tremendous results were reported, with the athletes experiencing a 216 percent increase in work output during the gelatin period. The nonathletes experienced a 52 percent increase and the females also increased their output. The major criticism of this study was the absence of a placebo or control group.

Chaikelis (1941) did employ a placebo group as he studied the effect of glycine upon the strength of some college athletes. Six g glycine was given daily to the forty experimental subjects over a ten-week period; a glucose-lactose placebo was given to the nineteen control subjects. The criterion measures were the Rogers Strength Index, consisting of strength measures for the grip, back and legs, and the McCloy Endurance Index, a ratio of 60-yard to 220-yard performance times. The results indicated a significant increase in the Rogers Strength Index for the glycine treatment, but no effect upon the endurance index. Although the author reported a significant benefit due to the glycine, the mean values for the strength scores seem to be in error. The mean grip strength scores were 253 to 310 pounds, while the back and leg strength levels were only 267 to 397 pounds. It is difficult to conceive that these values represent true forces by these divergent muscle groups.

Many of the older reports, plus a relatively recent study, suggest that gelatin or glycine are not ergogenic foods. Maison (1940) studied the effect of 15 g aminoacetic acid/day or the equivalent amount in 60 g gelatin upon fatigability of a small muscle group in two different experiments. A limited number of subjects, only six, finished the experiments. The results revealed no effect of the supplements on performance. However, no placebo group or control group was used in either experiment. Hellebrandt and her associates (1940) reported that women who were trained for severe physical work did not experience any gains in performance on an anaerobic task following dietary supplementation with gelatin. King and others (1942), using a double-blind placebo experimental protocol, studied the effect of aminoacetic acid upon bicycle ergometer work to exhaustion. The workload created exhaustion in three to five minutes. The experimental group received approximately 6 g aminoacetic acid/day, and the placebo group received lactose-saccharose. After three weeks, the groups reversed dosages. The subjects were in training for football, and the results revealed no effect of the aminoacetic acid upon performance.

Robinson and Harmon (1941) trained 9 nonathletic college men on a running program over a period of twenty-six weeks. Following the first eight weeks, 60 g gelatin was administered daily to some of the subjects. During the course of the experiment a number of performance variables were tested, including treadmill run to exhaustion, maximal oxygen uptake, and several track runs from 880 yards to 1.5 miles. Although training increased performance capacity, no significant difference was noted between the experimental and control subjects. Horvath and others (1941) gave varying amounts of glycine to eight men over an eight-week period of time and evaluated the effect upon muscular strength. They concluded that glycine does not increase strength or modify the course of the training curve.

Karpovich and Pestrecov (1941), in a series of five experiments, studied the effect of gelatin upon various physical performance parameters. In one experiment, a controlled blind-placebo design was used with prison inmates doing bicycle ergometer work. No special effect was attributed to gelatin. Addition of gelatin to the controlled diet of the inmates did not improve performance, nor did the withdrawal make it worse. The study was conducted over a six-month period. The other experiments included college students undertaking ergometer work similar to the prison inmates, campers involved in a swimming program, and two different groups of weight lifters. The duration of the experiments and amount of gelatin supplementation varied in these groups, but no group experienced any beneficial effect due to the gelatin added to their diet. In a more recent study, Hilsendager and Karpovich (1964) investigated the effect on endurance capacity of glycine, and glycine in combination with niacin. Eighty-six subjects were tested on either a bicycle or a forearm ergometer. The medication consisted of either 750 mg glycine, 75 mg niacin, or a combination of the two. All medicaments were given in a rotation order, which was repeated twice, so that each subject had eight experimental sessions. During the session, forty subjects undertook the bicycle ergometer task, while forty-six did the forearm ergometer workload. Three different time schedules were utilized for the administration of the supplements; sixty-six subjects received the medicaments two hours and again one hour prior to the trial, ten took it five minutes before, and ten subjects took it immediately before the trial. The statistical analysis revealed no significant effect upon either of the endurance tasks.

After reviewing the literature, it is concluded that gelatin, or its constituent amino acid glycine, exert no beneficial effect upon physical performance capacity when utilized as a supplement to the normal diet.

LECITHIN

Lecithin is a phosphatide found in many animal tissues, and supposedly possesses the therapeutic properties of phosphorus. Staton (1951) noted that soya lecithin is allegedly effective in increasing muscular strength, based on the assumption that its constituents play a significant part in the functional efficiency of muscle and nerve tissue. Several early German accounts reportedly found a beneficial effect of lecithin. Atzler and Lehmann (1935) evaluated the effect of 22 to 83 g lecithin daily for several days upon the power and endurance in both static and dynamic work in five subjects. They indicated increased values in most individuals following the lecithin treatment. However, Boje (1939) attributed their effects to training and suggestive factors rather than the physiological effect of lecithin. Dennig (1937) also mentioned some favorable effect of soya lecithin in one report, but the details were not clear. The report was primarily concerned with alkaline salts, which are discussed later.

Staton (1951) studied the effect of soya lecithin upon grip strength. Thirty subjects were divided into three equal groups. The control group received no supplement for the eight-week experimental period. The lecithin-placebo group received 30 g soya lecithin daily for weeks five and six, and a placebo for weeks seven and eight; the placebo-lecithin group reversed this procedure. In this rather good experimental design, Staton noted that the addition of soya lecithin to the normal diet does not significantly increase strength, nor does the withdrawal of the supplement cause a decrease.

Although the research with lecithin upon physical performance parameters is brief, Staton's study provides the most recent uncovered evidence relative to its ineffectiveness as an ergogenic aid.

PHOSPHATES

Phosphates are the salts of phosphoric acid. The salts of alkaline metals, such as sodium phosphate and potassium phosphate, have been ascribed ergogenic qualities. Embden and others (1921) reported that working capacity could be increased through the administration of phosphates, and indicated that they were used to alleviate fatigue in German soldiers during World War I. Riabuschinsky (1930) also reported that phosphates increase the physical working capacity of humans, and that the effect is greater in some individuals than in others. He noted that since phosphate is involved in the energetics of muscular activity, special attention must be paid to phosphate in the diet. Although his work revealed an ergogenic effect upon PWC, the mechanism was not determined. Flinn (1926), in a brief report of his work, indicated that the ingestion of sodium phosphate does not appear to increase muscular efficiency.

In 1939, Boje (1939) noted that the German research during the previous twenty years showed a beneficial effect of phosphates on mental and physical performance. He discredited the research due to unsound conclusions, yet noted that phosphates were in great demand by athletes in Germany, probably due to the intense advertising of their beneficial qualities. However, even after noting the limitations in the research, he concluded that phosphates, taken in quantities exceeding the amounts found in the normal diet, could probably increase human work output.

Karpovich and Sinning (1971), basing their conclusion on the early research with phosphates, noted that although the preponderance of evidence seems to favor the idea that phosphate preparations are beneficial, there is no definite proof that the administration of phosphates per se was responsible for improved performance in sports and athletics. They hinted that there may have been placebo effects involved.

On the other hand, Keller and Kraut (1959) reported that as late as the 1950's, phosphates still held a certain reputation among sportsmen in their ability to increase performance. They cited some experimental evidence by Rogoskin that athletic performance in a diverse number of events, ranging from a metric mile run to swimming distances of 100 m to 1500 m, was enhanced profoundly by the ingestion of 2 g sodium phosphate taken one hour before the event. The dosage was compared to a number of athletes not taking the phosphate.

It appears that this latter study may also be open to the charge of a placebo effect. Nevertheless, perusal of the literature revealed very few recent studies investigating the effect of phosphates on physical performance capacity. Further research appears warranted in this area.

MULTIPLE SUPPLEMENTS

Several investigators have studied the effect of combined nutrient substances upon athletic performance, and have reported no significant beneficial effect. Nelson (1960) evaluated the effect of an unnamed well-advertised vitamin-mineral supplement upon performance in a 10-yard sprint, the vertical jump, and maximal revolution speed on a bicycle ergometer. Football players and physical education students were assigned to either a placebo or experimental group. No indication was given as to the dosage or contents of the vitamin-mineral supplement, but the study was conducted over a twelve-week period. The performance tests were taken five times during the experiment, and the statistical analysis revealed no significant difference between the experimental or placebo group for any of the criterion tests.

Arterbury (1971) tested the effect of a multiple ergogenic aid upon strength, muscular endurance and recovery. The aid consisted of 300 mg citrated caffeine, 1000 mg sodium citrate, 500 mg sodium phosphate, 370 mg dextrose, 75 mg ascorbic acid, and 5 mg thiamine. Ninety-five male subjects were pretested for strength and endurance on a cable tensiometer and arm ergometer, respectively. Subjects were then randomly assigned to three groups: experimental, placebo and control. Dosages were administered for ten days and post-tests were then taken. A double-blind procedure was utilized. Arterbury concluded that the multiple ergogenic aid had no significant effect upon strength, endurance and recovery.

WHEAT GERM OIL

During the past twenty-five years, wheat germ oil has purportedly been one of the most popular nutritional ergogenic aids in the United States. It has been touted by many national and international athletes as an essential component of their dietary regimen, and several noted athletes attributed part of their outstanding success to wheat germ oil supplementation (Cureton, 1959). Cureton (1972a), citing the performance of four American swimmers in the 1956 Olympics at Melbourne, inferred that six months of wheat germ oil supplementation helped their swimming performance at the games. Wheat germ oil has been advertised as an ergogenic food for athletes. The Viobin corporation advertised that Viobin Wheat Germ Oil® or Prometol® (Viobin Oil Concentrate) improves endurance, stamina and vigor. Although not citing any objective data, their advertising brochure is replete with comments from coaches and trainers relative to the increased capacity of individual swimmers or track men. Cureton's research in this area is also a major component of their advertising campaign. Energol, a combination of vital oils including wheat germ oil, has recently been advertised with the implication that it will help to provide energy and build endurance. Indeed, wheat germ oil has been described as the "wonder" fuel for athletes (Cureton, 1955).

What are the magical properties of wheat germ oil, if any, that have been advertised to provide that additional ingredient to help an athlete become a champion? In the early years Percival (1951), in a report from the Shute Foundation for Medical Research, claimed that the alpha tocopherol, or vitamin E, in wheat germ oil was purported to reduce the oxygen requirement of the tissues, improve collateral circulation, and stimulate muscular power; the fatty acids were also used for energy in aerobic workloads. Cureton (1960) later reported it is reasonably certain that the endurance effect of wheat germ oil is not due to vitamin E. Cureton (1972b) attributed the ergogenic effect of wheat germ oil to octacosanol, not to vitamin E or the essential fatty acid, linoleic acid. Octacosanol is a solid white alcohol extracted from the germ, or embryo, of the wheat kernel.

The most vocal proponent of wheat germ oil has been Cureton, whose research with his associates over the years has been published in a single volume (Cureton, 1972a). Cureton has noted that wheat germ oil or octacosanol supplements have favorable effects in the same general direction as physical training effects themselves; but, over and above the physical training effects, the dietary supplements have induced additional improvements. However, as noted early in his research, Cureton (1955) reported that wheat germ oil needed to be combined with physical training; it was a supplement to training, as very little or no gains at all are made when it is used alone.

Wheat germ oil has been credited with the ability to increase capacity in a variety of physical performance tests, but the exact metabolic means whereby these capacity increases are mediated remains unclear. Zauner and Updyke (1973) reported that most endurance athletes take large daily dosages of wheat germ oil in an attempt to increase oxygen uptake in the heart and skeletal muscle. However, in their general article dealing with nutritional factors limiting human performance, they did not expound upon the underlying biochemical effects of wheat germ oil to elicit the increased oxygen uptake. In his book, Cureton (1972a) advanced several theoretical reasons relative to the ergogenic effect of wheat germ oil, but did not provide the explicit experimental research to support the contentions. He reported when wheat germ oil or octacosanol is used in conjunction with physical training, glycogen metabolism in the muscle is enhanced. As noted in Chapter Three, glycogen is a major substrate for energy during exercise of high intensity. Cureton also cited the review of the Russian literature by Brozek (1962), which covered the effects of nutrition upon activity of the central nervous system. Although not dealing specifically with nutrition for athletes, the Soviet studies indicated that the central nervous system is affected by such additional supplementary nutrients as vitamins and wheat germ oil, resulting in improved conditioned reflexes. Improved reflex activity would be beneficial in many athletic events involving quick responses, such as tennis, baseball and a multitude of others. Cureton (1972b) further reported that wheat germ oil adds resistance to stress and helps to stabilize the metabolism.

Although these several theories have been advanced relative to the beneficial psychological effects of wheat germ oil during physical activity, the literature does not appear to provide the necessary objective data to actually pinpoint the exact metabolic role of the wheat germ oil, much less the exact component of wheat germ oil that produces the alleged beneficial effect.

Since the majority of the research with wheat germ oil and physical performance has been generated by Cureton, it may be important to describe the composition of the substance used in his research. The wheat germ oil was extracted from the embryo of wheat and kept at 0°C until capsulated. Each capsule contains 175 mg of oil, high in linoleic acid; 0.44 mg vitamin E is also contained in each capsule, along with small amounts of choline, some naturally occurring vitamins and minerals, and plant sterols. Each capsule contained 3 minims, and the daily recommendation was 20 capsules; the total amount is equal to one teaspoonful, or about 4 ml.

The main research efforts relative to the ergogenic effect of wheat germ oil have emanated from Cureton and his associates, culminating in a book entitled *The Physiological Effects of Wheat Germ Oil on Humans in Exercise* (Cureton, 1972a). The book is a compilation of thirty-one group studies and eleven individual studies undertaken during a twenty-year period, 1950-1969. The studies encompassed three general age groups, including young boys between the ages of seven to thirteen, young men of college age, and adult men in the age range twenty-six to sixty. Many of the studies were master's theses and do not appear in the published literature, except in the book noted above. No attempt will be made to report the results of each study, but a general overview of his book and criticism of the published research in this area is presented below.

Although studying the effect of wheat germ oil on a variety of physical performance parameters, Cureton (1972a) has stressed the beneficial effect upon endurance. The general research design utilized by Cureton was sound, consisting of matched groups undergoing parallel treatment effects with the exception of the dietary supplement. Cureton noted that it was difficult to find a placebo substance of the same caloric value of wheat germ oil which did not have some biological value to humans. He generally used refined corn oil, cottonseed oil, or devitamized lard, with equivalent amounts of vitamin E. A variety of tasks were utilized to test cardiovascular and muscular endurance. Cardiovascular endurance was tested primarily by the 600-yard run and a treadmill run to exhaustion, whereas local muscular endurance was evaluated by all-out tests involving push-ups, sit-ups, pull-ups, parallel bar-dips, squat-jumps and others of a similar nature.

In one of his earliest published reports, Cureton (1954) reported a beneficial effect of wheat germ oil upon treadmill run time, reaction time and selected cardiovascular measures of middle-aged subjects in training. Using two matched groups, he found that although the training was instrumental in eliciting beneficial improvements, the experimental group improved more than the placebo group. In a similar published study with middle-aged subjects, Cureton and Pohndorf (1955) studied the interaction effects of wheat germ oil supplements and physical training upon treadmill run time to exhaustion in four groups of subjects. The results indicated a significant increase in performance time for the training groups, but again the wheat germ oil group did significantly better. In this study, 4 different groups were utilized, consisting of the combination of supplementation and no supplementation with training and no training. The interpretation of the results may have been affected if the data had been analyzed by ANOVA techniques, which may not have been in popular usage at that time.

In one of the more detailed studies, Cureton (1963) investigated the effects of wheat germ oil on thirty active men undertaking strenuous training five hours per day. Three groups of ten received one of the following supplements to their diet: octacosanol, placebo cottonseed oil, or whole fresh wheat germ oil. The men were evaluated on forty-three separate tests, consisting of seventeen physical tests, thirteen cardiovascular-respiratory tests, and thirteen motor fitness tests; the tests were administered before and after the experimental period. The interpretation of the results is rather confusing.

Cureton noted that of all the motor tests, the octacosanol group increased significantly on nine tests, the wheat germ oil group on five, and the placebo on four. He then concluded that the octacosanol group had the advantage. However, when comparing the differences between groups, the results become more obscure. For example, the octacosanol group reduced the mile time more than the wheat germ oil group, but was not significantly lower than the placebo group. Cureton noted that in the between group analysis, the improvement in the composite scores on the five dynamic muscular ability events (mile run, push-ups, squat-jumps, sitting-tucks and chin-ups) favor the dietary supplemental groups, but the difference between the groups was not significant. Thus, this finding would indicate the wheat germ oil or octacosanol is not effective in increasing cardiovascular or muscular endurance. However, the general implication of the report was that octacosanol and wheat germ oil were significantly better than the placebo treatments. Although Cureton noted that training is the major factor influencing the results, the dietary supplements were noted to be important secondary factors. It should be noted that Cureton disregarded much of the cardiovascular performance data in this experiment, as he reported the improvements in that area were hampered by insufficient sleep and fatigue during the training.

Cureton (1969b), in a periodical designed for swimming coaches, has indicated that wheat germ oil is effective in increasing endurance, based upon his research with the 600 yard run test and all-out treadmill runs. In a summarizing statement in his book, Cureton (1972a) reported that of the thireen studies conducted in which endurance was the main criterion, the dietary supplements improved performance in eleven of the thirteen experiments, ten times reaching statistical levels of significance. For endurance, wheat germ oil and octacosanol appeared to have identical effects whereas synthetic vitamin E had virtually no effect in the small amounts fed. In order for the supplements to be effective, Cureton noted that they must be taken over a four to five week period of time for statistically significant gains to occur. Thus, based upon his studies, and support from other research, Cureton has implied that wheat germ oil and octacosanol produce definite physiological changes in man conducive to increased performance capacity.

Several criticisms may be levelled at the reports by Cureton. First, he has utilized rather unconventional levels of significance, such as .07, .08 and even .13. In the ten endurance studies which have shown a beneficial effect of the wheat germ oil or octacosanol, he has used a significance level of .10. Cureton (1963) has rationalized these significance levels, indicating it is reasonable to accept a level of .15 for experiments with humans involving maximal exertion tests where the human motivation factor is so variable. This supposition is not commonly accepted by most investigators dealing with exertion in humans.

According to most exercise physiologists, the most important single test of cardiovascular endurance capacity is the maximal oxygen uptake test. Cureton (1972a), however, criticized the test, noting that it is too crude a test to show the changes due to the possible effects of the dietary supplements. He has criticized the test for being too variable even though he has justified the use of a .15 level of significance in studies involving maximal exertion tests because the human motivational factor is so variable. The two viewpoints appear to be contradictory. Cureton further discussed the difficulty in interpreting the results of the maximal oxygen uptake test due to the multitude of factors that contribute to its determination. He indicated that his research with wheat germ oil and octacosanol and their effect on maximal oxygen uptake is not very conclusive, for the placebo groups were not significantly different from the dietary supplemental groups.

Others (Poiletman and Miller, 1968) have criticized Cureton's work based on some of the parameters he utilized to evaluate fitness, such as the basal metabolic rate, breath holding, plethysmographic arterial pulse waves, and quick-standing blood pressure changes. The amplitude of the T wave was also used as a criterion measure of fitness.

The published research conducted outside Cureton's laboratory is rather limited, but in general is in contrast to his findings. Using highly-trained cross-country runners as subjects, 2 separate reports (Poiletman and Miller, 1968; Kennedy, 1973) revealed no significant effect of wheat germ oil supplementation upon T wave amplitude, thus conflicting with some of Cureton's research. However, it remains to be substantiated that the T wave itself may be used as a discriminating criterion of physical fitness.

Coulson (1969) assigned thirty-six prospective members of the University of Maryland lacrosse team to five experimental groups during an eight-week experiment involving intensive interval training. The groups consisted of a placebo and experimental group for the entire period, a control group, and two groups that took wheat germ oil for the first four weeks, one taking a placebo the final four weeks and the other receiving nothing during the final four weeks. During the experimental period, the groups undertook a bicycle ergometer ride to exhaustion five times. Although the training caused a significant increase in the ergometer riding time, the statistical analysis revealed no significant effect of the wheat germ oil supplementation. Fulton (1971) studied the effect of protein and wheat germ oil supplements upon the weight, arm strength, speed and endurance capacity of thirty-six junior high school athletes. Pull-ups, a 60-yard dash, and a one-minute test for squat thrusts were criterion tests. The experimental group received a protein-wheat germ oil supplement. A placebo and control group were also used in the twelve-week study. No significant differences were attributed to the wheat germ oil and protein supplements.

Since the evidence is conflicting, and not satisfactorily convincing that wheat germ oil supplementation is an effective ergogenic aid, further research is needed in order to investigate its purported merits. Cureton (1972a) has established a case in support of octacosanol and wheat germ oil, but the interpretation of the results is open to question.

ALKALINE SALTS

One of the theoretical contributing factors in the development of fatigue during exercise is increased acidosis, primarily due to lactic acid production during anaerobic work. Lactic acid is the anaerobic end product of glycolysis, and it may be produced in substantial quantities in the muscle during high intensity exercise; the lactate level then rises in the blood stream. During heavy exercise, the lactic acid component accounts for the majority of the oxygen debt, and deVries (1974) indicated that the magnitude of the oxygen debt which may be attained by an athlete may be a very important factor in heavy endurance work. He further noted that the size of the oxygen debt may be limited by the blood pH.

The blood pH is normally in the range of 7.35 to 7.45, but may decrease to 7.0 during exercise. The ingestion of alkaline salts, such as sodium citrate, sodium bicarbonate or potassium citrate, has been shown to displace the pH upwards during a resting state. The theory behind their use, therefore, is relatively simple. If the lowered blood pH during exercise is a contributing causative factor in the etiology of fatigue, then the use of alkaline salts will increase the normal alkaline reserve of the blood and help buffer the acid produced during exercise. This may keep the pH high in the muscle tissue as well as the blood, thus maintaining a more homeostatic condition for the functioning of the enzymes involved in muscular contraction. Astrand and Rodahl (1970) noted that the reduced alkaline reserve following acclimatization to altitude may be a factor behind decreases in anaerobic capacity; thus, it follows logically that an increased alkaline reserve may increase anaerobic capacity.

The primary alkaline salts which have been used as ergogenic aids are the citrates and bicarbonates of sodium and potassium. Upon oral ingestion they eventually elevate the blood pH. Other salts such as sodium phosphate and sodium sulfate would be effective, but they would have to be administered intravenously since they are not absorbed too well from the gastrointestinal tract. Organic compounds such as THAM (trometamol or trihy-droxymethylaminomethane) have been used medically to treat metabolic and respiratory acidosis, and thus are similar in action to the alkalinizers. However, THAM is also diuretic, and could have adverse effect on performance capacity by decreasing the blood volume.

The organic alkaline salts found in natural foods have been imputed with ergogenic qualities. Russian research (Unsigned, 1971a) has indicated that the intake of fruits and vegetables should be increased during training, possibly to the point where they comprised 12 to 20 percent of the total caloric value. They indicated that their studies have shown that fruits and vegetables, because they are alkaline, are beneficial in conditions that produce acidosis during muscular activity.

Although the increased pH would appear to confer a physiological advantage during exercise, it may also be disadvantageous. The increased pH, due to its effect upon the oxygen dissociation curve, will decrease the ability of hemoglobin to release oxygen at the tissue level. However, the primary use of alkalinizers may be in those events characterized by high levels of anaerobic work, i.e. maximal effort for two minutes or less. Thus, the effect on the oxygen dissociation curve may not be important.

The theoretical physiological rationale for the use of alkaline salts in athletics appears to be logical, and aside from the possible development of flatulence, there appear to be no serious side effects associated with normal dosages. However, only a few reported studies have been uncovered.

In the earliest investigation, Dennig and others (1931) indicated that a runner starting in a state of alkalosis, as compared to a normal state, may be able to accumulate a larger oxygen debt. However, they noted that their work rate was not severe enough to test their hypothesis. Dill and his associates (1932) reported that the ingestion of sodium bicarbonate did increase oxygen debt capability, noting an approximate 20 percent increase. Dennig (1937) later reported significant increases in treadmill and bicycle ergometer endurance times of subjects ingesting alkaline salts according to a specified regimen. His refined dosages included 5.0 g sodium citrate, 3.5 g sodium bicarbonate, and 1.5 g potassium citrate taken after each meal for two days prior to the event; no dosage should be taken five hours prior to exercise. Dennig stressed the importance of this time schedule since the body may otherwise adjust to the salts. One of the limitations of this study was the fact that only moderately-trained subjects were used. Karpovich and Sinning (1971), although not divulging too many details, reported that Dennig's formula had no significant effect on performance of college swimmers.

Hewitt and Callaway (1936) studied the effect of blood alkalinizing substances, namely tomato juice, orange juice and several commercial alkalinizers, on performances of college swimmers. A variety of strokes and distances were utilized, the maximal distance being 440 yards. The authors suggested that alkaline treatment, either in the form of organic salts of bases in foods or in a concentrated form, improved swimming performance. A habitual acidic diet also seemed to reduce performance capacity. However, they did note that the limited number of subjects precluded any general conclusions relative to the efficacy of alkalinizing agents. Karpovich (1941), in his own research, indicated that the liberal use of grapefruit, orange and tomato juices exerted no effect upon the muscular performance capacity of twenty-eight bicycle riders, nor was any change effected in the buffer alkalines of other men who consumed 3 quarts of juice in four hours.

In a field study, Johnson and Black (1953) studied the effects of alkaline salts and glucose on the performance of champion high school cross-country runners during a competitive season. The athletes, ranging in ages from sixteen to nineteen, ran the same 1.5 mile course eight times competitively during the season. They received either a placebo or experimental compound four hours prior to all meets except one; in the one exception, the dosage was administered 2.5 hours before competition. The rotation was such that each subject was tested twice with each of the following substances: (a) glucose, 2 ounces, (b) sodium citrate, 5 g, (c) sodium bicarbonate, 3.5 g, and potassium citrate, 1.5 g, and (d) sodium acid phosphate, 3 g, and glucose, 2.4 ounces. It should be noted that this procedure does not adhere to the regimen, either in dosages or time factors, that is advocated by Dennig. Subjects were unaware of the nature of the study and the criterion measure was time to run the course. The results indicated no significant effect due to the experimental drugs. However, Johnson and Black stated that the temperature range throughout the fall season (39 to 91°F) may have influenced the results.

More recently, Simmons and Hardt (1973) studied the effect of alkali ingestion upon the performance of highly-trained sprint and/or distance swimmers. However, since only two distance swimmers completed the experiment, no analysis was made regarding their performance. The five sprinters were tested on a 100-yard swim four times during the experimental phase of the study, with a one-week intertrial period. There were three experimental and two placebo subjects. The subjects consumed a mixture of 0.715 g sodium citrate, 0.50 g sodium bicarbonate, and 0.215 g potassium citrate. The placebo dose was 1.43 g sucrose. The alkalies were administered two days prior to and on the day of the test. The results indicated that the supplemental alkali, in contrast to the placebo, produced significant improvement in the performance of the swimmers. However, the limited number of subjects posed a major limitation. Rather than a separate experimental and placebo group, a repeated measures design including a placebo dose would possibly have been more appropriate.

As indicated previously, alkalinizers may be more effective in work which is primarily anaerobic in nature, i.e. maximal work capacity in events of two minutes or less. Astrand and Rodahl (1970) indicated a 50 to 50 percent derivation of energy from aerobic and anaerobic sources at maximal work for two minutes. The percentages become, respectively, 70 to 30 for maximal work of four minutes, and 90 to 10 for ten minutes. Thus, alkalinizers would appear to confer a physiological advantage primarily in events of short duration at maximal work rates. Examples would be the 800 meter or half-mile runs.

With this concept in mind, Margaria and his associates (1971) recently studied the effect of 3.24 g sodium bicarbonate, sodium citrate and potassium citrate upon supramaximal exercise performance (10 m.p.h. with 10% grade) of twelve normal men; there were four athletes, four active men, and four with no sports activity. Time to exhaustion was the criterion measured. The alkali salts had no significant effect upon performance. Blood lactic acid levels also were not affected. A few additional tests with massive doses of alkaline salts (12 g sodium bicarbonate) were conducted, and although endurance time increased up to 5.8 percent, this finding was not statistically significant. Therefore, the authors concluded that the alkaline salts had no appreciable influence on performance capacity of a supramaximal type.

In summary, the results indicate that alkaline salts are ineffective as ergogenic aids with trained athletes. However, more objective evidence is needed. Since these substances are relatively harmless, further research may be desirable.

ASPARTATES

Potassium and magnesium aspartate are salts of asparaginic acid, a dibasic nonessential amino acid. Consequently, they are classified as a food. They have been ascribed pharmacological actions to help prevent fatigue, since they are used therapeutically to relieve the general fatigue syndrome, and fatigue resulting from long marches. Fujioka and his colleagues (1963b) indicated that aspartates could have wide application to sports as a routine means to counteract fatigue.

Although aspartates have been utilized to counteract the fatigue developing from physical work, their mode of action is still unclear. Ahlborg and others (1968) suggested that aspartates may accelerate the resynthesis of ATP, phosphocreatine, and glycogen in the muscle, and may also exert a glycogen-sparing effect; these factors may enhance endurance capacity.

On the other hand, the Council on Drugs of the American Medical Association (1963) indicated that although several reports have engendered the idea that aspartic acid salts are useful in the management of fatigue, no objective evidence is available to substantiate that claim. The additional limited research conducted within the past ten years would resubstantiate this statement, especially in relationship to exhausting fatigue as experienced in athletic endurance events.

Several reports have indicated an ergogenic effect of aspartates on human physical work capacity. Fujioka and others (1963a) indicated that the degree of physiological fatigue encountered in a 30 kilometer full-pack march was decreased due to the ingestion of aspartic acid salts. Fukui and others (1962) suggested K and Mg aspartates were effective in the recovery from muscular fatigue, but the design of these studies with only an N = 3 and questionable methods for objectively determining muscular fatigue renders their conclusions doubtful. Using field tests, Fujioka and others (1963b) studied the effects of aspartates on the performance of military personnel in the 500-meter run, 1000-meter run, marathon running and Ranger training. They noted that the accumulation of fatigue, particularly that which leads to a state of exhaustion, was prevented by the administration of the aspartate preparation. However, it was not revealed whether the actual time performance of the various running events were significantly improved by aspartates.

In more controlled laboratory research, the general results indicate that aspartates will not benefit the trained subject who is motivated for work. Ahlborg and his coworkers (1968), using six subjects with average physical fitness levels for Sweden, studied the influence of aspartates on the capacity for prolonged standardized physical exercise. The subjects were tested four times on a bicycle ergometer workload that was designed to elicit exhaustion in about ninety minutes. A double-blind placebo design was used. Tablets were taken every sixth hour during the study. Placebo tablets were taken on days one, two, and four; aspartates (1.75 g tablets) were consumed on day three. The aspartates appeared to increase the capacity for prolonged exercise as the mean value for the aspartate was 128 minutes as compared to 93.7, 85.3, and 88.3 minutes for the three placebo days. The authors suggested the increase was due to the effect of aspartates upon the various sources of energy in the skeletal muscle, thus enhancing the resynthesis of ATP, creatine phosphate and glycogen. The increase due to aspartates was approximately 40 to 50 percent greater than on placebo days, a finding that is difficult to digest. It is conceivable that the nature of the workload, i.e. submaximal since the recorded heart rates were only 150 to 160, may have been subject to modification through psychological processes. If the subjective effects reported earlier were noted by these subjects, it may have influenced their performance. In addition, a counterbalanced design would have been more appropriate. Nevertheless, the design was good and the results are suggestive of an ergogenic effect of aspartic acid salts.

Nagle and his colleagues (1963) tested the effects of aspartates on fatiguing running exercise. Four subjects, two trained and two untrained, undertook three work tests on a treadmill: rested, following a sixty-minute cross-country run, and again following an additional forty-minute run. The subjects were trained to the task and then placed upon a Spartase regimen consisting of 2000 mg K and Mg aspartate daily for two weeks; one subject received the dosage for one week. The results indicated that the treatment had no effect on the trained subjects, but did appear to increase the performance capacity of the untrained men. However, the authors did note that limitations, such as the small number of subjects and possible training effect, precluded any generalizations concerning the antifatigue effects of Spartase.

Using a treatment by subjects design, Evans and Caldwell (1962) subjected five highly motivated subjects to a physical work test of strength and endurance involving the use of an arm dynamometer. Each subject undertook the test eight times, four with placebo and four following the administration of 2000 mg K and Mg aspartates/day for four days. A double-blind procedure was used. Although all the subjects were able to identify the subjective effects of the aspartates, the analysis revealed no significant effect upon strength or muscular endurance. The authors indicated that the aspartates were ineffective because highly motivated subjects were used. They also suggested that the salts may be effective with low motivated groups, possibly because the conversion of aspartates to glutamic acid may have an effect on the central nervous system (CNS) and increase motivational levels.

In a controlled study in which inmates in the Maryland State Penitentiary were subjects, Fallis and her colleagues (1963) studied the effect of aspartates upon the performance of twenty-six experienced weight lifters. The subjects were athletically inclined and considered to be in peak condition. Half the subjects were given placebos for ten days while the other half received 1 g/daily of K and Mg aspartic salts. This procedure was reversed for a second ten-day period. On the tenth day of each treatment session, maximal endurance scores were obtained on squats, bench press, military press and grip ergograph performance. The subjects's subjective evaluation of his condition and perception of time needed for recovery were also noted. The results indicated no significant differences between the aspartate and placebo conditions for any of the parameters, except the subjective perception of their physical condition was higher under the placebo treatment; this would contradict previous findings relative to subjective feelings of enhancement following aspartates.

The results of the two previous studies may be due to the nature of the induced fatigue. Both studies appeared to have studied local muscular fatigue with a heavy resistance, whereas the hypothetical benefit from aspartates would be in more moderate prolonged aerobic tasks. However, their results do support the viewpoint that aspartates are not effective ergogenic aids.

Consolazio and others (1964b) studied the effects of aspartates (500 mg K and Mg salts twice daily) upon oxygen uptake, oxygen debt and physical working capacity. Twelve men were randomly assigned to either a placebo or aspartate group and underwent two weeks of training, five weeks of aspartate therapy, and two weeks of recovery. All subjects exercised thirty minutes daily at 4 m.p.h. with a 3.5 percent grade on a treadmill. Towards the end of the aspartate period, subjects were exposed to a maximal test on the treadmill (7.0 m.p.h., 8.0% grade). The results indicated no significant differences in oxygen consumption, oxygen debt, or physical fitness levels. The authors concluded that aspartates are not beneficial to human endurance performance, at least as determined by their run to exhaustion test. However, no runs to exhaustion were reported and it appears that the physical fitness level was determined by the Harvard scoring system, which apparently uses recovery pulse rates to assess fitness.

In summary, aspartates do not appear to elicit any significant increase in the physical working capacity of trained men. However, as noted by deVries (1974), more research, especially with highly trained athletes, is warranted since aspartates appear to produce no serious adverse side effects.

ALCOHOL

Alcohol is legally a drug, and yet it is so often consumed as a component of various beverages, such as beer and wine, that accompany a meal, that it ofttimes may be considered as a food. Its use by athletes has been condemned by coaches for the past century, and even scientists have proscribed alcohol for athletes during training because of its deleterious effects upon coordination (Bullen and others, 1959). In a recent issue of a popular coaches' magazine, Jensen (1972) classified alcohol as detrimental to health. He cited several reasons against the use of alcohol in athletics, and there was some truth to them, primarily as they might relate to the acute effects or to the developing alcoholic, but not to the athlete who might consume several beers as a relaxant during the training season. He also helped to perpetuate the myth that alcohol is detrimental to athletes, noting that it saps energy and greatly increases fatigue by slowing the removal of lactic acid from the cells. This contention is unsupported by any substantial experimental evidence, especially as it pertains to an exercising athlete. On the other hand, some have contended that alcohol may exert an ergogenic effect, and is useful in certain athletic events. Is alcohol beneficial or detrimental to athletic performance?

Ethyl alcohol is not a foreign substance to the body, as it can be isolated in small amounts from any animal tissue or organ. Although exogenous sources of alcohol may be taken into the body in a variety of ways, the oral route is the most common. It is absorbed directly from the stomach and small intestine into the blood stream, with maximum concentration occurring in less than one hour. Alcohol is distributed in the water of the body, and its concentration in each tissue depends upon the water content of that tissue. Thus, the distribution of alcohol in the body is essentially a process of dilution. The elimination of alcohol proceeds at a constant rate, approximately three quarters of an ounce per hour. It is oxidized in three stages, with the first rate-limiting stage occurring primarily in the liver; alcohol dehydrogenase converts alcohol into acetaldehyde. The acetaldehyde is transformed to acetic acid, which is subsequently oxidized to carbon dioxide and water. In the process, 1 g alcohol yields 7 calories.

The alcohol content in the body may be detected through blood or breath analysis. Blood alcohol levels (BAL) are expressed in milligrams (mg) per 100 milliliters (ml) of blood. Thus, a BAL of 40/mg 100 ml blood would be expressed as .04 percent or 40 mg percent. BAL's up to .05 percent are not usually intoxicating, and the effect above the .05 level is dependent upon the individual. Many states interpret the .10 level as being legally intoxicated, whereas at the .15 to .20 level, most individuals are definitely drunk.

The effect of alcohol on physical performance has been covered in detail elsewhere (Williams, 1974). The highlights as it affects human performance are presented in the next few paragraphs.

Alcohol affects all cells of the body, with the most dramatic results of ingestion as the effects on the brain. Gould (1970) indicated that in spite of the long use of alcohol as a stimulant, it is actually a central nervous system depressant. The apparent stimulation is evinced because of the depressive action of ethanol on the reticular activating system. The inhibitory control mechanisms are decreased, and this results in unrestrained activity of many areas of the brain with loss of the integrating control of the cerebral cortex. A biphasic hypothesis regarding the effects of alcohol has been advanced, indicating that it may produce a transitory sensation of excitement followed by depressive effects. Thus, the application of alcohol may be based upon two paradoxical effects. In some cases, it may be used for the apparent stimulating effect, while in others for the depressive or tranquilizing effect on reducing excessive tension.

Boje (1939) indicated that in cases of extreme athletic exertion, or in events of brief maximal effort, alcohol has been given to athletes to serve as a stimulant by releasing inhibitions and lessening the sense of fatigue. As an illustration, Jokl (1968) reported evidence that alcohol was in wide use in European athletics at the turn of this century. He reported cases of a cyclist imbibing rum and champagne throughout a twenty-four-hour race, jockeys pouring champagne down the throats of their horses before the race, and marathon runners and walkers consuming considerable quantities of cognac or beer during competition. Rationale for their use was ascribed to their refreshing effect or the ability to restore the athlete's strength. On the other hand, Shephard (1972) noted that in some events, anxiety may disrupt performance by inducing excessive arousal of the cerebral cortex. In this case, the sedative action of alcohol may be beneficial. Marty Liquori, one of the top milers in the United States, reportedly consumes several beers the night before competition in order to relax and have sound sleep.

Although alcohol is a common beverage, and is part of the normal menu in several European countries, Ulmark (1963) indicated that alcohol should be forbidden to all athletes in training and during competition. Prior to 1968, it was proscribed as a doping agent by the IOC, and Shephard (1972) noted that two pistol-shooters were disqualified during the 1968 Olympics due to the alleged use of alcohol in an attempt to increase their competitive ability. Fischbach (1972), however, noted that alcohol, although called goldwater by athletes involved in shooting competition, was not listed as a specific doping agent for the 1972 Munich Olympics.

An abundance of studies has been been conducted in order to document the effect of alcohol on psychological processes. A number of these have dealt with the acute effects of intoxication, but they are not pertinent to this discussion as it is highly unlikely that an athlete would become intoxicated just prior to an event. Coopersmith (1964) succinctly summarized current knowledge regarding the effect of small amounts of alcohol upon behavior in normal subjects. He noted that both popular impressions and the clinical and anthropological evidence suggest that alcohol reduces feelings of insecurity, tension and discomfort, and thereby permits a freer and less constrained behavioral expression. Thus, as Shephard (1972) has noted, alcohol may elicit greater self-confidence in the athlete.

Sollman (1956) stated that the physical symptoms of ethanol ingestion show individual differences according to temperament and circumstances, but with increasing doses they tend to run a descending course on a continuum from euphoria to coma. Motor symptoms follow a similar, but not necessarily parallel, course.

Extensive research has been conducted relative to the effect of alcohol on psychomotor performance, especially in the realm of driver skills. No comprehensive coverage of these studies is offered here, since it falls outside the scope of this presentation, and Carpenter (1962) has succinctly summarized the findings. In a critical review of studies from 1940 to 1961 concerning the effects of alcohol on some psychological processes, including reaction time, Carpenter has noted in general that motor performance is impaired at low and moderate blood alcohol levels. In a series of tests during the same time period, Hebbelinck (1961) also noted in tests of physical performance that neuromuscular performance was adversely affected at BAL's lower than .05; he later concluded that neuromuscular incoordination and poorer reflexive control appeared to be responsible mainly for the deteriorative effects of alcohol on the basic components of physical performance (1963). Nelson (1959) reiterated these viewpoints, indicating that highly coordinated skills seemed to decrease most in efficiency following alcohol injection. He observed deteriorative effects of 2 and 3 ounces of pure ethanol upon reaction time and accuracy.

In summary, the evidence overwhelmingly supports the conclusion that alcohol does adversely affect fine psychomotor performance. However, Shephard (1972) interjects the intriguing thought that the greater self-confidence produced by alcohol may override the loss of skill and slowing of body reactions.

The effect of alcohol upon physiological adjustments to exercise, including cardiovascular, respiratory and metabolic changes, has been investigated recently. Williams (1974) has summarized the literature relative to acute effects of alcohol upon heart rate, cardiac output, blood flow, respiratory dynamics, and oxygen uptake during submaximal and maximal exercise. He summarized the data by noting that the acute ingestion of ethanol elicits neither favorable nor unfavorable physiological modifications in the cardiovascular, respiratory or metabolic responses to exercise, particularly if it is maximal exercise. Apparently the various physiological changes produced by alcohol during a resting state are abrogated by the various neural and hormonal adjustments associated with the onset of exercise.

Since alcohol has been a common beverage for thousands of years, and its behavioral effects well-known by medical personnel, it was one of the first substances investigated regarding its ergogenic effect. Most of the early research dealt with its effect upon local muscular strength and fatigue, while later studies included tests of general endurance capacity. The early reports were confounded by inadequate experimental methodology, and results ranging from tremendous increases to modest decreases in local muscular strength and endurance have been reported. In more recent years, research has indicated that the acute effects of alcohol do not increase muscular strength or local muscular endurance.

Hebbelinck (1959) reported no significant effect of 0.6 ml/kg absolute alcohol upon muscular strength; however, he did report a slight decrease in power. In a subsequent study (1963), although several individuals did better on strength and power tests under the influence of alcohol, he concluded that static strength as measured by a manuometer and back dynamometer was not changed after consumption of a small dose of alcohol. On the other hand, dynamic strength showed a decrease of 5.8 percent.

Nelson (1959) indicated that 2 and 3 ounces of pure alcohol elicited a decrease in isometric grip strength. Of the various gross motor tests involved in his study, he concluded that strength was one of the most adversely affected.

In a well-controlled study, Ikai and Steinhaus (1961) evaluated the effect of alcohol on measured tension in the right forearm flexors, using one maximum contraction per minute for thirty minutes. An increase of 3.7 pounds, or 5.6 percent, was attributable to alcohol. However, this increase was not statistically significant.

Williams (1969) studied the interaction effects of a control, small, moderate and large dose of alcohol with variant elapsed time periods following ingestion, allowing thirty minutes for complete absorption, elapsed time periods were zero, fifteen, thirty and sixty minutes. Thirty-five male university subjects were exposed to the control, small and moderate dose, while an experimental subgroup of nine also took the criterion test following the large dose. The standardized workload consisted of intermittent maximal contractions of the forearm flexors at the rate of thirty per minute for six minutes. Parameters studied included initial strength, maximal strength, steady state or final strength, total work, fatigable work and the mathematical rate of fatigue.

The results of the statistical analysis revealed no significant main or interaction effects, and Williams concluded that the alcohol doses utilized in his study had no effect upon the strength or endurance variables under investigation.

In summary, the general results of contemporary research indicate that the acute ingestion of alcohol has little or no effect on subsequent tests of local muscular strength or endurance.

The research regarding the effect of alcohol upon general, or cardiovascular endurance capacity is more limited. In one of the earliest studies, Asmussen and Boje (1948) investigated the influence of alcohol on the ability to perform maximal muscular work and concluded that the effect was not significant. Two tasks on the bicycle ergometer were utilized, simulating a 100-meter dash and a 1500-meter run. They found that alcohol in small doses (25 g pure ethanol) had no effect, and alcohol in larger doses (75 g pure ethanol) had only a diminishing effect on the ability to perform maximal work. Although Nelson (1959) noted a decrease in performance on seven gross motor tests following the intake of 2 and 3 ounces of pure ethanol, bicycle ergometer work time was one of the tests to show least change in efficiency when compared with control. Highly coordinated skills seemed to decrease most.

In a more recent investigation, Williams (1972) studied the effect of a moderate dose (0.4 ml/lb) of pure ethanol upon time to exhaustion on a progressive bicycle ergometer work task. Ten conditioned male subjects underwent four test trials, two with a control dose and two with alcohol. He concluded that a moderate dose of alcohol neither adversely nor beneficially affected maximal endurance performance.

The results of these studies suggest that alcohol would not be a very effective ergogenic aid in athletic events characterized by all-out general muscular endurance.

In tests duplicating actual athletic events, both Hebbelinck (1963) and Nelson (1959) reported detrimental effects of alcohol upon speed. Hebbelinck found that a small dose decreased speed in the 80-meter dash almost 10 percent. No details were reported concerning the actual conduct of the test, but the difference may have been due to reaction time changes at the start. Aside from these two reports, no other literature was uncovered which directly studied the effect of alcohol on field tests of athletic performance.

When interpreting the results of experimentation involving the acute effects of alcohol on human performance, such as in single or double dose administration studies, one must be cautious not to generalize the findings to include the effect of chronic ingestion on performance. In experimentation regarding the acute effects, it appears that the possible limiting physiological manifestations mediated by alcohol during rest are abrogated during an exercise situation. However, the chronic ingestion of alcohol may produce certain physiological changes resulting in decreased endurance capacity.

In summary, although alcohol may elicit subjective symptoms in some individuals which may make them believe they can perform physical activity at a higher level, the literature does not support the efficacy of alcohol as an ergogenic aid. Moreover, in events characterized by fine neuromotor control, slight excesses in alcohol consumption may prove to be detrimental to performance. Small to moderate doses do not appear to have any significant effect on tasks involving maximal strength, local muscular endurance or general cardiovascular endurance.

CAFFEINE

Caffeine is found in a variety of flora throughout the world, and like alcohol, is legally a drug. In contrast to alcohol, however, it is a central nervous system stimulant affecting the cerebral cortex, medulla oblongata and spinal cord. Resultant subjective symptoms include increased wakefulness and mental activity. Caffeine may also stimulate the cardiac muscle, and increase respiratory rate and depth. Shephard (1972) indicated that it produces an ergogenic effect. Although caffeine may be purchased in powder or tablet form, it is a natural constituent of coffee, tea, kola nuts and cocoa beans. Preparations made from these plants contain varying amounts of caffeine; an 8-ounce cup of regular coffee may contain 150 mg, whereas tea and cola drinks may average approximately half as much. Some aspirin compounds contain 15 to 30 mg caffeine per tablet, while the various "stay-awake" preparations contain approximately 100 mg/tablet. A normal therapeutic dose of caffeine is 100 to 300 mg.

The role of caffeine in athletics has been covered by Williams (1974) in some detail; a synopsis of that review follows. The hypothetical beneficial use of caffeine as a doping agent in athletics is predicated on its action as a CNS stimulant, creating an increased alertness. This behavioral effect has been known empirically for centuries, and has been substantiated experimentally. Physiologically, caffeine has increased urinary adrenalin secretion possibly indicative of a stimulating effect on the adrenal medulla. If this could augment the natural release of adrenalin during exercise, it could possibly produce a potentiating effect.

Since caffeine is a natural ingredient of some common everyday beverages and foods, there is some controversy regarding its use in athletics. Several reports have indicated that caffeine is commonly used in an attempt to increase athletic performance. However, Kourounakis (1972) contended that in order to obtain a reaction equivalent to amphetamine, caffeine would have to be administered in a toxic dose. In 1939, Boje (1939) stated the use of pure caffeine or preparations with a high caffeine content should be prohibited in connection with athletic competition. Yet he did indicate that coffee, tea or chocolate should not be forbidden altogether. More recently, Mustala (1967) reported that caffeine was one of the few known drugs that may enhance athletic performance and Kourounakis (1972) would classify it as a doping agent. In 1962, the Federation Internationale de Sports Medicine undertook a study among Italian athletes, and reported that caffeine was one of the most used doping agents; subsequently, its use was forbidden in conjunction with athletic competition. However, the Medical Commission of the 1970 British Commonwealth Games did not regard caffeine, in the quantity normally found in a cup of coffee, as a doping agent. No evidence has been uncovered to indicate that it is banned by the NCAA, AAU, or IAAF. However, the statement relative to the use of any substance designed to facilitate performance may be interpreted to include caffeine. On the other hand, Fischbach (1972) advocated the removal of caffeine from the doping list of the IOC and was successful in having it eliminated as a doping agent prior to the 1972

Olympics.

The problem relative to the use of caffeine in athletics is succinctly stated by Leake (1958):

> There seems to be no public condemnation of the use of coffee by athletes, either before an athletic contest, or in ordinary living. Nevertheless, caffeine produces the same general sort of central stimulation and reduction of fatigue that is characteristic of the amphetamines, the only difference being that the effects of caffeine are commonly less than those of the amphetamines, and coffee is an anciently used and long established social beverage. No one seems ever to have raised the question about athletes taking a large drink of coffee before an athletic contest or game. In contrast to public indignation at the use of amphetamines to increase physical performance, the situation regarding caffeine is an interesting commentary on what constitutes social acceptability. It seems that what has long been used, what is well established in social custom, and about which people think they know the facts generally are sufficient to assure social acceptability.

What are the facts relative to caffeine and athletic performance?

A number of older studies reported conflicting results relative to the effect of caffeine upon reaction time. In these dated reports, methodological problems existed due to the lack of control over interfering variables which are known to affect reaction time. In more recent studies with more sophisticated recording equipment and experimental methodology, results are controversial. Wenzel and Rutledge (1962) used a rather intricate experimental design to study the influence of 0, 100, 200 and 300 mg caffeine upon several motor and psychomotor tests. In general they noted that caffeine induced a significant dose-related improvement in simple visual reaction time, but an inverse relationship was found between dose and effect on complex reaction time. Three hundred milligrams elicited a modest, although insignificant, decrease in performance. The authors concluded that if caffeine is to be used for the improvement of performance, at least in the simple tasks they used, then the dose should not exceed 100 mg. It is interesting to note that the average cup of coffee contains more than this dose. In an equally well-designed study, although also studying the effects of alcohol, Carpenter (1959) found that three different caffeine dosages (0, 1.47, and 2.94 mg/kg), when interacting with zero dosages of alcohol, did not significantly affect simple reaction time. Lovingood and his coworkers (1960) reported that 324 mg caffeine had no effect upon simple visual reaction time. In an effective review of the literature relative to the effect of caffeine upon motor control, Weiss and Laties (1962) concluded that the drug had little or no effect upon reaction time.

Although the last three reports indicate no significant effect of caffeine upon reaction time, the findings of Wenzel and Rutledge may warrant further investigation.

The history of caffeine is full of empirical reports that it can increase work capacity. Catton in *The Army of the Potomac,* noted that the coffee ration kept the Union army going. In a 1939 report from the Health Organization of the League of Nations, Boje (1939) indicated that although there is no direct proof as to the beneficial effect of caffeine on athletic performance, it must be expected that its use as a doping agent is dangerous and therefore should be prohibited. On the other hand, Fischbach (1970; 1972) contended that normal doses will not affect athletes who are accustomed to coffee drinking, whereas high doses may cause a loss of sports performance ability. He also noted that normal doses may adversely affect those who are not accustomed to coffee.

Although several major books dealing with exercise physiology and pharmacology have indicated that caffeine may be a useful ergogenic aid for athletics, their conclusions appear to be based upon rather dated research. In these older studies, erroneous generalizations were often made due to methodological irregularities not known during the early era of drug experimentation with physical exertion in humans. Based primarily on these older reports, Weiss and Laties (1962) indicated that caffeine could prolong the amount of time an individual may perform physically exhausting work. However, more contemporary research would appear to contradict their statement.

Ganslen and his colleagues (1964), using five subjects, found that 200 mg caffeine had no effect upon work or aerobic capacity as determined by the Balke treadmill test. Margaria and others (1964a) administering 100 and 250 mg caffeine in five separate trials to three trained subjects, found no significant effect on maximal oxygen uptake or performance time on a treadmill run to exhaustion. Using twenty-five subjects, Bugyi (1969) studied the effect of 167, 324 and 500 mg citrated caffeine upon the strength and endurance of the right forearm flexors; the workload consisted of maximal contractions at the rate of 30/minute for six minutes. The statistical analysis revealed that all dosages had no effect on initial strength, final strength, fatigable work or total work.

In the most recent report, a double-blind placebo experiment, Perkins and Williams (1975) found that a small, medium or large dose of caffeine had no significant effect on a variety of performance parameters, including submaximal and maximal exercise HR, submaximal and maximal rating of perceived exertion, and maximal endurance capacity on a bicycle ergometer.

In summary, although older research may support the use of caffeine as an ergogenic aid, more recent research under controlled conditions indicate that it is relatively ineffective in strength and endurance type activities.

CHAPTER **TEN**___

WEIGHT CONTROL
AND PHYSICAL ACTIVITY

MAN IS CONSTANTLY harnassing and expending energy through the intricacies of his bodily metabolism. The energy content of the food he eats is constantly being transformed into other utilizable forms of energy, such as that expended during muscular contraction. Although Durnin and others (1973) noted that nutritionists are still ignorant about the mechanisms by which energy balance is maintained, Passmore and Durnin (1967) have indicated that there is no evidence that the behavior of living matter is not covered by the laws of physics, i.e., laws of thermodynamics. Hence, excess intake or expenditure of energy will create either a positive or negative energy balance. An excess energy intake would represent a state of positive energy balance and would result in an increased body weight; excess energy expenditure would decrease body weight, a negative energy state. When energy intake and expenditure are in balance, maintenance of body weight is attained.

In certain athletic events, increased body mass may be advantageous. Heavyweight and suma wrestling, certain positions in football and other contact sports, weight lifting, and long-distance swimming in cold water such as channel swimming are examples where increased body mass may contribute to stability, force development, protection or thermal insulation. However, in other sports, excess body weight which is not functional may not be advantageous to performance. Examples of such sports include gymnastics, long distance running, wrestling, boxing, high jumping, pole vaulting, boxing, riding and others. For most types of sports, Mayer and Bullen (1974) suggested that a male athlete in top condition carries no more than 7 percent of his body weight in fat. Buskirk and Haymes (1972) recommended that female athletes should be below 20 percent body fat, but even lower values should be attained in those events where the excess weight could be a serious disadvantage.

Unless the athlete is satisfied with his present weight, he is faced with the choice of gaining or losing excess tissue, depending upon the needs of the particular sport in which he participates. Both choices involve an alteration in the energy balance of the body. In a weight-gaining program, the desired increases should be in muscle, not body fat; in weight reduction programs, fat losses are of major importance.

In this chapter, brief attention will be given to weight-gaining programs, whereas obesity will be discussed at greater length. The principles underlying prevention and treatment of obesity are applicable to the athlete as well as the nonathlete in the regular physical education class, who may need guidance more than the athlete.

THE CALORIE CONCEPT IN WEIGHT CONTROL PROGRAMS

The concept of the calorie as a measure of energy was discussed in Chapter Two. The daily caloric expenditure may be approximated through appropriate charts, and the daily caloric intake may be estimated from food calorie tables. As an oversimplification, weight gains will occur when daily calorie intake exceeds daily caloric expenditure; weight loss will occur with the reverse situation. Heald (1972) has noted that a pound of adipose tissue (454 g) is about 87 percent, or 395 g, fat. Since each gram of fat has a caloric value of 9.5 calories/g, a pound of body fat would approximate 3,750 calories. Mayer (1968) has noted that each gram of body fat equals 8 cal/g since water is also contained in the fat cell; therefore, one pound of body fat would approximate 3,630 calories (8 x 454 g). Klafs and Arnheim (1973) utilized 7.7 calories/g body fat, or approximately 3,500 calories/pound. It would appear that a value of 3,500 calories/pound body fat would be a fair approximation of the energy storage in adipose tissue, and is the most used value in the literature. Thus, in order to lose one pound of body fat in a week, approximately 500 calories/day must be decreased from the dietary intake or expended through increased physical activity.

How many calories does a growing athlete need per day? The actual amount would depend upon the type of activity in which he or she participates, but several guidelines for maintenance of normal weight have been established. The National Research Council (1974) reported that after age ten, the caloric requirement for males in adolescence eventually drops to 45 cal/kg body weight; for females, the average is 38 cal/kg. A more discriminating chart was presented by the American Alliance for Health, Physical Education and Recreation (1971).

TABLE 10-I

DAILY CALORIC INTAKE NECESSARY TO MAINTAIN

DESIRABLE BODY WEIGHT

| | MALE | | FEMALE | |
Age	Cal/lb	Cal/kg	Cal/lb	Cal/kg
10-12	32	70	29	64
12-14	24	53	23	51
14-18	23	51	21	46
18-22	19	42	19	42
Adult	17	37	17	37

*Reprinted from *Nutrition for Athletes,* with the permission of the American Alliance for Health, Physical Education and Recreation, 1201 Sixteenth Street, N.W., Washington, D.C. 20036.

Table 10-I represents the caloric intake per pound body weight necessary to maintain desirable body weight in growing adolescents. For example, a fifteen-year-old girl who weighed 110 pounds (50 kg), would need 2310 calories/day to maintain her desirable weight (110 x 21). Notice that as the individual gets older, the calories needed per pound decrease, indicating that the anabolic developmental period of life is ending.

Needless to say, if an individual wanted to gain or lose weight, the caloric values in Table 10-I would have to be adjusted upward or downward accordingly. If an obese boy of fourteen weighed 200 pounds, his predicted daily caloric intake to maintain that weight would be 4800 calories (200 x 24). Thus the intake could possibly be reduced to a value like 15 cal/pound, or an equivalent of 3000 cal/day. Although this table may be applied to control of body weight in the average individual, the overly obese person should be under the guidance of a physician throughout his weight control program.

BODY COMPOSITION

A number of different methods have been developed to assess the ideal body weight of humans, some being very simple to apply and others being more complex. Theoretically, all techniques are designed to measure the amount of body fat in comparison to the lean body mass that an individual possesses, the latter being composed of muscles, bone and organ weight. Some techniques are more accurate than others, but these usually involve rather extensive laboratory procedures.

To assess the amount of body fat, several simplified practices have been utilized throughout the years. The simple pinch test involves grabbing a fold of fat between the thumb and forefinger on the back of the arm; normal values approximate .5 to 1.0 inch. The ruler test has the individual lying flat on his back and relaxed. The surface of the abdomen between the ribs and the pubis is normally flat or slightly concave. A ruler placed on the abdomen parallel with the vertical axis of the body should touch both ribs and pubis. The beltline or circumference test involves measurement of the girth of the chest at the level of the nipples and the abdomen at the level of the navel. The chest should be larger than the abdomen by several inches. This test is sex biased, of course for males. Probably the ultimate test is to look at yourself, nude, in a full length mirror, i.e. the mirror test. Use both a front and side view. Analyze what you see as objectively as you can relative to body configuration. Although these tests are simple, and may help you be more aware of your body structure, especially if you are becoming obese, they do not accurately detect body composition.

Data collection throughout the years has revealed some normal body weight values for a given body height. Leaders in the field were life insurance companies, who recognized the relationship between obesity and mortality. Consequently, selected tables were developed relative to age-height-weight norms, and these have been used as criteria for issuing insurance policies. One of the more popular tables for adult men and women has been developed by the Metropolitan Life Insurance Company and is presented as Table 10-II.

Appendix E represents norms for school age boys and girls. Although the utilization of small, medium and large frames is useful in recognizing differences in body build, there is still some doubt to the validity of this method in assessing body composition because the proportions of bones, fat and muscle are not totally considered. Single charts without body frames are even more misleading. However, as a general screening device, they may be useful.

Other techniques for assessing general growth and development changes in children are the Wetzel Grid and the Meredith age-height-weight chart. Both techniques follow a child's development throughout the school years, and may be effective in detecting deviations from normal growth and development patterns.

The more sophisticated techniques offer fairly accurate estimates of the amount of adipose tissue in the body. Underwater, or hydrostatic, weighing techniques have been commonly used. By weighing an individual on land and under water, in conjunction with measures of his residual lung capacity, accurate determinations of his body fat may be made. This technique is based upon Archimedes principle, noting that a body immersed in a fluid is acted upon by a buoyancy force in relation to the amount of fluid the body displaces. Since fat is less dense than water, it will displace a greater volume of water and the subject experiences a greater buoyancy force and weighs less under water than a person of equal weight but more muscle mass. A second method involving underwater techniques is the volumetric technique. A person

TABLE 10-11

DESIRABLE WEIGHTS FOR MEN AND WOMEN AGE 25

AND OVER

Weight in Pounds According to Frame (In Indoor Clothing)

	HEIGHT (with shoes on) 1-inch heels		SMALL FRAME	MEDIUM FRAME	LARGE FRAME
	Feet	Inches			
	5	2	112-120	118-129	126-141
	5	3	115-123	121-133	129-144
DESIRABLE	5	4	118-126	124-136	132-148
WEIGHTS	5	5	121-129	127-139	135-152
FOR MEN	5	6	124-133	130-143	138-156
of ages 25	5	7	128-137	134-147	142-161
and over	5	8	132-141	138-152	147-166
	5	9	136-145	142-156	151-170
	5	10	140-150	146-160	155-174
	5	11	144-154	150-165	159-179
	6	0	148-158	154-170	164-184
	6	1	152-162	158-175	168-189
	6	2	156-167	162-180	173-194
	6	3	160-171	167-185	178-199
	6	4	164-175	172-190	182-204

	HEIGHT (with shoes on) 2-inch heels		SMALL FRAME	MEDIUM FRAME	LARGE FRAME
	Feet	Inches			
	4	10	92- 98	96-107	104-119
	4	11	94-101	98-110	106-122
DESIRABLE	5	0	96-104	101-113	109-125
WEIGHTS	5	1	99-107	104-116	112-128
FOR WOMEN	5	2	102-110	107-119	115-131
of ages 25	5	3	105-113	110-122	118-134
and over	5	4	108-116	113-126	121-138
	5	5	111-119	116-130	125-142
	5	6	114-123	120-135	129-146
	5	7	118-127	124-139	133-150
	5	8	122-131	128-143	137-154
	5	9	126-135	132-147	141-158
	5	10	130-140	136-151	145-163
	5	11	134-144	140-155	149-168
	6	0	138-148	144-159	153-173

For girls between 18 and 25, subtract 1 pound for each year under 25.

*Courtesy of the Metropolitan Life Insurance Company.

is submerged and the amount of water he displaces is accurately measured. Other techniques involve the determination of total body water by the hydrometric technique, and the determination of total body potassium. Both techniques involve rather extensive laboratory procedures.

Probably the best compromise between practicality and accuracy for the determination of body fat is the skinfold test. Dozens of body fat prediction formulae from skinfold measurements have been formulated over the past three decades, many of them being specific to a given population. Damon and Goldman (1964) indicated that if fat prediction formulae are tested against subjects other than those from whom the formulae were derived, the formulae simply describe rather than predict. In a study of a number of fat prediction formulae, Damon and Goldman indicated that the closest predictions of densitometrically-determined fat were obtained from two standard skinfold sites, the triceps and subscapular. Thus, they noted that for skinfold determination of fat, the simplest was the best. They reported that the formulae developed by Brozek and Keys (1951) and Pascale and others (1956) were the most accurate for young men. The prediction formulae are available in those references. The Committee on Nutritional Anthropometry also recommended the triceps and subscapular sites.

Mayer (1968) has reported that the triceps skinfold is the easiest to measure and most representative skinfold of total body fatness. Minimum triceps skinfold thicknesses indicating obesity are presented in Table 10-III. However, others have proposed lower levels for determination of fatness. For young males, skinfold thickness has been utilized to classify leanness (< 7 mm), average fat content (7-13 mm), and overfat (> 13 mm). Buskirk and Haymes (1972) have set comparable standards for young females as leanness (< 10 mm), acceptable (10-15 mm) and overfat (> 15 mm).

The above discussion relative to body composition is extremely limited, as it was not considered a major topic within the context of this book. Excellent reviews are presented elsewhere. A prediction formula for both young men and young women is found in Appendix F. Detailed explanations of the more elaborate

TABLE 10-III

OBESITY STANDARDS FOR CAUCASIAN AMERICANS,

REPRESENTED BY MINIMUM TRICEPS SKINFOLD THICKNESS

IN MILLIMETERS

Age (years)	Skinfold measurements	
	Males	Females
5	12	14
6	12	15
7	13	16
8	14	17
9	15	18
10	16	20
11	17	21
12	18	22
13	18	23
14	17	23
15	16	24
16	15	25
17	14	26
18	15	27
19	15	27
20	16	28
21	17	28
22	18	28
23	18	28
24	19	28
25	20	29
26	20	29
27	21	29
28	22	29
29	23	29
30-50	23	30

*From Jean Mayer, OVERWEIGHT: Causes, Cost, and Control (c) 1968. Reprinted by permission of Prentice-Hall, Inc., Englewood Cliffs, N.J.

techniques, such as underwater weighing, may be found in some of the excellent exercise physiology laboratory manuals on the market.

WEIGHT GAINING

For the individual who desires to gain weight for sports competition, the increased mass should preferably represent muscles rather than fat. Simply adding body weight will not be an advantage in most sports, unless the tissue can be utilized for production of force. Thus, the athlete should be encouraged to initiate a progressive resistive exercise (PRE) weight training program in conjunction with increased caloric intake.

Methods for gaining body weight were presented in Chapter Five, along with some of the limited research in this area. For the role of protein supplementation in weight-gaining programs, the reader is referred to that chapter. The following discussion is a summary of the salient points which should be observed by the individual attempting to increase his body mass.

1. From the table in the first part of this chapter, calculate your energy needs daily. Evaluate your daily food intake in order to determine if you are meeting your caloric needs. The reason for underweight may be that the current caloric intake does not meet the recommended daily allowance.

2. Check the general composition of the food you eat. There should be a substantial percentage of protein in the diet, averaging about 15 to 20 percent.

3. Check your living habits. Are you getting enough sleep and rest?

4. When initiating your weight gaining program, set a reasonable goal within a certain time period. Get the advice of your coach or physical education teacher relative to the design and implementation of a sound PRE program. All the major muscle groups of the body should be stressed, as this will facilitate overall total body weight gains. The weight-training program will serve as a stimulus for the anabolic synthesis of muscle tissue.

5. Take careful and exacting measurements of your body weight, height and muscle girths at various reference points. These points should include the neck, upper and lower arm, chest, abdomen, thigh and calf. This is to insure that body weight gains are proportionately distributed. If available, use skinfold measurements for evaluation of body fat.

6. Increase your caloric intake. Many individuals have advised the utilization of protein supplement tablets or powders, but they may be unnecessary if the increased caloric intake is high in protein. The generally recommended protein allotment for a developing weight gaining athlete is on the order of 2 to 2.5 g/kg

body weight/day. By increasing the amount of cheese, milk, meat, and other animal products in the diet, increased levels of protein intake may be assured. If an average fifteen-year-old boy would increase his caloric intake from 3000 to 3500 calories/day, and consume about 20 percent of the caloric intake as protein, he would average over 2 g protein/kg body weight. The protein content of the diet would approximate 700 calories, or about 140 g. Thus, protein tablets or pills, which are relatively expensive sources of protein, would be unnecessary. However, they would not be harmful.

7. There are several high caloric supplements which are commercially available in most supermarkets. These usually are a good source of protein also. For example, a can of Nutrament contains 375 calories, with a composition of 25 g protein, 44 g carbohydrate and the remainder as fat. A can with each meal, along with the normal dietary intake, would be an effective means to increase both caloric and protein intake. The industrious athlete could, however, concoct his own high calorie-protein drink out of milk and appropriate ingredients. There are several reports (Sims, 1970; Blanchard, 1972) that the utilization of these dietary supplements may be useful adjuncts to weight-gaining programs.

8. If protein tablets or supplements are utilized, Crooks (1975) recommends that they be of high biological value, such as 65 percent utilizable protein. If you use a 90 percent protein powder supplement, Crooks noted that it should also contain a natural enzyme in order to facilitate digestion. However, as noted in Chapter Three, the utilization of these supplements is unnecessary if protein content of the daily diet is increased.

9. Certain drugs have been utilized for their weight-gaining properties. The anabolic steroids, patterned after the male sex hormone testosterone, may effectively increase muscle mass if used in conjunction with PRE, caloric and protein supplementation. However, they are not recommended for the developing athlete as there are some possible inherent medical risks associated with their use. Nevertheless, they appear to be popular with athletes participating in sports where body mass is an advantage.

Another drug which has been utilized as a weight-gaining

agent is Periactin®. Although Periactin is primarily used as an antihistamine, one of its side effects appears to elicit gains in body weight and it has been used successfully with young males who were underweight.

In summary, weight gaining for athletic performance necessitates a concerted effort by the individual, and it may be as difficult for some athletes to gain weight as it is for others to lose weight. The prospect is a little more pleasant, however, since man is almost always eager to increase his food intake, but does not like to restrict it. Nevertheless, knowledge relative to the disadvantages of excess body weight, in the form of fat, should be conveyed to the athlete, especially if he is of a mesomorphic-endomorphic somatotype. If the athlete follows the proper exercise and dietary regimen, increased muscle mass should accrue. As an important side point, although aerobic exercises expend calories, they should be a part of the training regimen because of the implications for the athlete in later life. He should be aware of the different roles of PRE training and aerobics training as they relate to the prevention of coronary heart disease.

OBESITY

One of the major health problems in the United States and many industrialized nations is excess body weight. Indeed, Durnin and others (1973) made the interesting comment that maybe the 70 percent of the world's population who are assumed to be undernourished may not be; the 30 percent who are adequately fed may be overnourished, and may be obese or overweight. Obesity is a body condition marked by excessive generalized deposition and storage of fat, and is to be distinguished from the condition of overweight. Overweight usually means that the individual weighs more than the normal value for his age and height. However, as noted in the section on body composition, a person with high muscular density may be overweight, but not obese. Conversely, a person may be of normal weight, but may be obese if he has a large percentage of his weight as fat.

Obesity affects both children and adults, and Mayer (1968) has noted that one out of five adolescents in the United States weighs more than he should for good health and appearance. However, the greatest increase in obesity is the twenty to thirty age group. Since it is a prevalent health problem, obese individuals are prime targets for medical quackery. The American Medical Association has estimated that over 100 million dollars per year are squandered on quick cures, even though it is a well-established fact that the two main means to decrease body fat is to diet and increase physical activity. Thousands of years ago, Socrates noted that one should eat only when hungry and never to leave the table with a feeling of satiety, while Hippocrates recognized the relationship between activity and leanness.

When is man obese? Mayer (1972b) has indicated that when the male is 25 to 30 percent above his ideal weight, he is considered obese; the corresponding precentage for females is 30 to 35. However, as noted previously, there are problems associated with the utilization of ideal weight tables, although these values may serve as a useful guide. The other simple body composition techniques, such as the pinch test, mirror test and circumference tests may be applied, or a skinfold analysis may be undertaken. A brief description of these tests was presented earlier in this chapter.

For the interested reader, a thorough discussion of obesity and overweight has been presented by one of the world's leading nutritionists, Jean Mayer (1968), in his book *Overweight: Causes, Cost and Control.*

Disadvantages of Obesity

There are a number of disadvantages associated with obesity, not only to the physical health of the individual but also to his socio-emotional health. Obesity exerts four different hazards to the health of the individual, not to mention disadvantages in most physical activities. It may change a variety of normal bodily functions, including increased stresses on the cardiovascular system. Secondly, obesity may exert a detrimental effect upon established diseases such as hypertension. The risk of incurring certain other diseases is associated with obesity, and lastly, adverse psychological reactions may occur.

Hippocrates recognized the fact that persons who are naturally fat are apt to die earlier than those who are slender. Clarke (1975) cited reports that the mortality rates were 79 percent for men markedly overweight, and 42 percent for men moderately overweight, above-standard risk groups; comparable figures were presented for women also. The excess mortality rates were attributed to the greater number of deaths from degenerative diseases among obese people.

Weinhaus (1969) has reported that for each five pounds above ideal weight, life expectancy is reduced by about one year. Obesity has been statistically associated with such disorders as kidney disease, cirrhosis of the liver, diabetes and cardiovascular disorders including hypertension and coronary atherosclerosis. Winick (1974), discussing childhood obesity, noted that coronary heart disease begins in childhood and is associated with childhood obesity and hypercholesteremia. Mayer (1960a) has indicated that although there are difficulties in establishing a causal relationship between obesity and coronary heart disease, it would be prudent to return to simple virtues such as dietary restriction of fats and increased physical activity.

For the developing adolescent, the major adverse effects of obesity are the psychological overtones. Heald (1972) noted that among the complex psychological aspects of adolescence, one of particular importance is body image. He indicated that body image tends to solidify during adolescence, and persists into adulthood. Any distorted feelings about body image may have undesirable psychological ramifications. Mayer (1972b) has noted that the onset of obesity in childhood is more disruptive personality-wise than if the onset occurs during adulthood. Mayer (1968) has suggested that obese individuals in the United States comprise a minority group, which suffers from prejudice and discrimination. Although the nature and extent of the myriad effects that prejudice will produce are difficult to determine, the sense of inferiority and self-blame imposed upon the obese individual by society are not conducive to development of a sound self-concept.

In the area of physical activity, Riendeau and others (1958) reported that excess body fat exerted an adverse effect upon several running and jumping events, thus imposing a limitation to motor fitness in general. If the obese child is unsuccessful in play activities, he will refrain from participation, thus eliminating an important avenue for the elimination of excess calories. A vicious cycle may be created, the withdrawal symptoms and absence of the socializing aspect of play contributing to improper psychological development at a critical stage in life, and further alienating the child from play.

The obese or overweight child and adult needs the attention of the physical educator and allied medical personnel. In the school situation, the educator should be aware of the etiology, prevention and treatment of obesity and overweight. Successful treatment programs have been developed in the public schools and will be discussed later in this chapter.

Etiology of Obesity

According to some individuals, the cause of overweight or obesity, by the simplest explanation, is an excessive caloric intake beyond that required for energy expenditure. However, the mechanisms which regulate food intake are complex, and lead to a multiple causality thesis relative to the etiology of obesity. Mayer (1968), after nearly thirty years of research into the causes of obesity, has provided evidence to support a multicausal etiology, and noted that it is an oversimplification to say overeating is the sole cause. There are a multiplicity of interactions leading to caloric imbalance. Of the various factors which may influence the development of obesity, Mayer implicated the following: genetic predisposition or heredity, endocrine imbalance, damage to the hypothalamus, nature of the diet, psychological trauma, social customs and physical inactivity. Mayer notes there is still an inadequate supply of knowledge related to obesity, but that the interaction of the above factors may create an energy imbalance, and since the cells cannot utilize the excess energy, will store it in the tissues usually in the form of fats. Mayer (1972b) generalized the etiology of obesity into two areas. In regulatory obesity the primary impairment is in the central control mechanism regulating food intake, probably in the hypothalamus. A feeding center and satiety center have been located in the hypothalamus, and Mayer has proposed a glucostatic theory relative to control of food intake. In general, the theory notes that the hypothalamus reacts to the rate of passage of glucose or related ions. If an inborn error of the hypothalamus precludes optimal functioning, food intake may be out of balance. Metabolic obesity is a state reflected by a biochemical error in the animal's metabolism other than in the regulatory center. Mayer has noted abnormal carbohydrate metabolism and adipose tissue functions as possible disorders leading to increased obesity.

A discussion of fat metabolism was presented in Chapter Four, and the reader may wish to review that section. Excess dietary fats and carbohydrates may be stored in the adipose tissue. The lipid is deposited in the adipose cell by one of two means, either by the direct incorporation of the preformed lipid from the circulation or the *de novo* synthesis of lipid from carbohydrate in the adipose cell itself. When the body needs the fat for energy, it may be mobilized by appropriate enzymes.

Hirsch (1972) has noted that obesity is achieved through both an increased number and fat content of adipose cells. Winick (1974), reviewing a 1973 conference on childhood obesity, also noted that the fat in the adipose tissue may be packaged in a large number of small cells, or in a smaller number of large cells. The former is hyperplastic obesity while the latter is hypertrophic obesity. Winick commented that early onset, or childhood, obesity is primarily hyperplastic, whereas late onset or adult obesity is hypertrophic. However, some overlap is acknowledged, and the theory is not totally accepted by others.

Whatever the cause, whether it is hyperplasia or hypertrophy of the fat cell, it may be important to consider the time in life when obesity may be treated and prevented. Van Itallie and Hashim (1970) noted that obesity had its roots in either one of three phases of childhood: the latter part of infancy, the time of starting school, and during adolescence. Hirsch (1972) indicated that the critical periods in man are not completely known yet, but the first three years of life and adolescence are important periods. There would appear to be some important implications here for parents and physical educators, as both may be able to influence dietary and exercise habits at critical periods for the development of obesity. Since obese children are likely to be obese adults, prevention is important. The condition known as creeping obesity also may afflict the young adult who ceases his active physical activities as he enters his twenties.

As previously noted, there are multiple causes of obesity. The teacher or coach should be aware of the genetic and environmental factors which may predispose the individual to excess body fat. Obesity tends to run in families, and Mayer (1968) has documented genetic influence in both man and animals. However, cultural patterns may also influence the familial tendency, as large and frequent meals may be a family custom. Glandular disturbances and psychological-emotional problems may also be involved in the etiology of obesity, and merit attention by medical personnel. However, in uncomplicated obesity, or with clearance from the physician, effective dietary and exercise programs may be implemented by physical educators. Even with hereditarial or genetic predispositions, these two mechanisms may be effective in reducing excess body fat. As Mayer (1968) has noted, genes may make one susceptible to obesity, but overeating and underexercise have to accompany it. The constitutional factors operating in the predisposition to obesity do not detract from the positive caloric balance concept.

As a nation, we are poorly educated in basic principles of nutrition and exercise. The average citizen does not know the caloric values of foods, or the calorie values of various physical activities, and hence cannot plan an adequate diet and exercise regimen. It is incumbent upon those involved with the food habits and physical activity of our youth, notably parents and health and physical educators, to instruct and motivate them towards sound habits. As with many other aspects of health, prevention is easier than treatment. Winick (1974) has noted that in order to control the increased number of fat cells in obesity, prevention must begin early in life, and thus is under the jurisdiction of parents. The other critical periods relative to the onset of obesity may be more under the influence of educators, who may teach the values of physical activity as a means to control body weight.

Prevention and Treatment of Obesity

When dealing with obese youngsters, it is more important to

stress immediate benefits of weight reduction, such as improved appearance, better social acceptance, and increased levels of physical fitness rather than the future benefits of lessened chances of coronary heart disease. With older individuals, the same factors are important, but health concerns may also be intrinsic motivational factors. For the individual who is obese and concerned about his health, whether young or old, a checkup with a physician is appropriate. He may check for endocrine imbalances and analyze dietary and activity habits, recommending appropriate therapy. For the adult or adolescent who is gradually becoming a victim of increased body weight, knowledge and application of sound principles underlying dieting and exercise may be effective in maintaining normal weight.

Dieting Principles

A tremendous amount of research has been devoted to the construction of sound diets, both for the individual who simply wants to lose weight or for the patient who must restrict the intake of certain nutrients due to some metabolic disorder. Diabetes and hypertension are pertinent examples. However, the focus of this section is on basic dietary principles for weight reduction. The literature is voluminous, for hardly a month passes without a new miracle diet being revealed in some leading magazine. Needless to say, for the normal healthy individual the principles of dieting are rather basic. One must reduce the caloric intake in order to effect a negative caloric balance and hence, lose weight. At the same time, essential nutrient intake must be assured. Nevertheless, many diets have been advanced purporting to have some special quality, such as a fat-mobilizing hormone which would facilitate catabolism of fats.

No detailed analysis of the various diets will be presented here. Although it is a very important topic, it is beyond the scope of this text. For the interested reader, the most comprehensive analysis available has been documented by Berland (1974) in an excellent book, *Rating the Diets*. Berland and the editors of *Consumer Guide* evaluated the vast majority of the popular diets, including Dr. Stillman's, Dr. Atkins', low carbohydrate, high fat, drinking man's, one food, the real and unreal Mayo clinic diets and many others. The book is well-grounded in nutritional principles and is highly recommended.

The following discussion centers upon the essential points and suggestions relative to the construction, implementation and maintenance of a dietary regimen. These principles apply to the overweight individual, or for the normal weight student who may wish to lose weight for a particular sport such as wrestling. The following chapter also contains some supplemental material.

1. If you decide to lose weight without the guidance of a physician, Mayer (1968) recommended that the maximal value be 2 pounds/week. For growing boys, Gregg (1970) recommended 1 pound/week. A diet should be planned for a prolonged period of time, with anticipation of forming life long habits.

2. Contrary to the title of a popular diet book, calories do count. In order to lose body fat, you must achieve a negative balance of approximately 3500 calories for every pound of fat. Consequently, to lose 1 pound/week, you must incur an average daily deficit of 500 calories. This may be achieved by diet alone, exercise alone, or a combination of the two.

3. A balanced diet has been recommended by Mayer (1968), consisting of 15 percent protein, 30 percent fat and 55 percent carbohydrate. However, there may be some small advantage to a high protein diet, as the specific dynamic action (SDA) of protein will help utilize extra calories by elevating the metabolic rate. The complexity of the protein molecule needs increased energy to catabolize it. However, a high protein diet must be judiciously selected, as it may prove to contain large quantities of fat if certain animal meats are selected. Also, a high protein diet will be relatively expensive, and it may be difficult to get the protein content of the diet above 30 percent. A slight increase in the protein content of the diet, with a concomitant decrease in fat and carbohydrate, may be a practical advantage.

4. The high fat-low carbohydrate diets are not recommended. The Council on Foods and Nutrition of the American Medical Association has condemned these general diets, indicating they are for the most part without merit, and may be potentially dangerous.

5. Water is a major source of body weight, and may mask real

losses. Some have advocated a starvation diet, or low carbohydrate diet, in order to release excess body water. Thus, the individual may lose several pounds in a couple of days, but it will primarily be water losses. On the other hand, Gordon and his associates (1963) noted that water retention may be enhanced during dieting due to increased secretion of the antidiuretic hormone. Thus, to the dismay of the dieter, he may not lose an appreciable amount of weight for ten to fourteen days due to the increased retention of body water. This may be particularly true of those on a gradual diet.

6. Drastic diets such as dehydration or complete fasting should be avoided. The body has a normal water level, and avoiding water may help you lose a few pounds of water weight, but homeostatic mechanisms will restore the water to normal levels upon resumption of fluid intake. Starvation is an effective means to lose weight, but it is rather drastic. However, some athletes practice nearly complete fasting in attempts to lose weight. This topic will be covered in a later section of this chapter.

7. Reducing drugs should be avoided if possible. There are several types available, including benzocaine to deaden taste buds, methylcellulose to expand the stomach for a sensation of fullness, and general anorectics such as amphetamines. Their chief value is the psychological support needed during the early stages, helping the individual to become re-educated to a proper diet.

8. The most useful adjunct to dieting is a concerted exercise program. Principles of establishing such a program are included in the following section.

9. A number of suggestions may be helpful in the battle against calories:

a. CHECK YOUR WEIGHT DAILY, SINCE SMALL WEIGHT GAINS ARE EASIER TO ADJUST.

b. KNOW THE CALORIC VALUES OF COMMON FOODS. PURCHASE THE HANDY DIET GUIDES AND BRAND NAME CALORIE BOOKS AVAILABLE IN MOST SUPERMARKETS. RESTRICT HIGH CALORIE FOODS FROM THE DIET.

c. CALCULATE YOUR CALORIC INTAKE FOR A WEEK. COMPARE THIS AGAINST YOUR RECOMMENDED INTAKE.

d. Instead of 2 to 3 large meals/day, eat 5 to 6 smaller ones. There is some evidence this may be a partial solution to the problem of obesity (Leveille and Romsos, 1974).

e. Use diet drinks or water at meals. Use saccharin or other sugar substitutes.

f. Avoid alcohol as much as possible. Alcohol is high in calories, low in nutrients. One gram of alcohol equals seven calories.

g. Trim the fat from meats; buy lean meats and broil or bake them. Avoid frying in butter.

h. Use low calorie margarines, salad dressings and similar products.

i. Bulk foods such as apples, celery and carrots may give a sensation of fullness without many calories.

j. The low calorie formula diets, such as Metrecal® may be useful to replace one meal a day during the early stages of the diet

k. Although Heald (1972) noted that conventional weight control methods are relatively unsuccessful with adolescents, he indicated that cutting food portions to prevent further fat accumulation is a realistic approach. Only cook small portions of food for meals; the temptation to overeat may be removed.

l. Exercise just before meal time; it may help curb the appetite.

m. If you need moral support, join a group such as Overeaters Anonoymous, Weight Watchers or TOPS (Take Off Pounds Sensibly). They appear to be relatively successful approaches. (Stunkard, et al. 1970).

In summary, it should be noted that these are only some of the suggestions available to help the dieter. Some of them are designed for the early stages of dieting, to help the individual lose weight initially. What is really needed is a solid education relative to sound nutritional principles, so that once the optimal weight is attained, a diet with nutritional and caloric balance may be made palatable to the individual. In addition, to complement the dietary program, a re-evaluation of activity habits should be made, with the intent of increasing energy expenditure through a concerted aerobics exercise program.

Exercise and Weight Reduction

Earliest observers in physiology and medicine have noted the relationship between inactivity and obesity. As early as the fifth century B.C., Hippocrates recognized the value of physical labor in preventing excessive body weight. Studying the evolution of man, Montague (1966) indicated that it is quite unlikely that obesity ever had any adaptive value, and on the whole, has always been handicapping. He noted that under natural conditions, primates such as gorillas and orangutans do not become obese, and yet they do get fat under captivity due to inactivity. Thus, he concluded that exercise is a helpful, if not a necessary, factor in the avoidance of obesity. As for humans, Mayer (1968) noted that men and women are using their bodies for purposes which they were not designed, i.e. inactivity. Man is meticuously designed for activity, and yet the mechanical age has denuded us of the need to get continuous, moderate exercise. The regulation of food intake was never designed, through the evolutionary process, to adapt to the highly mechanized conditions in modern society. Thus, the combination of overeating and inactivity leads to obesity. Mayer (1972b) reported that inactivity is one of the main health problems in the United States, while Grenier (1974) has characterized hypokinetism, or inactivity, as the disease of the century. These statements are directed at the relationship between inactivity and obesity, with the resultant health problems previously discussed.

Although inactivity prevails in the adult population, it is a phenomenon of children and adolescents as well. Mayer (1968) has reported that no single factor is more frequently responsible for the development of obesity in adolescents than lack of physical exercise. This viewpoint has been documented in reports by Huenemann and her associates (1967; 1972) who noted that the overall activity level of adolescents was extremely low, with approximately 90 percent of the boys' and 95 percent of the girls' time being spent in sleeping or light activity. They noted that these inactive teenagers may be expected to become less physically active as adults and thus experience obesity. Other studies

(Corbin and Pletcher, 1968; Bullen and others, 1964) utilized film analyses of children at play, and reported the relative inactivity of the obese child as compared to the nonobese.

There are implications here for the educator. Children and adolescents need to be encouraged to participate in activities which involve high degrees of energy expenditure, and which might be of social significance to them. These recommendations are especially important for those children who show a tendency towards obesity.

MECHANISMS AND MYTHS OF EXERCISE. When man exercises, body weight is lost from two main channels, body water and energy stored in the form of carbohydrates or fat. Therefore, body weight losses do not necessarily reflect total caloric expenditure, as the body mass lost during exercise may be primarily water, which has no caloric value. As noted in Chapter Eight, 10 to 15 pounds of body weight may be lost during prolonged exercise in a hot environment, the vast majority being water via the sweating mechanism in an attempt to control body temperature. One of the myths among weight watchers is that a good way to lose weight is to sweat as much as possible. However, sweating is an indication of water depletion, not fat depletion. Mitchell and others (1972) have also noticed water weight losses via the respiratory tract during exercise on the order of 2 to 5 g/minute, which could average approximately .5 pound/hour. Thus, when evaluating the effectiveness of exercise as a means of losing body weight, one must evaluate the chronic effects rather than acute effects.

To be precise, even over the long haul, changes in body weight might not accurately reflect losses in body fat. Since exercise is anabolic in nature for muscular tissue, the individual may experience increased concentration of muscle tissue while also experiencing a concomitant decrease in body fat during a training program. As muscle tissue has a greater density than fat tissue, the total body weight may not change appreciably while the body fat would decrease. In cases such as this, body composition analysis would be more appropriate to detect actual changes in body structure. In the case of the obese, exercise would almost assuredly cause a decrease in total body weight. Grande (1968) has indicated that the methods of body composition used to assess caloric deficits need to be studied carefully so that no erroneous conclusions are made relative to the effectiveness of certain techniques, dietary or exercise, in decreasing body fat.

The major mechanism whereby man loses body fat through exercise is the increased energy requirement. As explained in Chapter Two, man may increase his energy metabolism manifold above the resting level, and, once conditioned, maintain the high level of energy expenditure for a considerable period of time. For example, while the average man may expend only 70 calories/hour during rest, this value may approach 1000/hour during sustained high level activity such as running. Fat is mobilized from the adipose tissue to supply energy and hence body fat may be reduced, provided the individual does not overeat to compensate for this energy expenditure. An hour/day of running at 1000 cal/hr would equal two pounds per week. There are some fringe benefits also. First, during exercise the obese or overweight individuals definitely have a greater energy expenditure than the lean individual since they are moving more weight. Thus, for a given distance, the overweight subject will utilize more calories, thereby helping in the catabolism of body fat. Secondly, Mayer (1972b) has noted that as the body temperature is elevated, the feeding center may be depressed. The close anatomical relationship of the temperature and hunger centers in the hypothalamus may provide rationale for this effect. Exercise does elevate the body temperature, and may be effective in temporarily curbing the appetite. Finally, deVries and Gray (1963) have noted some metabolic aftereffects of exercise. They reported an elevated resting metabolic rate for nearly six hours following a forty-five minute exercise session. The authors indicated that the individual would utilize 53 cal/day above the metabolic cost of the activity itself. However, there were only two subjects in this study and the authors did suggest confirmation by independent research. Nevertheless, the elevated temperature and adrenalin levels following prolonged activity could keep the metabolic rate elevated for a period of time, thus expending excess calories.

Mayer (1968) has noted several misconceptions about exercise, existing in the minds of many adults and youth, which may deter them from initiating an exercise program for weight control. The first misconception is that exercise is a poor means to lose weight because it expends so few calories. One has to walk thirty-five miles to lose a pound of body weight. Since the average person utilizes approximately 100 cal/mile, there is some truth to that statement; however, one must think in terms of the future. Two miles a day will equal slightly less than a loss of two pounds/ month. If the individual can train to running five mile/day, a pound/week may be lost. Over a year's time, the loss may be substantial. Overweight people will expend even more energy while exercising, and hence be more efficient in losing weight.

The second misconception is that increased energy expenditure through exercise is counterbalanced by increased food intake. This is true to a large degree and it is the mechanism whereby normal weight is controlled. However, Mayer's research has indicated that this is not necessarily true with sedentary individuals, those most likely to be obese; their appetite might actually decrease.

This point has been recently resubstantiated by Jankowski and Foss (1972), who followed the energy intake of sedentary men for twenty-four hours after a bout of exercise. Compared to control days, the amount of food consumed following exercise was slightly less, but not significantly so. Also, appetite does not normally decrease with a decreased activity level. Thus, if one is active in sports or otherwise, attention should be directed to curtailing food intake upon the cessation of regular activity. Thus, according to Mayer, exercise may be an effective means to control body weight. Emphasis needs to be equally placed on caloric expenditure as well as caloric intake in weight control programs.

SUMMARY OF RESEARCH WITH PHYSICAL ACTIVITY AND WEIGHT REDUCTION. Numerous studies have been conducted to investigate the effect of physical activity upon body composition. Varient groups of subjects have been used, including senior citizens, middle-aged men and women, college-age men and women, high school boys and girls and elementary school children. The studies are too numerous to replicate here, but several recent reviews have succinctly summarized the general findings.

Following a review of the literature, including his own respected research, Oscai (1973) concluded that exercise may elicit favorable changes in body composition in both children and adults, preventing increased body fat and increasing lean body mass. Even if body weight does not change, the body composition reflects increased muscle mass and loss of fat. Oscai noted that the most appropriate approach to weight reduction in obese individuals would be a combination diet-exercise program, even though exercise alone is effective in expending excess calories and hence body fat.

Parizkova (1973) also concluded that systematic physical activity and athletic training could modify body composition, with the proportion of lean body mass increasing significantly at the expense of body fat. This is true of both children and adults. Parizkova indicated that inactivity reduces the utilization of fatty acids in the muscles and also produces a slower release from fat depots, with a resultant greater accumulation of fat. The reverse apparently occurs during periods of increased physical activity. Several of his longitudinal studies produced conflicting evidence relative to the effect of prepubertal exercise programs upon the body fat deposition of girls. In a three-year study with girl swimmers, he reported that the increase in body fat which normally occurs in girls with the development of clinical puberty was not prevented by the training program. On the other hand, in a similar study, female gymnasts, in comparison to controls, had less subcutaneous fat at the end of a five-year training period. Overall, Parizkova indicated that physical activity leads to a leaner individual.

In the most recent review, Clarke (1975) analyzed the data from the most pertinent studies done with humans. He noted that exercise is not a cure-all for obesity, but that the relevant literature revealed some important implications for physical fitness practices in the control of obesity and overweight. The most frequently studied exercise program to elicit fat reduction involves a walk-jog-run-type activity. Due to the nature of this activity, an appreciable number of calories may be expended in moderate activity of long duration, and thus contribute to weight loss. In general, the summary by Clarke reiterated the conclusions noted by Oscai and Parizkova above. Moreover, Clarke noted that intensive progressive weight training programs resulted in desirable changes of body composition, reflecting decreased body fat and increased lean body mass.

Bloom (1968) addressed himself to the question of whether it is better to fast or exercise. Although he noted the values of both techniques, Bloom recommended exercise as the choice to lose weight and reduce obesity because of the concomitant benefits of exercise upon the cardiovascular system. Several studies (Zuti, 1973; Dudleston and Bennion, 1970) have compared the relative effectiveness of diet and exercise upon weight loss, and reported no significant differences between the conditions if the negative caloric balance for each treatment was similar. Thus, probably the most effective approach, as noted by Oscai (1973), would be a combination of both diet and exercise.

Spot Reducing. The effectiveness of spot reducing, as a method of losing body fat in the specific exercised area, is controversial. Several earlier studies by Schade and associates (1962) and Roby (1962) did not support the thesis of fat reduction in the most active areas. However, the studies by Mohr (1965), Olson and Edelstein (1968), and Simka and others (1974), have found favorable effects of spot-reducing techniques. Clarke (1975) summarized the current viewpoint by stating that reduction of body fat in body areas is most likely to occur where fat deposits are the most conspicuous, regardless of the exercise format. Although both general and localized exercise programs may both be beneficial in reducing fat stores, a general exercise program is recommended because larger musculature areas are involved. Nevertheless, spot reducing may be effective for specific areas.

Practical Physical Education Programs for the Obese. Since one of the major health problems of public school-age children is obesity, it may be incumbent upon school authorities to implement programs to help alleviate the problem. Moody (1971) has suggested that it is the responsibility of physical educators to develop a program for the obese student, possibly patterned after an organization like Weight Watchers®, with regular meetings, maintenance of appropriate records, and provision of appropriate materials and advice. Indeed, no less an authority than Mayer (1968) is convinced that an effective program consisting of increased physical exercise, dietary education, and psychological support can be incorporated into the public school system. Obese students may desire such a program. Canning and Mayer (1968) studied the attitudes and knowledges of weight control in obese and normal weight adolescent girls. The obese had a more realistic awareness and interest in the issues of obesity and weight control, and had more positive attitudes towards exercise. These factors appeared to be irrelevant, since the girls still remained obese. Canning and Mayer suggested these interests and attitudes be exploited by the physical educator, and help the obese initiate and maintain an effective dieting and exercise program.

Several reports have documented the effectiveness of such programs. Christakis and others (1966) studied the effect of a combined program of physical fitness and nutritional education upon the degree of obesity in ninety high school boys. An experimental and a control group were utilized over an eighteen-month period, and the results indicated that the program was very effective in reducing the obesity of those boys who had been grossly obese at the start. The experimental group averaged an 11 percent decrease in their average degree of overweight. Seltzer and Mayer (1970) undertook a study whose purpose was to ascertain whether or not a program for obese youngsters could be successfully instituted in a large public school system. The obese elementary and junior high school students were placed into experimental (n = 189) and control (n = 161) groups. Special physical activity programs for the obese were conducted five days/week, instead of the usual two days. Special physical education teachers were hired for the project, stressing vigorous exercise with constant motion. No attempt was made to place the obese children on low calorie diets, although nutritional information was discussed. The results indicated that the program was effective in reducing obesity, and the authors suggested that such a program should be an integral part of all public school systems. As Seltzer and Mayer point out, at the present time public school physical education programs are not designed to handle these programs properly. For those individuals administering physical education programs in the public schools, it is time to devote increased attention to the specific physical needs of this segment of the school population — the obese — as well as other handicapped children. Some school systems already have well developed adapted physical education programs, but the practice is the exception rather than the rule.

IMPLEMENTING A WEIGHT REDUCTION PROGRAM THROUGH EX-
ERCISE. For the individual who desires to initiate a weight reduction program, several principles should be followed.

1. First, it would be advisable, especially for adults, to check
with a physician to ascertain the cause of the increased body
weight. If it is an uncomplicated caloric balance problem, then
diet and exercise may be effective.

2. Both dieting and exercise should be utilized. A low calorie
diet may be designed by a physician, or from one of the leading
medically approved diet manuals. Several low calorie diets which
provide the essential nutrients are contained in Appendix D. The
principles underlying dietary practice, which were discussed in a
preceding section of this chapter, should be reviewed.

3. One should be aware of the energy costs of various forms of
exercise. Reference to Table 2-IV in Chapter Two provides the
individual with the metabolic costs of most general activities. The
caloric cost of each activity may be calculated. An interesting
concept has been advanced by Konishi (1973) in his book, *Exercise
Equivalents of Foods.* He has calculated the energy cost of a given
activity against the caloric content of a given food, indicating the
type and amount of physical activity which was needed to counteract the caloric value of that food. For example, a large apple
with 101 calories has an energy equivalent of either of the following activities: nineteen minutes walking, twelve minutes bicycle
riding, nine minutes swimming, five minutes running, or 78
minutes resting (Konishi, 1965). This book may be illuminating
relative to developing a conscious awareness of the caloric values
of different foods, especially for the individual who is exercising
to expend those calories.

4. The recommended exercise program should be centered primarily around aerobic endurance-type activities supplemented by
a weight training program for the upper body. The main goal is
to lose body fat and to increase muscle tone. The endurance-type
exercises, such as distance jogging, swimming or bicycling will
be effective in expending calories. The weight-training program
for the upper body will help develop the musculature in the
chest, arms and shoulders. An excellent reference book for the

individual who desires to plan his own endurance exercise program is *The New Aerobics* by Kenneth Cooper, M.D. Cooper provides the individual with a structured program, and incorporates sound principles relative to exercise tolerance, overload and progression. The individual is advised to start slowly, and gradually increase the intensity and distance of the exercise bout. The benefits are not only reduced body fat, but increased cardiovascular fitness as well.

5. Parents should be encouraged to initiate exercise and endurance programs for their preschool children. Oscai and his associates (1974a; 1974b), although using animals, reported that exercise during youth is effective in significantly reducing the rate of adipose cell accumulation in epididymal fat pads and hence a significant reduction in body fat in later life.

For the obese and the overweight, changes in body composition necessitate changes in the general life style. Moderate physical activity should become a daily habit, and dietary behavior should be modified to eliminate excess empty calories and concentrate on nutritious low calorie foods. Both modifications take effort, but they may supplement each other very effectively. Art Buchwald stated that the word *diet* comes from the verb, to die. For those individuals who savor eating, exercise may provide a palatable alternative to strict dieting as the sole means of losing excess body fat.

WEIGHT LOSS FOR SPORTS COMPETITION

There are a number of sports in which a lower body weight may confer some advantage, but the most striking example with young men in the United States is amateur wrestling. If an athlete can maintain his strength and endurance following a weight reduction program which allows him to compete in a lower weight class, he may have a decided advantage in force and leverage provided his opponent has not also undergone similar weight reduction. Empirically, wrestlers have learned this concept over the years, and have lost prodigious amounts of body weight in order to participate in a certain weight class. As the wrestlers become coaches, they impose weight control on their charges. In a survey of leading high school wrestling coaches throughout the United States, Frederick (1968) reported that in most cases, successful coaches imposed stringent regulations relative to both fluid and food intake. Needless to say, the practice of imposing restrictions upon the fluid and food intake of growing boys in order to make weight for wrestling has received considerable attention from medical groups. Nonetheless, the practice of making weight is still universal in this sport.

The wrestler utilizes two approaches to making weight. One involves a rather long period of food restriction in order to lose as much body fat as possible, and levels as low as 5 percent body fat have been recorded in competitive wrestlers. The wrestler may come within 5 to 10 pounds of his desired weight class by this method, and then, during the competitive season, uses intermittant periods of acute partial or complete starvation along with dehydration for several days immediately prior to the weigh-in for the match in order to lose those final pounds. It is primarily these latter actions which draw criticism from medical authorities.

Dehydration techniques are utilized extensively to reduce those final 7 to 8 pounds of body weight before a match. The physiological and performance effects of dehydration have been treated in Chapter Eight, and generally speaking, dehydration may exert a detrimental effect upon prolonged performance. In an article condemning this practice among wrestlers, Slocum and others (1967), representing the American Medical Association Committee on Medical Aspects of Sports, indicated that excessive dehydration, on the order of 3 percent of the body weight, could impair performance, maybe not in a single match, but over the duration of a tournament it could be hazardous. On the other hand, other reports with experienced wrestlers showed no adverse effects of rapid weight reduction. Weiss and Singer (1967) studied ten college wrestlers after they lost 7 percent of their body weight over a five-day period. They studied this effect upon parameters associated with wrestling, i.e. strength, cardiovascular endurance and total body response. No significant effect was noted on the first two parameters, but a significantly faster total body response time was found. They noted that a wrestler may improve his performance by dropping down one weight class. However, they did note that other factors, primarily the age of the participant, should be considered by coaches, wrestlers and parents. Their study was conducted with college age males. The results might be different for high school boys. In an earlier study, Tuttle (1943) found no effect of a 5 percent reduction of body weight on various physiological responses in five wrestlers.

College wrestlers normally have five hours following the weigh-in until match time; for high school wrestlers, the corresponding time is usually one hour. Thus, there is some time available to replenish fluids lost during the dehydration period. Several studies have been cited in Chapter Eight, and the general consensus is that rehydration may effectively restore any decrement in physical working capacity. Most of these studies, however, were conducted with college wrestlers and involved a three to five hour rehydration period. In addition, the tests were submaximal, and usually monitored heart rate response to a submaximal workload. Dehydration would adversely affect this response, and rehydration restore normalcy. An example of this type of study, showing beneficial effects of rehydration, was presented by Ribisl and Herbert (1970).

In reality, it is not proven that acute dehydration will adversely affect the performance of a wrestler. The American Medical Association (1973) has concluded that rapid weight loss by dehydration over a forty-eight hour period is detrimental to aerobic capacity. This is true if one talks about prolonged activity, especially in the heat. But wrestling is not a completely aerobic type activity. It is characterized by intermittant periods of moderate activity with sudden spurts of anaerobic energy expenditure. Thus, the anaerobic nature of the performance may not be adversily affected by dehydration per se.

Starvation Techniques

Aside from dehydration, complete or partial starvation is used by wrestlers as a weight control method. As is obvious, complete fasting would create a substantial negative caloric balance, and indeed, the practice has been utilized with a high percentage of success in a hospital situation with obese individuals who have not been successful with other techniques; it should be stressed that the patient is under strict medical supervision (Mayer, 1968). Passmore and Durnin (1967) reported that a healthy man or woman can fast completely for two weeks and suffer no permanent ill effects. They noted that during starvation, the exhaustion time for body carbohydrate is less than one day, whereas protein and fat have sufficient reserves for up to forty days.

When an individual fasts, he may lose weight rapidly, including water, carbohydrates, fats and proteins. Hypoglycemia may develop in twenty-four to forty-eight hours, with adverse effects upon the nervous system. As the glucose and glycogen stores are utilized during the first day, a large quantity of water is also lost. The individual may lose close to 3 pounds in one day of complete fasting if he has expended approximately 3500 calories. He would lose a pound of body tissue and approximately two pounds of water. The water was bound to the carbohydrate and some of the protein that was lost (Mayer, 1972b). Passmore and Durnin indicated that approximately 60 g protein would be lost per day. Some of it would be converted into glucose by the process of gluconeogenesis, since some glucose may be needed by the central nervous system. During prolonged starvation, however, the brain begins to utilize ketone bodies, intermediate products of fat metabolism, for its energy source. Thus, after the first day, protein and fat supply the energy for bodily functions. In a resting average man, about 1600 calories will be utilized per day. Protein will supply about 250 calories, or 60 g, and fat 1350 calories, or 150 g (Passmore and Durnin, 1967).

Starvation is a complex topic by itself, and has been a subject of considerable research. The early research with the whole subject of subnutrition is well documented by Keys and his associates (1950) at the University of Minnesota in *Human Starvation*. Only some highlights of their research, and several contemporary reports, will be discussed.

In a most thorough study on semistarvation, covering a year, Keys and his colleagues (1950) studied thirty-two subjects throughout several phases, including a twenty-four week period on a diet of 1570 cal/day. Following this period of time, the subjects experienced significant decreases in maximal aerobic power, reflected by a 25 percent decrease in maximal oxygen uptake/kg body weight. A decreased oxygen debt capacity was indicative of decreased anaerobic capacity; speed of leg movement and strength also declined. Studying four men on a 2.5-day fast and twelve men on a five-day fast, Henschel and others (1954) evaluated the effects of acute starvation. They noted a loss of speed and coordination on the second day. This loss appeared to be dependent upon the blood sugar level, and could easily be reversed by the administration of 100 g sugar. Although they reported no effect upon strength and maximal oxygen uptake, the capacity to do anaerobic work decreased. However, they noted that the general deterioration in performance was reversed by three days of refeeding.

Consolazio and others (1967a; 1967b) recently conducted several studies concerning the metabolic effects of acute starvation in normal humans for ten days. The general physiological effects included great body water losses leading to hypohydration, fairly large losses of nitrogen, indicating metabolism and excretion of body protein, and large mineral losses concomitant with the large water losses. The subjects appeared to be weak physically and had apathy towards physical work. When studying the subjects' reaction to daily submaximal and maximal tests in a subsequent phase of the study, they reported no significant decrease in the maximal oxygen consumption, but a significant decrease in the maximal oxygen debt. However, endurance, as measured by time to exhaustion, did not change significantly over the starvation period. Nonetheless, they did note that some interference in the study was created by a training effect, even though the starvation period was preceded by two weeks of training. Although they concluded that physical performance was not significantly impaired during a ten-day starvation period, they did not recommend complete fasting.

The general findings of the studies above appear to provide some evidence against the use of complete fasting, as a decrease in anaerobic performance may occur. However, in an earlier study, Taylor and others (1945) indicated that repeated exposure to fasting resulted in more effective physiological adaptations during the later trials. Several subjects were exposed to five successive 2.5 day fasts with five to six weeks between each fast.

In contrast to total starvation, several studies have investigated the effects of partial caloric restriction upon physical performance capacity. Taylor and his associates (1957) evaluated the effect of two dietary regimens against a normal diet; six men were on a 580 cal/day diet for twelve days, and thirteen men were on a 1010 cal/day diet for twenty-four days. The diet was pure carbohydrate with 4.5 g salt daily. In essense, both diets helped to maintain the capacity to perform aerobic and anaerobic work tasks, although the lower calorie diet did elicit some deterioration in the oxygen debt during work. The authors noted that if sufficient calories, along with sufficient minerals and vitamins, are given to prevent ketosis, dehydration and hypoglycemia under conditions of moderate energy output, performance capacity may be well maintained up to a weight loss of 10 percent of the original body weight.

Consolazio and others (1968) compared the effects of different caloric diets upon body weight losses. In eight men who were limited to 420 cal/day for ten days, with an energy expenditure of 3200 cal/day, it was observed that the limited number of calories was more beneficial than complete starvation. However, body weight losses were still substantial, being 8 percent in a group without mineral supplementation and 5 percent in the group with mineral supplements. The complete starvation group lost 9.6 percent body weight.

Daws and his associates (1972) studied the physiological work performance of eight subjects who received 420 and 500 cal/day for ten days in separate studies. In each study, four of the men received the daily adult mineral allowance recommended by the National Research Council. All subjects took maximal and submaximal tests, and in the 500 cal study, a stamina test. The 420 cal diet was composed of liquid carbohydrate, whereas the 500 cal diet consisted of 85 g sucrose and 40 g egg albumin. They reported no significant decreases in maximal oxygen consumption during the period of starvation, nor did performance on the stamina test decline significantly. They concluded that in short term caloric restriction, physical performance at three work levels was not significantly impaired, but there were implications of some abnormalties such as hypohydration and protein catabolism. The weight losses were below 10 percent of the body weight and the subjects were able to maintain the capacity to perform both aerobic and anaerobic work.

With appropriate minerals, vitamins and proteins in the diet, it would appear that a limited number of calories would enable a wrestler to lose body weight effectively and yet still maintain high levels of aerobic and anaerobic activity. A recommended diet for wrestlers is presented in the following chapter.

Theoretical Health Hazards of Making Weight

There are many unanswered questions relative to the effect of chronic intermittant starvation and dehydration, as practiced by wrestlers, upon their general health. The Committee on the Medical Aspects of Sports of the AMA has condemned the practice, noting that it is not only unethical but might seriously affect his health (Slocum and others, 1967). Cooper (1966) also theorized that by putting a boy on a starvation diet, and severely dehydrating him, may do some permanent harm to his health. Tcheng and his associates (1975) noted that weight loss through dehydration may cause kidney problems, and Taylor and others (1954) noted some signs of temporary liver damage in some subjects who underwent acute starvation combined with hard work. However, the signs of liver damage were not presented in all series of experiments they conducted. At the end of 4.5 days of complete starvation, one man showed unequivocal evidence of jaundice, and liver function tests revealed definite malfunction. However, all liver function tests returned to normal by the third day of recovery. Paul (1966) added to this list of the health hazards of crash dieting by also citing possible complications as acute pancreatitis, ulceration and chronic nephritis. One bright note, however, Amundson (1973) noted that the boy who is overfed or overweight is doing more damage to his health than the young man who is exercising hard to lose weight.

Although severe starvation and dehydration may pose some acute health problems to the individual, they have not been extensively documented as they relate to the different weight control methods and the ultimate health of the growing youth. Mayer

(1972b) has posed some interesting questions, which have not been adequately researched as of the present. What is the effect of current weight reduction practices on growing and developing youngsters? Are there any pathological consequences of hyperketonemia and dehydration? What are the long-term effects on the liver and other organs of alternating total fasting and refeeding?

In general, it may appear unwise to restrict caloric intake during a developmental period of a boy's life. Yet individuals in impoverished countries subsist on a much lower caloric intake than the normal American, and still can maintain high levels of activity. We are products of our historical evolution, the development of body fat as a compact means to store energy was one of man's advantages in the survival of the fittest. Thus, in earlier days, man was able to subsist for days at a time between successful hunting forays, literally living off his fat. Since we still have a substantial amount of body fat, which appears to be an increasing problem as mentioned previously, it would appear that man still has the ability to undergo successive periods of fasting without any permanent damage.

The potential health problems are incurred when a youngster sets an unrealistically low body weight goal for himself, and utilizes a number of techniques, including starvation, dehydration, diuretics and appetite suppressant drugs to accomplish his goal. Everyone who has been involved in wrestling has known individuals such as these, and in most cases, no apparant harm is immediately done. Unfortunately, we do not know the long-range effects, if any.

With these thoughts in mind, many attempts have been made to devise a method to control body weight losses of high school wrestlers, but as Amundson (1973) noted, the path to the moon is clearer than the path to proper weight control in wrestling. The American Medical Association recommended that the boy should undertake an intensive training program for four to six weeks without any emphasis on body weight. At the end of this period, he should record the weight in a prebreakfast, posturination state and consider that weight as the minimal effective weight for competition as well as certification purposes. The only problem is that the wrestlers would probably undergo dehydration and other techniques for this preliminary weigh-in.

Tcheng and Tipton (1973) recently developed a minimal weight prediction equation for wrestlers, based on the assumption that finalists in a state wrestling tournament were the best examples of well-conditioned athletes who were effectively competing at their minimal body weights. From their anthropometrical data, they recommended that the lowest possible body weight permissable without medical approval is one that contains a fat content of 5 percent. They proposed that anthropometrical measurements be obtained six to eight weeks prior to the wrestling season, and that the minimal weight be predicted. If an individual wished to compete at a lower level, he could do so only with the

TABLE 10-IV

TCHENG-TIPTON EQUATIONS FOR PREDICTING A

MINIMAL WRESTLING WEIGHT

A. LONG FORM:

```
Minimal
Weight  =      1.84 Height (inches)
        +      3.28 Chest Diameter (cms)
        +      3.31 Chest Depth (cms)
        +      0.82 Bi-iliac Diameter (cms)
        +      1.69 Bitrochanteric Diameter (cms)
        +      3.56 Both Wrists (cms)
        +      2.15 Both Ankles (cms)
        -281.72
```

r = .933 with a standard error of estimate of 8.7 pounds

B. SHORT FORM:

```
Minimal
Weight  =      2.05 Height (inches)
        +      3.65 Chest Diameter (cms)
        +      3.51 Chest Depth (cms)
        +      1.96 Bitrochanteric Diameter (cms)
        +      8.02 Left Ankle (cms)
        -282.18
```

r = .923 with a standard error of estimate of 8.9 pounds

*From Tcheng, T. and Tipton, C., Iowa Wrestling Study: Anthropometric measurements and the prediction of a "minimal" body weight for high school wrestlers. *Med Sci Sports,* 5:1-10, 1973

consent and approval of the physician. Their prediction formula is presented in Table 10-IV. Clarke (1974) field tested the Tcheng-Tipton method in a state wrestling meet and found that the method was valid, if the basic assumption of their study can be accepted.

There are some difficulties in establishing effective weight control methods for young wrestlers, and the AMA Committee on Medical Aspects of Sports has indicated that a minimal weight figure cannot be definable by formula or edict (Slocum and others, 1967). Professional judgment of the coach and physician needs to be exercised. However, many coaches, and wrestlers, still remain unconvinced that current weight control practices pose any immediate or future health hazard. The available objective data is limited, and this general area is in dire need of longitudinal research to either substantiate or reject some of the contentions being made.

CHAPTER **ELEVEN** ____

FEEDING THE ATHLETE

THE BASIC PURPOSES of food for humans are to provide energy, build and repair tissue, and supply substances to help regulate the various metabolic functions in the body. These functions and the related nutrients and foods are presented in Figure 11-1.

Although these functions are important to the sedentary individual, they become increasingly important to the athlete who may elevate his metabolic rate more than ten-fold through exercise and maintain that high rate for an hour or more. The performance of an athlete may be seriously hampered by an improper or faulty diet, and Naughton and Hellerstein (1973) have indicated that a number of experimental studies on man have shown that undernourishment reduces the maximal aerobic power. The converse, however, has not been substantiated. Overnutrition has not been proven to be effective in increasing athletic performance. Examples throughout this book have documented the value of certain nutritional practices upon physical performance, i.e. glycogen storage and hyperhydration, but they are usually related to a specific event and cannot be applied across the board due to the diverse nature of the myriad of physical performance activities.

Most authorities agree that there is no basic difference in feeding an athlete as contrasted to a nonathlete. The basic nutritional principles apply to both, except that the athlete may need more calories for his increased energy expenditure. During training, Bensley (1951) noted that if the athlete consumed his extra calories in the form of all ordinary types of food, such as milk, meat, vegetables and grain products, he would satisfy his increased demand for protein and the regulatory vitamins and minerals. Blix (1965) has reported a linear relationship between caloric intake and the content of many nutrients such as protein, vitamins and minerals. However, Bobb and others (1969), in a study of the diet of college athletes, concluded that when left on their

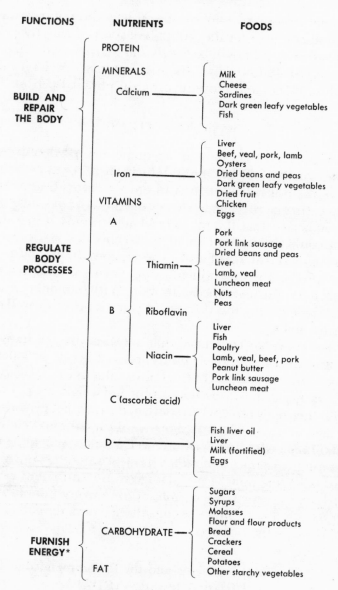

FUNCTIONS   NUTRIENTS   FOODS

PROTEIN

MINERALS

BUILD AND REPAIR THE BODY

Calcium —
- Milk
- Cheese
- Sardines
- Dark green leafy vegetables
- Fish

Iron —
- Liver
- Beef, veal, pork, lamb
- Oysters
- Dried beans and peas
- Dark green leafy vegetables
- Dried fruit
- Chicken
- Eggs

VITAMINS

A

REGULATE BODY PROCESSES

B

Thiamin —
- Pork
- Pork link sausage
- Dried beans and peas
- Liver
- Lamb, veal
- Luncheon meat
- Nuts
- Peas

Riboflavin

Niacin —
- Liver
- Fish
- Poultry
- Lamb, veal, beef, pork
- Peanut butter
- Pork link sausage
- Luncheon meat

C (ascorbic acid)

D —
- Fish liver oil
- Liver
- Milk (fortified)
- Eggs

FURNISH ENERGY*

CARBOHYDRATE —
- Sugars
- Syrups
- Molasses
- Flour and flour products
- Bread
- Crackers
- Cereal
- Potatoes
- Other starchy vegetables

FAT

*Although carbohydrate and fat are the principal sources of energy, protein also provides energy. This, however, is not the major function of protein.

Figure 11-1   Functions of food in nutrition. Courtesy of National Live Stock and Meat Board.

own to buy and prepare foods, the athletes did not have a well-balanced diet geared for the demands of sports. Thus, the principles of basic nutrition will be briefly summarized in the first part of this chapter, followed by a discussion of some special considerations for athletes and those involved in physical performance.

BASIC NUTRITION

When does a person have an adequate diet? By definition, an adequate diet would be one in which all nutrient and caloric needs of the individual are met in order to provide good nutritional health and prevent deficiency disease. Astrand and Rodahl (1970) indicated that if a man could adjust himself to a simple diet, he could feed himself for about 60 cents/day. A formula diet consisting of cereal, dried milk powder, corn oil margarine, and sugar with vitamin and mineral supplements would provide all the necessary nutrients needed by man. With economic inflation as it has been during this decade, the price is probably well over a dollar by now.

White (1974) has contended that a well-nourished individual has a general appearance of vitality and well-being, feels alert and has the energy to perform normal physical activities. His appetite should be good, and growth in height and weight are normal for his inherited body build when compared with other persons of the same age and sex. Clinical signs would involve a well-shaped skeletal frame with good posture, well-formed teeth and healthy gums, well-developed musculature, clear smooth skin, and adequate bodily functioning such as digestion, elimination, physical endurance, nervous stability and rapid recovery from fatigue or other stresses. Everything else considered equal, the balanced diet should ensure these things.

Essential Nutrients and the Recommended Dietary Allowances (RDA)

Man has an essential requirement for water, some inorganic ions and a host of organic compounds. Table 11-I represents the nutrients, with the exception of water, which are known to be or

TABLE 11-I

NUTRIENTS REQUIRED BY MAN

Amino Acids	Elements	Vitamins
Established as Essential		
Isoleucine	Calcium	Ascorbic acid
Leucine	Chlorine	Choline
Lysine	Copper	Folic acid
Methionine	Iodine	Niacin
Phenylalanine	Iron	Pyridoxine
Threonine	Magnesium	Riboflavin
Tryptophan	Manganese	Thiamine
Valine	Phosphorus	Vitamin B_{12}
	Potassium	Vitamins A, D, E, and K
	Sodium	
	Zinc	
Probably Essential		
Arginine	Fluorine	Biotin
Histidine	Molybdenum	Pantothenic acid
	Selenium	Polyunsaturated fatty acids

*From White, A., Handler, P., and Smith, E., PRINCIPLES OF BIO-
CHEMISTRY, 1973. Courtesy of McGraw-Hill Book Company, New York.

are probably essential to man.

Linoleic acid, a fatty acid, has been deemed an essential nutrient by Krause and Hunscher (1972). Based primarily upon

epidemiological data, a decrease in dietary fiber has been associated with a broad spectrum of diseases involving the gastrointestinal tract and some metabolic disorders. The physiological mechanisms remain to be identified, and at the present time no drastic change in the fiber content of the diet is advocated (National Dairy Council, 1975). However, for those who eat predominately refined and prepared foods, some effort might be made to increase the dietary fiber content.

The amounts of certain nutrients that man needs have been established by the Committee on Dietary Allowances of the National Research Council (National Research Council, 1974). These amounts have been established for protein and calories as well as sixteen different vitamins and minerals. The Recommended Dietary Allowances (RDA) are the levels of intake of essential nutrients considered, in the judgment of the Food and Nutrition Board on the basis of available scientific knowledge, to be adequate to meet the known nutritional needs of practically all healthy persons. The current RDA are found in Appendix B, the eighth revision since they were initiated in 1943.

Many individuals believe that the RDA is a recommendation for an ideal diet, and that the requirements must be ingested daily. Harper (1974) indicated that this is not so, that the RDA should be used as a tool for the assessment of the nutritional adequacy of the diet, and the daily RDA should average over a five to eight day period. Since the requirements of man for many nutrients have not been totally established, it is important that the individual select as wide a variety of food as possible in order to insure that the diet is adequate. The RDA exceeds the requirements of most members of the population, and yet the low energy expenditure of the people in the United States, together with a trend towards consumption of relatively large amounts of fats, sugars and alcohol in forms that provide only small amounts of many essential ingredients, is becoming a matter of concern to the Food and Nutrition Board (Harper, 1974). Thus, as indicated in previous chapters, certain nutritional deficiencies may exist in the United States, even among athletes on high caloric intakes. Of particular concern should be the dietary selection of wrestlers, who may be on extremely low calorie diets. The food should be carefully selected in order to provide the necessary nutrients.

Relative to the previous discussions of vitamins and minerals, the National Research Council (1974) noted that for the normal

Four Basic Food Groups

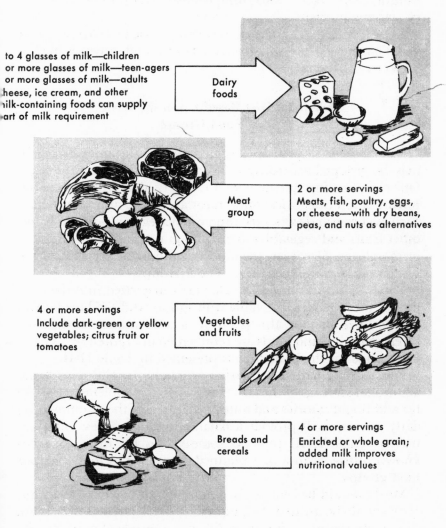

to 4 glasses of milk—children
or more glasses of milk—teen-agers
or more glasses of milk—adults
heese, ice cream, and other
ilk-containing foods can supply
art of milk requirement

Dairy foods

Meat group

2 or more servings
Meats, fish, poultry, eggs,
or cheese—with dry beans,
peas, and nuts as alternatives

4 or more servings
Include dark-green or yellow
vegetables; citrus fruit or
tomatoes

Vegetables and fruits

Breads and cereals

4 or more servings
Enriched or whole grain;
added milk improves
nutritional values

Figure 11-2   The four basic food groups. Courtesy of the National Dairy Council.

individual, it cannot be emphasized too strongly that although there are strong proponents of ingesting excessive amounts of certain individual nutrients, the Committee on Dietary Allowances is unaware of any convincing evidence regarding unique health benefits accruing from consumption of an excess of any one nutrient.

RDA for protein and calories were discussed in Chapters Five and Ten respectively, and for the vitamins and minerals in their respective chapters.

Adequate Diet Based Upon the Basic Four Food Groups

One of the basic principles of nutrition education is that foods may be grouped according to nutrients in which they are rich. One classification system, which is still used, consists of the following seven categories: milk; meat and other animal products such as cheese and eggs; green and yellow vegetables; citrus fruits; other fruits and vegetables; bread and grain products; and butter or margarine. However, the most commonly used classification system today is the Basic Four Food Groups.

Foods of similar nutrient value are categorized into the milk group, meat group, vegetable-fruit group, and the bread-cereal group. As is obvious, this is simply a condensation of the basic seven grouping and foods are represented in Figure 11-2. A daily food guide for the basic four is presented in Table 11-II.

Fats such as butter, margarine or salad oils, plus dessert and additional servings of the basic foods help to supplement the diet for additional calories and nutrients. Intake of the recommended daily servings will provide a balanced diet of the essential nutrients. Table 11-III presents some values for the most well-known nutrients in a diet planned according to the basic four food groups.

Meals should be centered around the four basic food groups. Milk should be utilized daily especially by children. It is the main source of calcium in foods, and is also a source of good quality protein, vitamin A and riboflavin. Skim milk is simply whole milk minus the fat and the fat soluble vitamin A, unless the skim

TABLE 11-11

DAILY FOOD GUIDE FOR THE BASIC FOUR FOOD GROUPS

FOOD GROUP	DAILY AMOUNTS	MAIN CONTRIBUTION
I. Milk and cheese or equivalents*	Children under 9: 2 to 3 cups Children 9 to 12: 3 or more cups Teenagers: 4 or more cups Adults: 2 or more cups	Calcium Protein Riboflavin
II. Meat: Beef, veal, pork, lamb, poultry, fish, eggs	2 or more servings Serving size: 2-3 ounces lean, boneless cooked meat, poultry, fish 2 eggs	Protein Thiamin Iron
Alternates: Dry beans, dry peas, lentils, nuts, peanut butter	1 cup cooked dry beans, dry peas or lentils 4 tablespoons peanut butter	Niacin Riboflavin
I. Breads and cereals (whole-grain or enriched)	4 or more servings Serving size: 1 slice bread 1/2 to 3/4 cup cooked cereal, macaroni, spaghetti, hominy grits, rice, noodles, 1 ounce (1 cup) ready-to-eat cereal 5 saltines or 2 Graham crackers	Thiamin Riboflavin Niacin Iron Protein
IV. Vegetables and fruits	4 or more servings Serving size: 1/2 cup dark green or deep yellow every other day 1/2 cup or 1 medium citrus fruit (or any raw fruit or vegetable rich in ascorbic acid) Other vegetables and fruit including potato (1 medium)	Vitamin A Ascorbic Acid Other vitamins and minerals
Water	6 or 8 glasses	

ilk equivalents: 1 cup whole or skimmed milk, 1 cup buttermilk, 1/2 cup evaporated
lk, 1/4 cup non-fat milk powder, 1 ounce cheddar cheese, 2 cups ice cream, 1-1/2
ps cottage cheese. (The amount given is figured on the basis of calcium content.)

rom Krause, M., and Hunscher, M., FOOD, NUTRITION AND DIET THERAPY, 1972. Courtesy
W.B. Saunders Company, Philadelphia.

	Grams	Approximate Measure	Energy (kcal)	Protein (gm)
Milk Group				
Milk or equivalent	488	16 oz or two 8 oz glasses (1 pint)	330	17
Meat Group*				
Meat, fish, or poultry	100	1 avg. serving, cooked, lean only	295	24
Egg	50	1 medium	80	6.5
Vegetable and Fruit Group				
Vegetables:				
Deep green or yellow†	100	1/2 cup, cooked	29	2.0
Potato	100	1 medium, baked	93	2.6
Other ‡	100	1/2 cup, cooked	42	2.1
Fruits:				
Citrus or tomato§	185	6 oz juice	55	1.1
Other‖	100	1 avg. serving	75	0.7
Cereal Group				
Bread, white, enriched	70	3 slices	180	6.0
Cereal, whole-grain or enriched	30 dry wt.	2/3 cup flakes	70	1.8
Total nutrients in foundation diet			1250	64
Recommended allowances:				
Man, 70 kg, mod. active, 22-25 yrs.			2800	65
Woman, 58 kg, mod. active 22-25 yrs.			2000	55

*Average of ten 100 gm servings of lean, edible portions of meats, in-
†Average of ten 100 gm servings, one each of asparagus, broccoli, spinach, yellow (winter) squash, and sweet potato.
‡Other vegetables: average of ten 100 gm servings of beets, cauli- turnip, and zucchini.
§Daily average based on three servings of orange juice, two servings of fresh raw tomatoes.
‖Other fruits: daily average based on one average serving each of sauce, apricots, peaches, and pineapple, plus one serving of dried
ʹIncludes niacin as such and from tryptophan conversion.

*From Bogart, L. J., Briggs, G. M., and Calloway, D. H., NUTRITION delphia.

DIET PLANNED ACCORDING TO

FOOD GROUPS

Calcium (mg)	Iron (mg)	Vitamin A (11')	Thiamin (mg)	Riboflavin (mg)	Niacin (mg)	Vitamin C (mg)
570	0.4	740	0.14	0.82	0.4	4
11	2.2	178	0.16	0.21	6.0	2
27	1.2	590	0.06	0.15	0.1	0
5	1.1	3900	0.07	0.11	0.6	29
9	0.7	Trace	0.10	0.04	1.7	20
22	0.8	220	0.07	0.06	0.7	13
20	0.7	519	0.09	0.04	0.7	50
13	0.7	550	0.04	0.05	0.5	11
57	1.8	Trace	0.18	0.15	1.8	Trace
5	0.6	Trace	0.09	0.03	0.6	0
740	10.2	6700	1.00	1.66	13.1	130
					Niacin Equiva-lents' mg	
800	10	5000	1.4	1.7	18	60
800	18	5000	1.0	1.5	13	55

cluding beef, lamb, pork, poultry, and fish.
brussel sprouts, carrots, green snap beans, green lettuce and romaine,

flower, celery, corn, green peas, lima beans, onions, summer squash,

of grapefruit juice, three servings of tomato juice, and two servings

fresh apple, banana, peach, pear: one serving each of canned apple-
or stewed prunes.

AND PHYSICAL FITNESS, 1973. Courtesy of W.B. Saunders Company, Phila-

milk is fortified. Milk may be consumed in several forms, including soups, puddings, custards and combined with other foods such as cereal. Foods in the meat group supply about 50 percent of the daily protein requirement. Animal products such as meat, fish, poultry, cheese, and eggs are excellent sources of the essential amino acids, but dried beans or peas, and peanut butter are also good sources of high quality protein. Eggs and meat are also good sources of iron and the B vitamins. For the vegetable-fruit group, a dark green leafy or deep yellow vegetable should be used four to five times per week for vitamin A. Citrus fruits or tomatoes, which are good sources of vitamin C, should be used every day. Other fruits and vegetables including potatoes, whether fresh, frozen or canned, should be included in the diet for variety as well as good sources of vitamins, minerals, and roughage. In the bread and cereal group, choices may be made from breads, ready-to-eat and cooked cereals, crackers, pasta products such as spaghetti and macaroni, and other baked goods made with whole grain or enriched flour. The bread and cereal groups are good sources of carbohydrate energy as well as B vitamins and some protein. The recommended number of servings and serving size for each of the four groups is contained in Table 11-II. Examples of the particular types of foods found in each group, plus substitute foods, are found in Appendix C.

Table 11-II provides some guidelines for the basic four food requirements of adults; in general, smaller servings should be utilized for smaller children, while larger servings may be used with teenagers. A more detailed allowance chart for the various components of the basic four is presented for different ages of children in Table 11-IV.

Daily Food Intake

Once you have determined from Table 10-I how many calories you need per day in order to sustain your optimal weight, the foods may be selected from the basic groups in order to meet the caloric need and yet provide a balanced supply of nutrients. The caloric value of various foodstuffs may be determined from the table on Nutritive Value of Foods found in Appendix A, or from

TABLE

FOODS INCLUDED IN A GOOD

FOOD	PRE-SCHOOL 3-5 YEARS OLD	EARLY ELEMENTARY 6-9 YEARS OLD
Milk	2 cups	2-3 cups
Eggs	1 whole egg	1 whole egg
Meat, poultry, fish	2 ounces (1/4 cup) (1 small serving)	2-3 ounces (1 small serving)
Dried beans, peas (Also an occasional replacement for meat, poultry or fish)	3-4 tablespoons	4-5 tablespoons
Potatoes (May occasionally be replaced by equal amount enriched macaroni, spaghetti or rice	3-4 tablespoons	4-5 tablespoons
Other cooked vegetables (Often a green leafy or deep yellow vegetable)	3-4 tablespoons at one or more meals	4-5 tablespoons at one or more meals
Raw vegetables (Lettuce, carrots, celery, etc.)	2 or more small pieces	1/4 cup
Vitamin C food (Citrus fruits, tomatoes, etc.)	1 medium-size orange or equivalent	1 medium-size orange or equivalent
Other fruits	1/3 cup at one or more meals	1/2 cup or more at one or more meals
Cereal, whole grain restored or enriched	1/2 cup or more	3/4 cup or more
Bread, whole grain or enriched	2 or more slices	2 or more slices
Butter or fortified margarine	1 tablespoon	1 tablespoon
Sweets	1/3 cup simple dessert at 1 or 2 meals	1/2 cup simple dessert at 1 or 2 meals
Vitamin D source		Enough to provide 400
Recommended allowances	1600 kcal. 40 grams protein	2100 kcal. 52 grams protein

*From Krause, M., and Hunscher, M., FOOD, NUTRITION AND DIET THERAPY, 1972.

11-IV

DAILY DIET FOR CHILDREN

LATER ELEMENTARY 10-12 YEARS OLD	EARLY TEENS 13-15 YEARS OLD
3 cups or more	3-4 cups or more
1 whole egg	1 or more whole eggs
3-4 ounces (1 serving)	4 ounces or more (1 serving)
5-6 tablespoons	1/2 cup or more
1/3 cup or more	3/4 cup or more
1/3 cup or more at one or more meals	1/2 cup or more at one or more meals
1/3 cup	1/2 cup or more
1 medium-size orange or equivalent	1 large orange or equivalent
1/2 cup or more at one or more meals	2 servings
1 cup or more	1 cup or more
2 or more slices	2 or more slices
1 tablespoon or more	1 tablespoon or more
1/3 cup or more simple dessert at 1 or 2 meals	1/2 cup or more at 1 or 2 meals
U.S.P. units of vitamin D daily	
Girls: 2200 kcal. 55 grams protein Boys: 2400 kcal. 60 grams protein	Girls: 2500 kcal. 62 grams protein Boys: 3000 kcal. 75 grams protein

Courtesy of W.B. Saunders Company, Philadelphia.

some of the popular calorie books found in most supermarkets and drug stores.

It may be a good idea for the coach to post a suggested dietary plan on a bulletin board, focusing attention upon the selection of proper foods. The table in Appendix A may be obtained from the Superintendent of Documents rather inexpensively, and may be a valuable tool in the training room. Menu plans may also be duplicated and distributed to the athletes for home use. The American Alliance for Health Physical Education and Recreation has developed a food scoreboard, which may be used to evaluate the distribution of foods within the daily intake. A one-day meal record should be accurately maintained, recording the amount and type of food ingested for breakfast, midmorning snack, lunch, afternoon snack, dinner, evening snack and munching during the day. From the total record, the data may be transferred to a score card individually designed dependent upon the recommended caloric intake. An example scoreboard for fourteen to eighteen-year-old boys is presented in Table 11-V.

By using this scoreboard, and knowing the approximate caloric value of the various foods within the groups, the individual may increase or decrease the caloric content primarily by altering the intake in the meat, bread and fat groups. When increasing the total daily caloric content, as many athletes in training must do in order to sustain body weight, the increased allotments should be distributed across all classes of foods in order to meet increased demand for the various nutrients. Empty calories, such as candy and carbonated beverages should be limited in the diet.

Low Calorie Diets

For the individual who desires to lose weight, total calories should be decreased without sacrificing the needed nutrients. In sports such as wrestling and boxing, where the athlete may lose a substantial amount of body weight in order to compete, it is imperative that he sustain necessary nutrient intake because he is still engaged in high levels of energy expenditure. The recommended weight reduction plan for wrestlers involves a gradual loss over the duration of precompetitive season training. This

TABLE 11-V

FOOD SCOREBOARD FOR BOYS, AGES 14-18

(APPROXIMATELY 3000 CALORIES)

To Score: *Use the totals on your one-day meal record*

Recommended Foods	Minimum Goal*	My Score
Milk (2% fat content)	4 cups	_____
Meat (fish, poultry, cheese or eggs)	7 ounces	_____
Dark green or deep yellow vegetables	1 serving (½ cup)	_____
Citrus fruit	1 serving (½ cup)	_____
Other fruits and vegetables	3 servings (1½ cup)	_____
Bread (enriched or whole grain bread, cereal, or potatoes)	18 servings	_____
Fats (butter, margarine, or other fat spreads)	10 teaspoons	_____
Plain dessert, sugar, or jelly, snacks, carbonated beverages, ades, etc.	2 small servings	_____

Take a look at your score. You may find that you have been leaving out important foods, and if so, you need to start including them. Or you may find that you have been taking too many "empty" calories such as carbonated beverages and candy.

Foods to Add   Foods to Cut Down On

_____   _____

_____   _____

_____   _____

_____   _____

*The amounts of each food, except milk, dark green or deep yellow vegetables, are guidelines. A person knowledgeable in nutrition and in food content can adapt these servings of food so as to obtain the same approximate calories and nutritive value.

may be accomplished by high levels of energy expenditure through exercise, and a well-balanced low calorie diet. The following may serve as a general daily guideline diet, totalling about

1200 to 1400 calories and yet meeting the nutrient needs as related to protein, vitamins and minerals. However, a vitamin-mineral supplement may be recommended to insure adequate intakes of those nutrients.

Skim Milk — 4 cups
Lean meat, fish, poultry, cheese or eggs — 6 ounces
Vegetables — 3 servings
Fruit — 1 serving
Bread or other grain products — 5 servings
Low calorie margarine — 2 servings

Most low calorie diets are designed to be used under the guidance of a physician. As Mayer (1968) has noted, if the individual plans to lose more than 2 pounds/week, he should consult a physician. Utilization of the above general diet plan, in conjunction with an exercise training program such as wrestling, might create a daily negative caloric balance of 2000 to 2500 calories, which could elicit a 4 to 5 pound weight loss in body tissue per week. Therefore, the team physician and family physician should be aware of the magnitude of weight reduction contemplated by these athletes.

Daily meal patterns for 1000-, 1200-, 1400- and 1800-calorie menus are presented in Appendix D, with some additional advice relative to increasing the variety and taste of the meals.

SPECIAL CONSIDERATIONS FOR THE ATHLETE

A number of suggestions relative to the feeding of athletes have been made throughout this text, dealing with such topics as salt and water replacement, protein supplementation for weight gaining programs, and glycogen storage for endurance athletes. No detailed review of that material is to be presented in this section, but other concerns of the athlete's general diet regimen will be covered.

Energy Requirement

A respected textbook in exercise physiology recently recommended that an athlete's daily diet should be comprised of some 180 g protein, 135 g fat and 730 g carbohydrate, with an approximate total caloric intake of 5000 cal/day. This is, of course, an oversimplification of the energy needs of an athlete, for there are different energy requirements for the diverse types of athletic activities. A baseball player and a distance runner in training should require different amounts of calories in their daily intake. Buskirk (1971) classified athletic activities by type of effort and the approximate daily caloric demands of that activity, along with the general percentual increase in the caloric requirement during training. His schema is presented in Table 11-VI.

Buskirk did note, however, that the table is an oversimplification since it was assumed that the body size and weight were

TABLE

CLASSIFICATION OF ACTIVITIES

DAILY CALORIC DEMANDS OF

LENGTH OF PRACTICE ON THE

Duration of activity Intensity of activity	Short Burst Maximum effort	Less than 1 Minute Strenuous effort	Sustained Low Intensity
Event:	Shot-put Javelin High jump Diving Ski jumping	Dashes including 440 yd Hurdles Long jump Hop, step, jump Pole vault Long horse vault 50 and 100 yd swimming events	Baseball Golf
Kcal/day:	3,000 to 4,000	3,000 to 4,000	3,000 to 4,000

Training Percent Increase in Daily Caloric Requirement over that Required			
<1 hr:	5	5	8
1-2 hrs:	10	10	17
>2 hrs:	15	15	25

Remarks: It is assumed that body weight and size were approximately equal gories. Such an assumption is an oversimplification, e.g., shot-putters are Note that an athlete in training requires at least 3,000 kcal/day, and that ment.
< denotes "less than or equal to."
> denotes "equal to or more than."

*Reprinted from *Administration of Athletics in Colleges and Universities* Education, 1201 Sixteenth Street, N.W., Washington, D.C. 20036.

approximately equal for the participants in the different categories. For example, he noted that shot putters are usually large while divers are smaller in stature and weight. The table may be useful as a general guideline, as the athletes are grouped in categories of increasing levels of energy expenditure. As noted, the percentage increase in their caloric intake is designed to accommodate increased amounts of time spent in training.

Since body size is an important determining factor in the caloric requirement of the athlete, it may be important to utilize the values presented in Table 10-I and increase them a certain percentage dependent upon the type of activity. For example, relative to their body weight, cross-country runners consume significantly more calories per day than do football players. Pargman (1971)

11-VI

BY TYPE OF EFFORT AND THE

THE ACTIVITY AND EFFECT OF

DAILY CALORIC REQUIREMENT

1 to 10 Minutes Sustained Effort	10 minutes or More Intense Repeated Effort	Endurance High Intensity
880 yd run	Football	Cross country running
1 & 2 mile runs	Basketball	6 mile run
Swimming events	Ice hockey	Soccer
over 100 yd	Lacrosse	Cross country skiing
Wrestling	Tennis	
Most gymnastic	Gymnastic all-round	
events	Fencing	
Downhill, slalom	3 mile run	
skiing		
3,000 to 5,000	3,000 to 6,000	4,000 to 5,000

during Day of Competition		
10	10	13
20	20	25
30	30	38

for the participants in the events referred to in the above cate-
usually very large men and divers are usually small men.
additional training can markedly increase his daily caloric require-

with the permission of the American Alliance for Health, Physical

utilized experienced nutritionists to tabulate the caloric intake of certain athletes. He noted that the distance runners consumed approximately 35 cal/pound/day, for an average total mean value of 5035 calories. Football players consumed 4334 calories per day, but the average was only 20 cal/pound. From Table 10-I, a sixteen-year-old boy would need 23 cal/pound/day. If he weighed about 150 pounds, his recommended total caloric allowance would be 3450 cal/day. Training one to two hours/day would increase this value by 25 percent, for a total recommendation of about 4310 calories. Similar computations may be made for the other activity categories. A good check on caloric sufficiency would be the maintenance of accurate daily records of body weight. Trends may be easily discerned from these recordings.

Endurance Athletes

Due to the nature of their event, cross country runners, most soccer players, and other endurance athletes are engaged in high levels of energy expenditure over prolonged periods of time, and therefore may need special dietary attention. The two main considerations include glycogen storage, and fluid and electrolyte replacement. The vastly increased caloric demands of the endurance athlete should be accommodated by a balanced increase in the foods in the basic four groups. However, in order to facilitate replenishment of glycogen stores, large quantities of high quality carbohydrates should be included in the diet. Enriched breads and other grain products will not only supply the necessary caloric intake, but also provide the concomitant necessary minerals, vitamins and substrate for glycogen storage. More detailed coverage of glycogen enhancement techniques and benefits is presented in Chapter Three. Fluid and electrolyte replacement should follow the principles set forth in Chapter Eight. These principles are especially pertinent to any athlete who does prolonged exercise in the heat.

The Female Athlete

Buskirk and Haymes (1972) have indicated that nutrition for female athletes differs little from that of male athletes, with the possible exception of small differences in the areas of caloric, B_6

and iron allowances. The total caloric requirements of boys and girls varies little up until puberty, because the body weights and structure are fairly similar. However, the difference in calories/pound body weight is not strikingly different, and actually becomes identical in early adulthood. Consult Table 10-I.

Buskirk and Haymes (1972) reported that little evidence is available to support the contention that the processes of energy turnover are qualitatively different for women as contrasted to men. Thus, the needs for thiamine, riboflavin, niacin and most other vitamins and minerals are not greatly different for the sexes. On the other hand, there may be some possible benefit from vitamin B_6 or iron supplementation. The female has lower hemoglobin levels than the male. Vitamin B_6, which is important in the formation of hemoglobin, myoglobin and the cytochromes and thus plays a role in the oxygen transportation schema in the body, may need to be increased in the diet during periods of increased protein intake, especially during the early periods of training. This may be related to the development of so-called "sports anemia" discussed in Chapter Five.

Although Haymes (1975) reported that the female athlete does not need more iron than the average American woman, there have been a number of reports that average American women may be iron-deficient. Thus, White (1974) contends that education programs are needed to encourage women to eat a greater variety of foods rich in iron. Meat, eggs, green vegetables, beans, nuts and whole-grain and enriched cereals are the best sources of iron. An iron supplement tablet may be recommended. A discussion of the role of iron in the diet of athletes was presented in Chapter Seven.

Since the nutritional requirements of the normal female are little different from that of the male, most of the recommendations for the athletes in this text would pertain to both sexes. Although not covered, it should be noted that the nutritional requirements of the pregnant or lactating woman are different from those of other women.

Vegetarian Athletes

Throughout history, many groups of people have subsisted primarily on vegetarian diets, either out of necessity or the belief that animal products were not beneficial to mind and body. McCollum (1957) reported that before the Christian Era, certain sects of pure minded and pious people, especially the Jewish sect known as Essenes, practiced vegetarianism. Ascetics in India and China also consumed diets with no meat. As indicated in Chapter One, diets of the early Greek athletes consisted primarily of fruits, vegetables and grain products, with very little meat; but, during the later era of Greek athletics, the meat diet was introduced as a distinct opposite to the prevailing diet. Since that time, there have been advocates of both types of diets for the athlete in training, one consisting primarily of high protein meat products, and the other being either a strict vegetarian or limited vegetarian diet.

There have been some very successful vegetarian athletes, Pavlo Nurmi, Finland's premier Olympic champion distance runner, being one of the most famous. Most recently, Bill Walton of the National Basketball Association (NBA) has been subsisting on a vegetarian diet, although Walt Frazier, another star of the NBA, questions the advisability of being a vegetarian and playing the rugged schedule of the professional basketball player. He noted that all the vegetarians he saw looked weak, and stated that you have to eat animal protein and animal fat (Unsigned, 1975b). The latter part of this statement is erroneous, for man can subsist without animal meats.

The term *vegetarian* has several meanings. A strict vegetarian, known also as a *vegan*, uses only plant sources for his food; he eats no animal products. The vegan may get all the nutrients he needs, except vitamin B_{12}, from plant sources. He will need a supplemental source of this vitamin or he may suffer from pernicious anemia. Another class of vegetarians are known as lactoovovegetarians, adding milk, dairy products and eggs to their plant sources. Other vegetarians may eat fish and other sea products.

The major problem with the vegetarian diet is the inclusion of the essential amino acids necessary for optimal protein metabolism in the body. Protein quality is dependent upon the amount and availability of the 10 essential amino acids, which are contained in protein foods of animal origin. The vegetarian must take special care to include a variety of whole grain cereals, dried peas and beans, nuts, and a variety of fruits and vegetables. He may get all the essential amino acids, but grain products are low in lysine and dried peas and beans are low in methionine; therefore, they are considered to be low quality proteins. However, when grain products and peas and beans are eaten together, an adequate balance is provided. Other nutrients such as calcium, iron and riboflavin may also be in short supply in a strict vegetarian diet. The addition of milk, dairy products and eggs to the diet greatly reduces the possibility of nutritional inadequacies.

There has been very little experimental research to support or negate the value of a vegetarian diet as a means of increasing physical performance capacity. Most of the reports are very dated, and would have no creditability today. McCollum (1957) reported a study in 1904, when twenty-five Belgian students were tested upon an ergograph. The students were divided into vegetarians and meat eaters, and the results indicated the vegetarians could produce more work on the ergograph. Caspari (1905) noted the most probable cause for the lack of endurance in meat eaters was due to toxic substances absorbed from the colon. However, he did note that vegetarians possessed a zeal not shown in meat eaters, and hence psychological factors may be a prevailing factor in the increased performance of the vegetarians. Fischer (1907) also noted that vegetarians had greater endurance, in a test with the arm held horizontally, than flesh eaters. He suggested that it may be due to the greater willpower of the vegetarians. Wishart (1934) studied a vegetarian long-distance bicyclist under several different dietary conditions, mainly varying the amount of protein in the diet. The protein, eggs, was of animal origin. Although the data may not be generalized due to the nature of the experiment, he concluded that in hard muscular exercise, the best performance is obtained on a high calorie diet rich in protein derived from animals.

The available evidence does not support either a beneficial or detrimental effect of a vegetarian diet upon physical performance capacity. Although an individual could get the required protein allotment through strict vegetable sources, animal products such as milk, cheese and eggs are good sources of high quality protein. Aside from the possible limitation of saturated fat intake, there appears to be no health benefit in completely removing meat from the diet. Moreover, poultry and fish may provide high quality protein with lower levels of saturated fats. For the developing athlete, increased levels of high quality protein have been recommended, and animal products are excellent sources of that protein. The choice of a vegetarian diet is the athlete's decision, but he should be knowledgable in nutritional principles before implementing such a dietary regimen.

Pregame Meals

Probably one of the most over-rated aspects of nutrition for athletic performance is the pregame meal. It is a well-known fact that the ingestion of food is not followed by an increase in physical efficiency, and yet a number of special meals have been utilized throughout the years because of their alleged benefits upon physical performance. Hirata (1973) has criticized the traditional pregame meal, which many times is mammalian meat, and indicated that American athletes have been exposed to unsound nutritional concepts relative to the pregame meal since their first competition in grade school. Many coaches and trainers do have idiosyncrasies about food, especially pregame meals, which are not in accord with current scientific information, and although the choice of a particular pregame meal is not likely to influence performance, there are certain principles to keep in mind when feeding the athlete prior to competition.

Pre-event nutrition should not be construed to mean the meal immediately before the game. Dietary advice should be given to the athlete the entire season in order to provide optimal nutritional health for his particular sport. In this light, sound advice relative to the composition of the pregame meal may be incorporated into the total nutritional education of the athlete. The wise coach should recognize individual preferences in diet, allowing the athlete to select pregame foods based upon his likes or dislikes and yet within the confines of sound scientific principles and empirical knowledge.

Two of the major points are the timing and size of the pregame meal. Hutchinson (1952) has indicated that long periods between meals may give rise to hunger, which is ofttimes associated with feelings of nervousness and weakness. On the other hand, pre-event emotional tension or anxiety may contribute to possible indigestion and a sensation of nausea, and may be very uncomfortable if the pregame meal is too close to competition time.

Rose and Fuenning (1960) studied gastrointestinal motility in four football players before a game. They were fed a heavy meal, and then consumed some barium sulfate in order that digestive processes could be studied. The meal was eaten about five hours prior to the game. In general, the athletes were two to three hours behind the normal digestive schedule, the reduced gastrointestinal motility being attributed to pregame emotional tension. Consequently, the food from this large meal was still undergoing digestion in the small intestine at game time. Some 25 to 50 percent of the food was still in the stomach 2.5 to 3 hours after eating. Thus, most authorities recommended against a large meal, and favor a rather small, easily digestible meal three to four hours prior to competition. A liquid supplemental meal about one to two hours prior to competition has also been recommended. A later section in this chapter includes some pertinent research relative to timing of the pregame meal.

Regarding the composition of pregame meals, a number of different foods have been criticized over the years. The athlete has been advised to restrict or eliminate intake of gas-producing foods, spicy ingredients, seedy vegetables, cellulose, roughage, proteins, tea or coffee, fats, milk and alcohol. On the other hand, others have recommended some of these substances, including tea and protein, as well as numerous other foods such as bread, potatoes, honey, raw meat, sugar, etc. Although no one food may be justifiably banned for every athlete, since there are many diverse individual preferences and many diverse types of athletic demands, there may be some rationale for selecting or restricting certain types of foods prior to athletic competition. Nevertheless, one will still probably read reports of the world class swimmer who consumed a lunch of two hamburgers, french fries, a root beer float, three brownies and a candy bar two hours prior to setting a new world's record in the 200-meter butterfly.

For a solid, instead of liquid, pregame meal, carbohydrate content should be stressed, while fat and protein intake should be restricted. Especially for endurance athletes, training should taper down a day or two prior to competition, and carbohydrate intake should be increased. This will help insure muscle glycogen storage, the principles underlying this advantage being discussed in Chapter Three. In essence, muscle glycogen is the preferred energy source at sustained high levels of energy expenditure. A high carbohydrate pregame meal is also recommended, as it is easily digested and readily absorbed. On the other hand, large quantities of concentrated sugars, in the form of honey, glucose, dextrose or sucrose, should not be consumed immediately prior to an event. Mayer (1972b) has noted that these forms of sugar may draw fluid into the gastrointestinal tract and may contribute to dehydration, while AAHPER (1971) noted that they may cause the body to rebel, creating cramps and nausea. A simple pregame carbohydrate meal, with about 500 to 1000 calories and a small amount of protein could consist of skim milk, a toasted sandwich, honey, cookies and a banana. A number of carbohydrate substitutes could be made. Although Horstman (1972) has indicated that a high carbohydrate meal results in a rapid rise of blood glucose, it is followed by a decline to below-normal level, probably due to a hypersecretion of insulin which clears the blood. However, if the liver glycogen supply is adequate, the secretion of epinephrine prior to competition should restore the blood glucose level to normal by its effect on glycogenolysis in the liver.

Fat content of the pregame meal should be restricted due to its slowing effect upon gastric emptying time and slow absorption time.

High protein content of pregame meals have been criticized on two points. First, they may increase the amount of fixed acid in the body and hence restrict performance, and secondly, they may add to the metabolic load. According to White (1974) foods may be classified as either neutral, acid forming or alkali forming, a property dependent upon the minerals in the food. For example, most fruits and vegetables include minerals such as sodium, potassium and calcium, which are alkali-forming, whereas meats and eggs with sulfur and phosphorus are acid-forming. Thus, a pregame meal high in protein may produce acid residues and contribute to acidosis. If this acidity adds to the metabolic acidity of exercise, it may theoretically compromise physiological capacity, as acidosis has been implicated as a possible cause in the etiology of fatigue. Horstman (1972) has indicated that the metabolism of protein to carbohydrate is an energy-consuming process, and thus might be detrimental to performance where most energy should go towards muscular activity. Simonsen (1951) also reported that high protein meals taken several hours prior to work may add substantially to the metabolic load, and also indicated that protein is not essential to work performance.

In essence, it is the responsibility of the coach and trainer to have knowledge relative to the adverse effects of certain foods in the pregame meal, and to educate athletes to sound nutritional principles so that wise food selections may be made.

The Liquid Pregame Meal

Although Hirata (1973) indicated that each individual athletic program must develop its own pregame meal pattern, he recommended that the liquid meal is the only ultimate answer to pregame feeding, an objective which all in athletic medicine should strive to attain. There may be inherent values to using a liquid pregame meal, for it may be economical, well-balanced in nutrient value and easily digested and assimilated. Several athletic team physicians have used liquid meals successfully, noting that they may be useful in preventing the adverse effects of pregame tension. Rose (1961) reported that the use of Sustagen did not differ from a conventional solid meal relative to subsequent hunger, diarrhea, vomiting or weight changes in athletes prior to a major football game. Rose recommended the liquid pregame meal because it did not have to be converted to a liquid state, it left the stomach almost immediately, and there would therefore be no competition, between the stomach and muscles, for the blood supply. Cooper (1962), although not conducting a controlled study, reported that a similar liquid meal, Nutrament, could be used effectively to control nausea in football players.

Aside from their possible value as a pregame meal, liquid meals may also be valuable supplements to the athlete who has problems maintaining body weight. Depending upon the brand selected, they may be good sources of extra calories and protein.

Macaraeg (1974a) reported the following composition for two popular brands: Sustagen contains 390 cal, with 66.5 g carbohydrate, 23.5 g protein and 3.5 g fat; Nutrament contains 375 cal, 50.3 g carbohydrate, 23.5 g protein and 8.9 g fat.

Some have contended that pregame liquid meals may provide an ergogenic effect. In a pamphlet relative to the composition of precompetition meals, the Carnation Milk company cited research relative to performance in a 100-yard free style swim, noting that athletes swam faster after eating Carnation Instant Breakfast or a placebo rather than no meal at all. Even more significant, the athletes swam faster after drinking the Carnation product than when the placebo was taken. Several other research reports were included in the pamphlet, implying that varsity runners performed better in the mile following consumption of Carnation Instant Breakfast as a pregame meal, supposedly due to some physiological and psychological energy edge. The report concluded that the carbohydrate content of the meal is almost immediately available for energy that could give the edge needed in competition at a given moment (Carnation Company, no date). As a criticism of this report, it may be sufficient to note that although the mean times for the 100-yard swim and mile run were slightly faster for the liquid meal condition, there was very little difference between them and no statistical analysis of the data was presented. Nonetheless, Macaraeg (1974a), in a paper presented to the Scientific Congress of the Twentieth Olympic Games in Munich, noted that liquid meals may be useful as a dietary supplement for added strength and stamina. However, he did not present any substantial data to support this contention.

There are several research reports available relative to the role of liquid meals as ergogenic aids. White (1968) studied the effect of Carnation Instant Breakfast and whole milk upon performance in a mile run. The liquid meal was comprised of 34 g carbohydrate, 17.5 g protein and 9.4 g fat. With the exception of the liquid meal, food intake was prohibited about four hours prior to the run. Ten male college track men each ran the mile forty times, ten times each under three experimental conditions and a control trial. The three experimental conditions consisted of intake of the liquid meal either thirty minutes, one hour, or two hours prior to the run. No meal was ingested in the control trial. The mean times for the mile run for each time period and the control were, respectively, 5:07.6, 5:05.1, 5:05.8, and 5:07.7.

The data from this study by White is strikingly similar to that contained in the pamphlet distributed by the Carnation Company. The pamphlet indicated that the consumption of the Instant Breakfast had a beneficial effect upon performance in the one-mile run, and the mean times given in the report would support this contention. However, White analyzed the data by analysis of variance techniques and found no significant differences between the experimental and control conditions. Thus, when proper statistical techniques were utilized, the liquid meal was found not to improve running time in the mile run as compared to no supplement at all.

Ryder (1971) also investigated the effect of a liquid meal, Nutrament, on performance times in the mile run of twelve varsity college distance runners. Each subject ran the mile twice under three conditions: Nutrament, a liquid placebo, and no supplementation. No significant differences were noted between the times. Wooding (1968) also found no significant effect of Nutrament upon the physiological performance of highly trained wrestlers. The liquid food, given at a volume of .24 ounces/pound body weight, had no significant effect upon exercise heart rate, ventilation, oxygen consumption, oxygen pulse or work capacity.

Liquid meals have no value as ergogenic aids; however, they may be useful as a convenient, easily digestible pregame meal or to help maintain weight in players throughout training. They may be purchased in most food stores, or can be prepared more economically at home. For approximately one quart of liquid meal, mix together .5 cup of water, .5 cup of nonfat dry milk, .25 cup of sugar, 3 cups of skim milk and a teaspoon of flavoring, such as cherry, vanilla or chocolate extract.

Research with Solid Pregame Meals

Although liquid meals may be recommended as pre-event food, a number of studies have reported no adverse effects of low calorie meals, primarily solid foods, consumed prior to performance. In an early study, Haldi and Wynn (1946) investigated the effect of four different pre-event meals upon performance in a 100-yard swim. The meals were eaten approximately 2.5 to 3 hours prior to performance, and consisted of either a heavy meal with 1051 cal or a light meal with 551 cal; two other conditions included the light meal plus either 50 or 100 g sugar. There was no difference between the performance times, and the sugar did not affect the performance. Youmans and others (1960) studied the effect of a small meal, consisting of milk, toast and cereal, upon the sprinting performance of runners in a 50- and 100-yard dash. They found that for six different time intervals (thirty, sixty, ninety, 120, 150 and 180 minutes) between eating and running, the consumption of the meal had no beneficial or adverse effects. Ball (1962), using the same time intervals, found no effect upon 100-yard swim time of a similar meal, 472 calories of cereal with skim milk, toast, sugar and butter.

In a series of experiments, Asprey and his associates studied the effect of a small meal upon a variety of performance tasks. The meal was low in calories, approximately 510, and consisted of cereal with whole milk, toast, butter and sugar. In each experiment, the meal was consumed either thirty, sixty or 120 minutes prior to performance. No beneficial or adverse effects of the meal or the time sequences were noted upon performance in the 440- and 880-yard runs (Asprey and others, 1963), the one-mile run (Asprey and others, 1964), the 200- and 400-yard free style swim (Asprey and others, 1965a), and the two-mile run (Asprey and others, 1965b), or the one-mile free style swim (Asprey and others, 1968).

Singer and Neeves (1968) used a similar experimental design with a larger meal, approximately 800 calories, and reported no significant effect upon performance in a 200-yard swim. They did report, however, several cases of nausea when the meal was eaten thirty minutes prior to performance. Although all of these studies demonstrated no adverse effects of the solid meal upon performance time, and in general no subjective effects such as nausea, they were conducted under noncompetitive conditions with apparently no emotional tension. Nevertheless, it would appear that a solid, low calorie, primarily carbohydrate meal could be utilized without any adverse effects one to two hours prior to competition.

Nonrecommended Foods for the Pregame Meal

A number of food products have been proscribed by coaches and trainers for pre-event consumption. Field (1966) undertook an interesting study to evaluate the effect of nonrecommended foods upon physical performance on a test battery consisting of strength, power, reaction time, local muscular endurance and general endurance. A list of nonrecommended foods was selected from training books and manuals. Among the listing were such foods as pork, gravy, pie, french fried potatoes, milk, pickles, mustard, potato chips, chili and coke. After baseline performance was obtained on the criterion tests, an experimental meal containing some of the above ingredients was fed to the subject two hours prior to performance. The author reported no significant difference between the treatments for any performance parameter, and he concluded that there appears to be no valid basis for the avoidance of certain foods before physical exertion. However, it should be noted that the performance tests may have been of such a nature as not to be adversely affected by fatty foods, such as gravy, in the stomach. All tests were rather short in nature, and the general endurance task did not involve maximal work time to exhaustion.

Milk has also been restricted during training and, by some coaches, as a pregame nutrient. Van Huss and others (1962) noted that various reasons have been advanced for this restriction, including the suppositions that milk contributes to the development of cottonmouth, curdles in the stomach, and elicits a lower respiratory quotient during exercise. However, in their study, they found that restriction of milk in the diet of the athlete has no scientific basis, and that milk does not hamper performance capacity. Indeed, they noted that when milk products are eliminated from the diet, nutrients such as calcium and riboflavin might fall below recommended levels. Nelson (1961), after conducting his own research and reviewing the literature, concluded that if an athlete likes milk and wants it in his pregame meal, there is no justifiable reason to eliminate it.

Breakfast and Physical Performance

Although reviewing the literature as it relates primarily to efficiency in industrial work, Haggard and Greenburg (1935) noted that muscular efficiency is lowest before breakfast, and remains low if the subject does not eat breakfast. Early research suggested this effect may be due to hypoglycemia, and consequently breakfast could help restore efficiency due to the readily available carbohydrates. Moreover, several nutritionists (Wilson and others, 1967; Addison and others, 1953) have recommended a breakfast high in protein, for it will be more effective than a breakfast primarily of carbohydrates in maintaining blood glucose levels throughout the morning. The gluconeogenesis from protein serves to provide glucose over a period of time, whereas the rapid increase in blood glucose from a high carbohydrate meal would increase insulin secretion and hence remove glucose from the blood more rapidly. To alleviate some of the midmorning effects of hypoglycemia, some protein may be recommended in the breakfast composition.

The research is limited relative to the effect that breakfast exerts upon physical performance. Karpovich and Sinning (1971) noted, in unpublished data on breakfastless days, that male college students experienced no significant decline in maximal bicycle ergometer endurance. On the other hand, Tuttle and his associates reported adverse effects of omitting breakfast in a series of experiments. In the first report (Tuttle and others, 1949b), they studied four breakfast conditions upon reaction time and maximal bicycle ergometer output for one minute. The conditions involved a heavy breakfast (800 cal), a light breakfast (400 cal), coffee and no breakfast. In general, they concluded that omitting breakfast caused a decrease in maximal work output and a slower reaction time, although individual differences in response to altered breakfast habits were noted. In a subsequent report, Daum and others (1950) compared the effect of four breakfast conditions, i.e. heavy (1000 cal), light (300 cal), a basic breakfast (600 cal), and no breakfast, upon the same criterion measures. They also found that the omission of breakfast resulted in a lower total work output. Similar findings were again reported by Tuttle and his associates (1950) in another report. Using different types of foods to comprise the breakfast, Tuttle and his colleagues (1951) found no significant difference between cereal or bacon and eggs if the caloric content was similar. However, in the same report, they noted that a heavy breakfast could be detrimental to maximal work output. This condition could be analogous to a heavy pregame meal.

In more recent research, Brannon (1971) noted that a 700-calorie breakfast elicited significantly better scores on six of the seven items on the AAHPER Physical Fitness Test when compared to a no breakfast condition. The subjects were fifty junior high school girls, who took the tests under the two conditions, with a two week intertrial period. However, there did not appear to be a counterbalancing design to the experiment, and hence a possible learning factor or other confounding variable may have affected the results.

Sage (1969) grouped thirty-six subjects into three different subgroups, those who ate light breakfasts, and those who habitually ate no breakfast. Using a step test as a criterion measure of endurance performance, each subject then ate either a heavy, light or a liquid breakfast during respective one week periods of time. The heavy breakfast consisted of eggs, bacon or sausage, toast and juice, and averaged about 500 calories. The light breakfast was about 200 calories, containing toast or rolls, coffee and juice. The liquid meal was an instant breakfast in 8 ounces of milk. The data indicated no significant differences between the groups; however, the liquid breakfast elicited a slightly significant increased performance in comparison to the heavy and light breakfasts. There may have been a psychological component operating, since there would be no physiological explanation for the results.

Although individual differences should be taken into account, it would appear worthwhile for an athlete in training to consume a good breakfast, not only as a substantial source of his needed extra calories, but protein as well. It may not be too surprising that some of these earlier studies revealed that omission of breakfast produced a detrimental effect upon performance, since going fifteen to sixteen hours without food could produce hypoglycemic symptoms, especially in subjects who habitually eat breakfast.

Myths, Misconceptions, and Education

As indicated in Chapter One, Durnin (1967) has noted that there is still no sphere of nutrition in which faddism and ignorance are more obvious than in athletics. It is hoped that some of the evidence presented in this text has helped to differentiate fact from fancy. There are some useful applications of dietary principles to athletics and physical performance, and some areas where there may be some beneficial effects, based upon theoretical considerations, that need to be substantiated or discredited through appropriate experimental research. However, the vast majority of claims relative to the ergogenic effect of certain foods are without merit. Protein is not the main energy food, meat does not build strength, honey is not a quick energy food in the sense the term is used, wheat germ oil is not essential to the trained athlete, milk does not cut the wind, there are no special properties of yogurt, blackstrap molasses, sauerkraut juice, gelatin, brewer's yeast, brown rice, or the so-called health foods that will turn a well-conditioned, well-nourished athlete into a champion. The list could go on *ad nauseum.*

The athletic world needs coaches and trainers who are grounded in sound nutritional principles, and will use their knowledge to educate the athlete about nutrition in general and as it applies to their particular athletic event.

BIBLIOGRAPHY

Abrahams, A.: The nutrition of athletes. *Brit J Nutr, 2*:266-69, 1948.

Addison, V., and others: Effect of amount and type of protein in breakfasts on blood sugar levels. *J Am Diet Assoc, 29*:674-77, 1953.

Ahlborg, B.: Human muscle glycogen content and capacity for prolonged exercise after different diets. *Forsvarsmedicin, 3*:85-99, 1967.

Ahlborg, H., and others: Effect of potassium-magnesium-aspartate on the capacity for prolonged exercise in man. *Acta Physiol Scand, 74*:238-45, 1968.

Ahlman, K., and Karvonen, M.: Weight reduction by sweating in wrestlers and its effect on physical fitness. *J Sports Med Phys Fitness, 1*:58-62, 1962.

Albrink, M.: Diet and cardiovascular disease. *J Am Diet Assoc, 46*:26-29, 1965.

Alcohol metabolism during rest and exercise. *Nutr Rev, 24*:239, 1966.

Alexander, M., and Stare, F.: Overweight, obesity and weight control. *Calif Med, 106*:437-46, 1967.

Alfin-Slater, R. and Aftergood, L.: *Nutrition for Today.* Dubuque, Brown, 1973.

American Alliance for Health, Physical Education and Recreation: *Nutrition for Athletes: A Handbook for Coaches.* Washington, D.C., AAHPER, 1971.

American Medical Association: *Comments in Sports Medicine.* Chicago, AMA, 1973.

American Medical Association: Dietary fat and its relation to heart attacks and strokes. *JAMA, 175*:389-91, 1961.

Amundson, L.: Sports medicine symposium: Weight cutting and wrestling. *South Dakota J Med, 26*:31-35, October, 1973.

Anderson, H., and Barkue, H.: Iron deficiency and muscular work performance. *Scand J Clin Lab Invest, 25*:Suppl. 114, 9-37, 1970.

An exercise induced protein catabolism in man. *Nutr Rev, 30*:108-110, 1972 (a).

Archdeacon, J., and Murlin, J.: The effect of thiamine depletion and restoration on muscular efficiency and endurance. *J Nutr, 28*:241-54, 1944.

Arnold, M.: Endurance and nutrition. *Swimming Technique, 8*:34-35, July, 1971.

Arterbury, T.: *The effects of a multiple ergogenic aid upon strength, muscular endurance and recovery.* Paper presented at National AAHPER Convention, Detroit, April, 1971.

Asmussen, E.: Muscular Exercise. In *Handbook of Physiology Respiration,* Washington, American Physiology Society, 1965.

Asmussen, E., and Boje, O.: The effects of alcohol and some drugs on the capacity of work. *Acta Physiol Scand, 15*:109-18, 1948.

Asprey, G., and others: Effect of eating at various times on subsequent performances in the one mile free style swim. *Res Q Am Assoc Health Phys Educ, 39*:231-34, 1968.

Asprey, G., and others: Effect of eating at various times on free style swimming performance. *J Am Diet Assoc, 47*:198-200, 1965(a).

Asprey, G., and others: Effect of eating at various times on subsequent performances in the 2-mile run. *Res Q Am Assoc Health Phys Educ, 36*:233-36, 1965(b).

Asprey, G., and others: Effect of eating at various times upon subsequent performances in the one-mile run. *Res Q Am Assoc Health Phys Educ, 35*:227-30, 1964.

Asprey, G., and others: Effect of eating at various times on subsequent performances in the 440-yard dash and half-mile run. *Res Q Am Assoc Health Phys Educ, 34*:267-70, 1963.

Astrand, P.: Something old and something new . . . very new. *Nutr Today, 3*:9-11, 1968(a).

Astrand, P.: Limiting factors in prolonged heavy exercise. *Theorie a Praxe Telesne Vychory, 16*:7-12, 1968(b).

Astrand, P.: Diet and athletic performance. *Fed Proc, 26*:1772-77, 1967(a).

Astrand, P.: Interrelation between physical activity and metabolism of carbohydrate, fat and protein. In Blix, G. (Ed.): *Nutrition and Physical Activity*, Uppsala, Sweden, Almqvist and Wiksells, 1967(b).

Astrand, P., and Rodahl, K.: *Textbook of Work Physiology*. New York, McGraw-Hill, 1970.

Athletes talk about nutrition. *Swimming Technique, 10*:20, April, 1973.

Atzler, E., and Lehmann, G.: Die wirkung von Lecithin auf Arbeitsstoffwechsel und Leistungsfahigkeit. *Arbeitsphysiologie, 9*:76-93, 1935.

Bailey, D., and others: Vitamin C supplementation related to physiological response to exercise in smoking and nonsmoking subjects. *Am J Clin Nutr, 23*:905-12, 1970.

Bair, G.: Chronic Vitamin A poisoning. *JAMA, 146*:1573-74, 1951.

Bajusz, E.: *Nutritional Aspects of Cardiovascular Diseases*. Philadelphia, Lippincott, 1965.

Baker, E.: Vitamin C requirements in stress. *Am J Clin Nutr, 20*:583-90, 1967.

Baker, E., and others: Ascorbic acid metabolism in man. *Am J Clin Nutr, 19*:371-78, 1966.

Baldwin, K., and others: Substrate depletion in different types of muscle and in liver during prolonged running. *Am J Physiol, 225*:1045-50, 1973.

Balke, B.: The measurement of physiological factors. In Larson, L. (Ed.): *Fitness, Health and Work Capacity*, New York, MacMillan, 1974.

Ball, J.: Effect of eating at various times upon subsequent performances in swimming. *Res Q Am Assoc Health Phys Educ, 33*:163-67, 1962.

Banister, E.: Energetics of muscular contraction. In Shephard, R. (Ed.): *Frontiers of Fitness*, Springfield, Thomas, 1971.

Banister, E., and Brown, S.: The relative energy requirements of physical activity. In Falls, H. (Ed.): *Exercise Physiology*, New York, Academic, 1968.

Banister, R.: Human beings are not the same. *Physician and Sportsmed, 2*:91-2, September, 1974.

Barborka, C., and others: Relationship between vitamin B complex intake and work output in trained subjects. *JAMA, 122*:717-20, 1943.

Barnes, F.: Vitamin supplements and the incidence of colds in high school basketball players. *North Carolina Medical J, 22*:22-6, January, 1961.

Basu, A., and others: The effect of exercise on the levels of nonesterified fatty acids in the blood. *Q J Exp Physiol, 45*:312-17, 1960.

Basu, N., and Ray, G.: The effect of vitamin C on the incidence of fatigue in human muscles. *Indian J Med Res, 28*:419-26, 1940.

Bell, C., and others: *The effect of glucose ingestion on perceptual responses during long term work.* Paper presented at National American College of Sports Medicine meeting, New Orleans, May, 1975.

Benade, A., and others: The significance of an increased RQ after sucrose ingestion during prolonged aerobic exercise. *Pfluegers Arch, 342*:199-206, 1973.

Bensley, E.: Feeding of athletes. *Canad Med Assn J, 64*:503-04, 1951.

Berg, K.: Body composition and nutrition of adolescent boys training for bicycle racing. *Nutr Metab, 14*:172-80, 1972.

Bergstrom, J.: Local changes in ATP and phosphorylcreatine in human muscle tissue in connection with exercise. *Cir Res, 20*:Suppl. 1, 91-8, 1967.

Bergstrom, J., and Hultman, E.: Nutrition for maximal sports performance. *JAMA, 221*:999-1006, 1972.

Bergstrom, J., and Hultman, E.: The effect of exercise on muscle glycogen and electrolytes in normals. *Scand J Clin Lab Invest, 18*:16-20, 1966.

Bergstrom, J., and others: Muscle glycogen consumption during cross-country skiing (The Vasa Ski Race). *Int Z Angew Physiol, 31*:71-5, 1973.

Bergstrom, J., and others: Effect of nicotinic acid on physical working capacity and on metabolism of muscle glycogen in man. *J Appl Physiol, 26*:170-76, 1969.

Bergstrom, J., and others: Diet, muscle glycogen and physical performance. *Acta Physiol Scand, 71*:140-50, 1967.

Berland, T.: *Rating the Diets.* Skokie, Illinois, Publications International, 1974.

Berry, W., and others: The diet, haemoglobin values and blood pressures of olympic athletes. *Br Med J, 1*:300, 1949.

Berryman, G., and others: Effects in young men consuming restricted quantities of B-complex vitamines and proteins, and changes associated with supplementation. *Am J Physiol, 148*:618-47, 1947.

Berven, H.: The physical working capacity of healthy children. Seasonal variation and effect of ultraviolet radiation and Vitamin D supply. *Acta Pediat, 148*:Suppl.1-22, 1963.

Best, C., and Partridge, R.: Observations on olympic athletes. *Proc R Soc Lond,*

105:323-32, 1930.

Bialecki, M.: Nicotinic acid after physical exertion. *Pol Tyg Lek, 17*:1370-75, 1962.

Bicknell, F., and Prescott, F.: *The Vitamins in Medicine.* London, Heinemann, 1953.

Bideau, D., and Pagliuchi, D.: *L' Alimentation du Sportif.* Paris, R. Lepine, 1955.

Bierring, E.: The respiratory quotient and the efficiency of moderate exercise with special reference to the influence of diet. *Arbeitsphysiol, 5*:17-48, 1932.

Blanchard, D.: How Stanford beat the weight loss problem. *Scholastic Coach, 41*:88, March, 1972.

Blank, L.: An experimental study of the effect of water ingestion upon athletic performance. *Res Q Am Assoc Health Phys Educ, 30*:131-35, 1959.

Blix, G. (Ed.): *Food Cultism and Nutrition Quackery: Symposia of the Swedish Nutrition Foundation.* Uppsala, Sweden, Almqvist and Wiksells, 1970.

Blix, G. (Ed.): *Nutrition and Physical Activity.* Uppsala, Sweden, Almqvist and Wiksells, 1967.

Blix, G.: A study on the relation between total calories and single nutrients in Swedish food. *Acta Soc Med Upsalla, 70*:117, 1965.

Bloom, W.: To fast or exercise. Am J Clin Nutr, 21:1475-79, 1968.

Blyth, C., and Burt, J.: Effect of water balance on ability to perform in high ambient temperatures. *Res Q Am Assoc Health Phys Educ, 32*:301-07, 1961.

Bobb, A., and others: A brief study of the diet of athletes. *J Sports Med Phys Fitness, 9*:255-62, 1969.

Bock, W., and others: The effects of acute dehydration upon cardiorespiratory endurance. *J Sports Med Phys Fitness, 7*:67-72, 1967.

Boddy, K., and others: Total body, plasma and erythrocyte potassium and leucocyte ascorbic acid in "ultra-fit" subjects. *Clin Sci Mol Med, 46*:449-56, 1974.

Bogart, J., and others: *Nutrition and Physical Fitness.* Philadelphia, Saunders, 1973.

Bohm, W.: *Opinions of experienced coaches and athletes in training track and field athletes.* Unpublished masters thesis, Springfield College, Springfield, Massachusetts, 1938.

Boileau, R., and others: Body composition changes in obese and lean men during physical conditioning. *Med Sci Sports, 3*:183-89, 1971.

Boje, O.: Doping: A study of the means employed to raise the level of performance in sport. *League Nat Bull Health Org, 8*:439-69, 1939.

Bolliger, A.: Schweissverluste und Trinkmengen von Tennisspielern. *Schweiz Z Sportmed, 201*:25-32, 1974.

Borisov, I., and Sluka, P.: Use of artificially ionized air and vitamins C and D for preventing increased capillary fragility in student athletes. *Gig Sanit, 38*:105-7, 1973.

Bosco, J., and others: Effects of progressive hypohydration on maximal isometric muscular strength. *J Sports Med Phys Fitness, 8*:81-86, 1968.

Bourne, G.: Nutrition and exercise. In Falls, H. (Ed.): *Exercise Physiology.* New York, Academic, 1968.

Bourne, G.: Vitamins and muscular exercise. *Brit J Nutr, 2*:261-63, 1948.

Bradfield, R.: A technique for determination of usual daily energy expenditure in the field. *Am J Clin Nutr, 24*:1148-54, 1971.

Brannon, D.: *Breakfast and breakfast omission: A comparison of performance on selected AAHPER youth fitness test items in junior high school girls.* Unpublished master's thesis, Boston University, 1971.

Bray, G.: The myth of diet in the management of obesity. *Am J Clin Nutr, 23*:1141-48, 1970.

Bray, G. and others: The acute effects of food intake on energy expenditure during cycle ergometry. *Am J Clin Nutr, 27*:254-59, 1974.

British Committee on Medical Aspects of Food: Diet and coronary heart disease. *Nutr Today, 10*:16, Jan/Feb., 1975.

Brooke, J., and Davies, G.: Nutrition during severe prolonged exercise in trained cyclists. *Proc Nutr Soc, 31*:93-4A, 1972.

Brooke, J., and Green, L.: Variations in available carbohydrate and physical work ability with repeated prolonged severe exercise. *Proc Nutr Soc, 32*:11A, 1973.

Brozek, J.: Soviet studies on nutrition and higher nervous activity. *Ann N Y Acad Sci, 93*:667-714, 1962.

Brozek, J.: Changes of body composition in man during maturity and their nutritional implications. *Fed Proc, 11*:784-93, 1952.

Brozek, J., and Keys, A.: The evaluation of leanness and fitness in man: norms and interrelationships. *Br J Nutr, 5*:194-206, 1951.

Bruch, H.: What makes people food cultists or victims of nutrition quackery. In Blix, G. (Ed.): *Food Cultism and Nutrition Quackery.* Uppsala, Almqvist and Wiksells, 1970.

Brunner, H.: Vitamin C und Armeesport. *Schweiz Med Wochenschr, 71*:715, 1941.

Bugyi, G.: *The effects of moderate doses of caffeine on fatigue parameters of the forearm flexor muscles.* Unpublished master's thesis, University of Maryland, College Park, 1969.

Bullen, B. and others: Physical activity of obese and non-obese adolescent girls appraised by motion picture sampling. *Am J Clin Nutr, 14*:211, 1964.

Bullen, B., and others: Athletics and nutrition. *Am J Surg, 98*:343-52, 1959.

Burt, J., and others: *An evaluation of four schedules of fluid replacement during physical activity under extremes of temperature and humidity.* Paper presented at National Convention of American College of Sports Medicine, Oklahoma City, May 5, 1962.

Burton, B.: *The Heinz Handbook of Nutrition.* New York, McGraw-Hill, 1965.

Buskirk, E.: Nutrition for the athlete. In Ryan, A., and Allman, E. (Eds.): *Sports Medicine.* New York, Academic, 1974(a).

Buskirk, E.: *Nutrition and athletic performance*. Presented at Art and Science of Sports Medicine. Charlottesville, Virginia, June 28, 1974 (b).

Buskirk, E.: Nutrition and college athletics. In Steitz, E. (Ed.): *Administration of athletics in colleges and universities*. Washington, NEA, 1971.

Buskirk, E., and Beetham, W.: Dehydration and body temperature as a result of marathon running. *Medicina Sportiva, 14*:493-506, 1960.

Buskirk, E. and Haymes, E.: Nutritional requirements for women in sport. In Harris, D. (Ed): *Women and Sport: A National Research Conference*. University Park, Penn State University, 1972.

Buskirk, E., and Mendez, J.: Nutrition, environment and work performance with special reference to altitude. *Fed Proc, 26*:1760-67, 1967.

Buskirk, E. and others: Work performance after dehydration: Effects of physical conditioning and heat acclimitization. *J Appl Physiol, 12*:189-94, 1958.

Byrd, O. and Byrd, T.: *Medical Readings on Nutrition*. San Francisco, Boyd and Fraser, 1971.

Cade, J.: Changes in body fluid composition and volume during vigorous exercise by athletes. *J Sports Med Phys Fitness, 11*:172-77, 1971.

Cade, J. and others: Effect of fluid, electrolyte, and glucose replacement during exercise on performance, body temperature, rate of sweat loss and compositional changes of extracellular fluid. *J Sports Med Phys Fitness, 12*:150-56, 1972.

Campbell, D.: Effect of controlled running on serum cholesterol of young adult males of varying morphological constitutions. *Res Q Am Assoc Health Phys Ed, 39*:47-53, 1968.

Campbell, D.: Influence of several physical activities on serum cholesterol concentration in young men. *J Lipid Res, 6*:478-80, 1965.

Campbell, R., and others: Studies of food intake regulation in man. *N Engl J Med, 285*:1402-07, 1971.

Canning, H., and Mayer, J.: Obesity: Analysis of attitudes and knowledge of weight control in girls. *Res Q Am Assoc Health Phys Ed, 39*:894-99, 1968.

Cantone, A.: Physical effort and its effect in reducing alimentary hyperlipemia. *J Sports Med and Phys Fitness, 4*:32-6, 1964.

Carlson, L.: Plasma lipids and lipoproteins and tissue lipids during exercise. In Blix, G. (Ed.): *Nutrition and Physical Activity*. Uppsala, Sweden, Almqvist and Wiksells, 1967(a).

Carlson, L.: Lipid metabolism and muscular work. *Fed Proc, 26*:1755-59, 1967(b).

Carlson, L., and Mossfeldt, F.: Acute effects of prolonged, heavy exercise on the concentration of plasma and lipoproteins in man. *Acta Physiol Scand, 62*:51-59, 1964.

Carlson, L., and Oro, L.: The effect of nicotinic acid on the plasma free fatty acids. *Acta Med Scand, 172*:641-45, 1962.

Carlson, L., and others: Effect of nicotinic acid on the turnover rate and oxidation of the free fatty acids of plasma in man during exercise. *Metabolism, 12*:837-45, 1963.

"How to solve the problems of pre-competition meals." Carnation Company, n.d.

Carpenter, J.: Effects of alcohol on some psychological processes. *Q J Stud Alcohol, 23*:274-314, 1962.

Carpenter, J.: The effects of caffeine and alcohol on simple visual reaction time. *J Comp Physiol Psychol, 52*:491-96, 1959.

Carpenter, T.: The fuel of muscular activity in man. *J Nutr, 4*:281-304, 1931.

Caspari, W.: Physiological studies with vegetarians. *Pfluegers Arch, 109*:478-595, 1905.

Causeret, J.: Nutrition et capacites physiques. *Bull Soc Scient Hyg Aliment, 45*:19, 1957.

Cavagna, G., and others: Mechanical work in running. *J Appl Physiol, 19*:249-56, 1964.

Celejowa, I., and Homa, M.: Food intake, nitrogen, and energy balance in Polish weight lifting during a training camp. *Nutr Metab, 12*:259-74, 1970.

Cerretelli, P.: Exercise and endurance. In Larson, L. (Ed.): *Fitness, Health and Work Capacity*. New York, MacMillan, 1974.

Chaikelis, A.: The effect of glycocoll (glycine) ingestion upon the growth, strength and creatinine-creatine excretion in man. *Am J Physiol, 132*:578-87, 1941.

Cho, M. and Fryer, B.: Nutrition knowledge of collegiate physical education majors. *J Am Diet Assoc, 65*:30-34, 1974(a).

Cho, M., and Fryer, B.: What foods do physical education majors and basic nutrition students recommend for athletes. *J Am Diet Assoc, 65*:541-54, 1974(b).

Christakis, G., and others: Effect of a combined nutrition, education and physical fitness program on the weight status of obese high school boys. *Fed Proc, 25*:15-19, 1966.

Christensen, E.: Das Essen und Trinken des Sportlers. *Sportmedizinische Schriftenreihe Wander*, Heft 6:7-34, 1958.

Christensen, E. and Hansen, O.: Arbeitsfahigkeit und Ernahrung. *Skand Arch f Physiol, 81*:160, 1939.

Christensen, E., and others: Investigations of heavy muscular work. *Q Bull League of Nations Health Org, 3*:388-417, 1934.

Christophe, J. and Mayer, J.: Effect of exercise on glucose uptake in rats and men. *J Appl Physiol, 13*:269-72, 1958.

Clarke, H.: Exercise and fat reduction. *Phys Fit Research Digest, 5*:1-27, April, 1975.

Clarke, H.: *Phys Fit Research Digest, 2*:1-14, 1972.

Clarke, K.: Predicting certified weight of young wrestlers: a field study of the Tcheng-Tipton method. *Med Sci Sports, 6*:52-57, 1974.

Clarke, K.: Quackery and sports. *Ohio State Med J, 64*:913-20, 1968.

Clausen, D.: *The combined effect of aerobic exercise and vitamin E upon cardiorespiratory endurance and measured blood variables*. Unpublished master's thesis, University of Wyoming, 1971.

Committee on Assay of Foods. II. Vitamin B Complex. *Am J Public Health,* 34:783-94, 1944.

Committee on Iron Deficiency: Iron deficiency in the United States. *JAMA,* 203:407-12, 1968.

Committee on Nutrition, American Heart Association: Diet and coronary heart disease. *Nutr Today,* 9:26-27, May/June, 1974.

Committee on Nutritional Misinformation, National Research Council: Water deprivation and performance of athletes. *Nutr Rev,* 32:314-15, 1974.

Connor, W.: Diet and coronary heart disease. *Modern Med,* 38:85-8, November 30, 1970.

Consolazio, C., and Johnson, H.: Dietary carbohydrate and work capacity. *Am J Clin Nutr,* 25:85-90, 1972.

Consolazio, C., and others: Metabolic aspects of caloric restrictions: hypohydration effects on body weight and blood parameters. *Am J Clin Nutr,* 21:793-802, 1968.

Consolazio, C. and others: Metabolic aspects of acute starvation in normal humans: performance and cardiovascular evaluation. *Am J Clin Nutr,* 20:684-693, 1967(a).

Consolazio, C., and others: Metabolic aspects of acute starvation in normal humans (10 days). *Am J Clin Nutr,* 20:672-83, 1967(b).

Consolazio, C. and others: Effects of octacosanol, wheat germ oil, and vitamin E on performance of swimming rats. *J Appl Physiol,* 19:265-67, 1964(a).

Consolazio, C., and others: Effects of aspartic acid salts (Mg and K) on physical performance of men. *J Appl Physiol,* 19:257-61, 1964(b).

Consolazio, C., and others: Environmental temperature and energy expenditure. *J Appl Physiol,* 18:65, 1963.

Cooper, D.: Nutrition in athletics. *J Amer Coll Health Assoc,* 14:261-64, 1966.

Cooper, D., and others: Use of a liquid meal in a football training program. *J Okla State Med Assoc,* 55:484-86, 1962.

Coopersmith, S.: The effects of alcohol on reaction to affective stimuli. *Q J Stud Alcohol,* 25:459-75, 1964.

Corbin, C., and Pletcher, P.: Diet and physical activity patterns of obese and non-obese elementary school children. *Res Q Am Assoc Health Phys Ed,* 39:922-28, 1968.

Costill, D.: Muscular exhaustion during distance running. *The Physician and Sportsmed,* 2:36-41, October, 1974.

Costill, D.: *Rapid fluid replacement during thermal dehydration.* Paper presented at ACSM national meeting, Philadelphia, May, 1972(a).

Costill, D.: Water and electrolytes. In Morgan, W. (Ed.): *Ergogenic aids and muscular performance.* New York, Academic, 1972(b).

Costill, D., and Fox, E.: Energetics of marathon running. *Med Sci Sports,* 1:81-6, 1969.

Costill, D., and Sparks, K.: Rapid fluid replacement following thermal dehydration. *J Appl Physiol,* 34:299-303, 1973.

Costill, D., and others: *Water and electrolyte replacement during repeated days of work in the heat.* Paper presented at ACSM national meeting, New Orleans, May, 1975.

Costill, D., and others: Glycogen depletion pattern in human muscle fibers during distance running. *Acta Physiol Scand, 89*:374-83, 1973(a).

Costill, D., and others: Glucose ingestion at rest and during prolonged exercises. *J Appl Physiol, 34*:764-69, 1973(b).

Costill, D., and others: Factors limiting the ability to replace fluids during prolonged exercise. *Med Sci Sports, 5*:57, 1973(c).

Costill, D., and others: Muscle glycogen utilization during prolonged exercise on successive days. *J Appl Physiol, 31*:834-38, 1971(a).

Costill, D., and others: Muscle glycogen utilization during exhaustive running. *J Appl Physiol, 31*:353-56, 1971(b).

Costill, D., and others: Fluid ingestion during distance running. *Arch Environ Health, 21*:520-25, 1970.

Coulson, L.: *The effects of forced withdrawl of an ergogenic aid (wheat germ oil) on the bicycle ergometer riding time of collegiate athletes.* Unpublished master's thesis, University of Maryland, College Park, 1969.

Council on Drugs, AMA: New drugs and developments in therapeutics: potassium and magnesium aspartates (Spartase). *JAMA, 183*:362, 1963.

Craig, F. and Cummings, E.: Dehydration and muscular work. *J Appl Physiol, 21*:670-74, 1966.

Creff, A.: *La Dietetique Sportive.* Paris, Amicale des Entraineurs Francais D'Athletisme, 1964.

Creff, A. and Berard, L.: *Sport et Alimentation.* Paris, La Table Ronde, 1966.

Crews, E. and others: Weight, food intake, and body composition: Effects of exercise and of protein deficiency. *Am J Physiol, 216*:359-63, 1969.

Crooks, M.: Protein supplementation and weight gain. *Scholastic Coach, 44*:62, April, 1975.

Csik, L., and Bencsik, J.: Versuche, die Wirkung von B-vitamin auf die Arbeitsleistung des Menschen Festzustellen. *Klin Wochenschr, 6*:2275-78, 1927.

Cureton, T. K.: *The Physiological Effects of Wheat Germ Oil on Humans in Exercise.* Springfield, Thomas, 1972(a).

Cureton, T.: *The physiological effects of wheat germ oil on exercise.* Paper presented at AAHPER National Convention. Houston, March, 1972(b).

Cureton, T.: The diet of schoolboy athletes can be improved. *Athletic J, 50*:71, September, 1969(a).

Cureton, T.: Nutritive aspects of physical fitness work. *Swimming Technique, 6*:44-49, July, 1969(b).

Cureton, T.: Improvement in physical fitness associated with a course of U. S. Navy underwater trainees, with and without dietary supplements. *Res Q Am Assoc Health Phys Ed, 34*:440-53, 1963.

Cureton, T.: Diet related to athletics and physical fitness. *J Phys Educ, 57*:104-107, May/June, 1960.

Cureton, T.: What about wheat germ. *Scholastic Coach, 29:*24-28, 1959.

Cureton, T.: Wheat germ oil, the "wonder" fuel. *Scholastic Coach, 24:*36, March, 1955.

Cureton, T.: Effect of wheat germ oil and vitamin E on normal human subjects in physical training programs. *Am J Physiol, 179:*628, 1954.

Cureton, T., and Pohndorf, R.: Influence of wheat germ oil as a dietary supplement in a program of conditioning exercises with middle-aged subjects. *Res Q Am Assoc Health Phys Ed, 26:*391-407, 1955.

Dagenais, G., and others: Hemodynamic effects of carbohydrate and protein meals in man: rest and exercise. *J Appl Physiol, 21:*1157-62, 1966.

Damon, A., and Goldman, R.: Predicting fat from body measurements: densiometric validation of ten anthropometric equations. *Hum Biol, 36:*32-44, 1964.

Darden, E.: Questions and answers on health foods for athletes. *Scholastic Coach, 44:*68, March, 1975.

Darden, E.: Food-fuel for energy. *Scholastic Coach, 44:*108-11, September, 1974.

Darden, E.: Nutrition and athletic performance. *Scholastic Coach, 42:*88, September, 1972.

Darden, E., and Schendel, H.: Dietary protein and muscle building. *Scholastic Coach, 40:*70, March, 1971.

Darling, R., and others: Effects of variations in dietary protein on the physical well-being of man doing manual work. *J Nutr, 28:*273-81, 1944.

Daum, K., and others: Effect of various types of breakfast on physiologic responses. *J Am Diet Assoc, 26:*503-09, 1950.

Davies, C., and Van Haaren, J.: Effect of treatment on physiological responses to exercise in East African industrial workers with iron deficiency anemia. *Br J Ind Med, 30:*335-40, 1973.

Davies, C., and others: Iron deficiency anemia: its effect on maximum aerobic power and responses to exercise in African males aged 17-40 years. *Clin Sci, 44:*555-62, 1973.

Davis, T., and others: Review of studies of vitamin and mineral nutrition in the United States (1950-1968). *J Nutr Educ, 1:*Suppl. 1, 41-54, 1969.

Daws, T., and others: Evaluation of cardiopulmonary function and work performance in man during caloric restriction. *J Appl Physiol, 33:*211-17, 1972.

Debigne, G.: *Alimentation du Sportif et de L'Homme Moderne.* Paris, Editions Amphora, 1970.

DeLuca, H.: Vitamin D — A new look at an old vitamin. *Nutr Rev, 29:*179-81, 1971.

Dempsey, J., and others: Work capacity determinants and physiologic cost of weight supported work in obesity. *J Appl Physiol, 21:*1815-20, 1966.

Dennig, H.: Uber Steigerung der korperlichen Leistungsfahigkeit durch Eingriffe in den Saurebasenhaushalt. *Deutsche med Wochenschrift, 63:*733-36, 1937.

Dennig, H., and others: Effect of acidosis and alkalosis upon capacity for work. *J*

Clin Invest, 9:601-13, 1931.

Denton, D.: Salt appetite. *Nutr Abstr and Rev, 39*:1043-49, 1969.

Depinto, A., and others: Salt in athletic training. *Scholastic Coach, 40*:62, February, 1971.

deVries, H.: *Physiology of exercise for physical education and athletics.* Dubuque, Brown, 1974.

deVries, H., and Gray, D.: Aftereffects of exercise upon resting metabolic rate. *Res Q Am Assoc Health Phys Ed, 34*:314-21, 1963.

deWijn, J., and others: Hemoglobin, packed cell volume, serum iron, and iron binding capacity of selected athletes during training. *J Sports Med Phys Fitness, 11*:42-51, 1971(a).

deWijn, J., and others: Hemoglobin, packed cell volume, serum iron and iron binding capacity of selected athletes during training. *Nutr Metab, 13*:129-39, 1971(b).

Diet and Heart Disease. *Nutr Rev, 25*:130-32, 1967(a).

Diet, exercise and endurance. *Nutr Rev, 30*:86, 1972(b).

Dill, D., and others: Blood sugar regulation in exercise. *Am J Physiol, 111*:21-30, 1935.

Dill, D., and others: Alkalosis and the capacity for work. *J Biol Chem, 97*:58-59, 1932.

Dorcher, N.: The effects of rapid weight loss upon the performance of wrestlers and boxers, and upon the physical proficiency of college students. *Res Q Am Assoc Health Phys Ed, 15*:317-24, 1944.

Dowdy, R.: Copper Metabolism. *Am J Clin Nutr, 22*:887-91, 1969.

Doyle, J.: Remediable precursors of coronary artery disease. *Ann Intern Med, 73*:131-33, 1970.

Drug abuse in athletics. Proceedings, California Assembly Interim Subcommittee on Drug Abuse and Alcoholism, October 20, 1970.

Drummond, G., and Black, E.: Comparative physiology: Fuel of muscle metabolism. *Ann Rev Physiol, 22*:169-90, 1960.

Dudleston, A., and Bennion, M.: Effect of diet and/or exercise on obese college women. *J Am Diet Assoc, 56*:126-29, 1970.

DuPain, R., and Loutfi, M.: Vitamin C et Courbatures. *Rev Med Suisse Romande, 63*:640, 1943.

Durnin, J.: The influence of nutrition. *Can Med Assoc J, 96*:715-20, 1967.

Durnin, J., and others: How much food does man require. *Nature, 242*:418, April 6, 1973.

Early, R., and Carlson, B.: Water soluble vitamin therapy on the delay of fatigue from physical activity in hot climatic conditions. *Int Z Angew Physiol, 27*:43-50, 1969.

Eaves, C.: *Effects of four liquids on the endurance of college wrestlers following dehydration.* Unpublished doctoral dissertation, Ohio State University, 1968.

Edgerton, V.: Iron deficiency anemia and physical performance and activity of rats. *J Nutr, 102*:381-99, 1972.

Edwards, H., and others. Metabolic rate, blood sugar, and the utilization of carbohydrate. *Am J Physiol, 108*:203-09, 1934.

Efremov, V., and Sakaeva, E.: Importance of vitamin E in intense physical exertions of sportsmen. *Vopr Pitan, 32*:22-4, September-October, 1973.

Egana, E., and others: The effects of a diet deficient in the vitamin B complex on sedentary men. *Am J Physiol, 127*:731-41, 1942.

Ekblom, B.: Temperature regulation during exercise dehydration in man. *Acta Physiol Scand, 79*:475-83, 1970.

Embden, G., and others: Increase of working capacity through administration of phosphate. *Zeit f Physiol Chem, 113*:67-107, 1921.

Engel, R.: Food Faddism. *Nutr Rev, 17*:353-55, 1959.

Ericsson, P.: The effect of iron supplementation on the physical work capacity in the elderly. *Acta Med Scand, 188*:361-74, 1970.

Ershoff, B., and Levin, E.: Beneficial effects on an unidentified factor in wheat germ oil on the swimming performance of guinea pigs. *Fed Proc, 14*:432, 1955.

Evans, W., and Caldwell, L.: The effects of the potassium and magnesium salts of dl-aspartic acid on human fatigue and recovery. *U. S. Army Med Res Lab Rep, 550*:5, August 16, 1962.

Eating at various times before exercise. *Nutr Rev, 21*:40, 1963.

Exercise and cholesterol catabolism. *Nutr Rev, 28*:211, 1970(a).

Exercise and gastrointestinal absorption in human beings. *Nutr Rev, 26*:167, 1968.

Exercise, nutrition and caloric sources of energy. *Nutr Rev, 28*:180-84, 1970(b).

Fallis, N., and others: Effect of potassium and magnesium asparates on athletic performance. *JAMA, 185*:129, 1963.

Falls, H.: *Exercise Physiology.* New York, Academic, 1968.

Fat and cholesterol in the diet. *Nutr Rev, 23*:3, 1965(a).

Feeley, R., and others: Cholesterol content of foods. *J Am Diet Assoc, 61*:134-49, 1972.

Field, E.: *Effect on non-recommended foods on performance.* Unpublished master's thesis, University of California, Los Angeles, 1966.

Fischbach, E.: Problems of doping. *Med Monatsschr, 26*:377-81, 1972.

Fischbach, E.: Coffee and sports. *Minerva Med, 61*:4367-69, 1970.

Fischer, I.: The influence of flesh eating on endurance. *Yale Med J, 13*:205-21, March, 1907.

Fleming, A.: *Super Food for Super Athletes.* Oakland, Sea Classics Press, 1968.

Flinn, F.: The so-called action of sodium phosphate in delaying onset of fatigue. *Pub Health Rep, 41*:1463, 1926.

Foley, P.: Effect of ingesting water in swimming. *Swimming Technique, 8*:34, July, 1971.

Foltz, E., and others: Influence of components of the vitamin B complex on recovery from fatigue. *J Lab Clin Med, 27*:1396-99, 1942.

Food and Nutrition Board: Recommendation for increased iron levels in the American diet. *Nutr Review, 28*:108-09, 1970.

Food for the athlete. *Lancet, 2*:152, 1948.

Fordtran, J., and Saltin, B.: Gastric emptying and intestinal absorption during prolonged severe exercise. *J Appl Physiol, 23*:331-35, 1967.

Fox, E., and Mathews, D.: *Interval Training.* Philadelphia, Saunders, 1974.

Fox, E., and others: Effects of football equipment on thermal balance and energy cost during exercise. *Res Q Am Assoc Health Phys Ed, 37*:332-39, 1966.

Fox, F., and others: Vitamin C requirements of native mine workers. *Br Med J, 2*:143-47, 1940.

Fox, S., and others: Physical activity and cardiovascular health. III. The exercise prescription: Frequency and type of activity. *Mod Concepts Cardiovasc Dis, 41*:25, 1972.

Frankau, I.: Acceleration of co-ordinated muscular effort by nicotinamide. *Br Med J, 2*:601-603, 1943.

Frazier puts meat in diet. Virginia Pilot, Norfolk, March 4, 1975(b).

Frederick, R.: *The practices of leading high school wrestling coaches with regard to dieting among amateur wrestlers.* Unpublished master's thesis, University of North Carolina at Greensboro, 1968.

Friedman, T., and Ivy, A.: Work at high altitude. *Quart Bull N W Univ Med School, 21*:31-44, 1947.

Froberg, O.: Medicine and Sport. In Poortmans, J. (Ed.): *Biochemistry of Exercise.* Basel, Karger, 1969.

Fuge, W., and others: Effects of protein deficiency on certain adaptive responses to exercise. *Am J Physiol, 215*:660-63, 1968.

Fujioka, H., and others: Inhibitory effects of 1-aspartic acid salts against fatigue resulting from march. *Nat Def Med J, 10*:525-28, 1963(a).

Fujioka, H., and others: On the anti-fatigue effects of potassium and magnesium salts of 1-aspartic acid as evaluated by several fatigue indexes. *Nat Def Med J, 10*:72-8, 1963(b).

Fukui, T., and others: The effect of potassium and magnesium aspartates on fatigue. *Tokushima J Exp Med, 9*:24-31, 1962.

Fulton, E.: *The effect of dietary supplements of protein and wheat germ oil on selected physical measurements of junior high school athletes.* Unpublished master's thesis, North Texas State University, 1971.

Ganslen, R., and others: Effects of some tranquilizing, analeptic and vasodilating drugs on physical work capacity and orthostatic tolerance. *Aerosp Med, 35*:630-33, 1964.

Gardiner, E.: *Athletes of the ancient world.* London, Oxford University Press, 1930.

Gardner, G., and Edgerton, V.: *Iron deficiency and physical work performance.* Paper presented at National ACSM Meeting, Philadelphia, May, 1972.

Gastineau, C., and Rynearson, E.: Obesity. *Ann Int Med, 27*:883-97, 1947.

Gemmill, C.: The fuel for muscular exercise. *Physiol Rev, 22*:32-53, 1942.

General Health and Fitness Corporation Report. Norwood, N. J., General Health and Fitness Corporation.

Giese, M., and Corliss, R.: *Exercise caloric expenditure and serum lipid levels.*

Paper presented at National American College of Sports Medicine Meeting, Knoxville, May 10, 1974.

Glatzel, H.: Sinn und Unsinn in der Diatek. VI. Sport. *Med Welt, 25*:16-20, 1974.

Godin, G., and Shephard, R.: Body weight and the energy cost of activity. *Arch Environ Health, 27*:289-93, 1973.

Goldberg, A.: Protein synthesis during work induced growth of skeletal muscle. *J Cell Biol, 36*:653-58, 1968.

Goldspink, G.: The combined effects of exercise and reduced food intake on skeletal muscle fibers. *J Cellular Comp Physiol, 63*:209-16, 1964.

Gollnick, P., and King, D.: Energy release in the muscle cell. *Med Sci Sports, 1*:23-31, 1969.

Gollnick, P., and others: Selective glycogen depletion patterns in human muscle fibers after exercise of varying intensity and at varying pedalling rates. *J Physiol, 241*:45-57, 1974.

Gollnick, P., and others: Diet exercise and glycogen changes in human muscle fibers. *J Appl Physiol, 33*:421-25, 1972.

Goode, R., and others: Effects of exercise and a cholesterol-free diet on human serum lipids. *Can J Physiol Pharmacol, 44*:575-80, 1966.

Gordon, B.: Sugar content of the blood in runners following a marathon race. *JAMA, 85*:508, 1925.

Gordon, E., and others: A new concept in the treatment of obesity. *JAMA, 186*:50-60, 1963.

Gould, L.: Cardiac effects of alcohol. *Am Heart J, 79*:422-25, 1970.

Gounelle, H.: Action de la vitamine B, dans l'exercise musculaire et la prevention de la fatigue. *Bull Soc Med Hop*, Paris, *56*:255-57, 1940.

Grafe, H.: *Optimale Ernahrungsbilanzen fur Leistungssportler*. Berlin, Academie Verlag, 1964.

Grande, F.: Energetics and weight reduction. *Am J Clin Nutr, 21*:305-14, 1968.

Green, J., and Bunyan, J.: Vitamin E and the biological antioxidant theory. *Nutr Abstr Rev, 39*:321-45, 1969.

Greenleaf, J.: Exercise and water electrolyte balance. In Blix, G. (Ed.): *Nutrition and Physical Activity*. Uppsala, Sweden, Almqvist and Wiksells, 1967.

Greenleaf, J., and Castle, B.: Exercise temperature regulation in man during hypohydration and hyperhydration. *J Appl Physiol, 30*:847-53, 1971.

Gregg, W.: *A boy and his physique*. Chicago, National Dairy Council, 1970.

Grenier, R.: Hypokinetism: The disease of the century. *Union Med Can, 103*:483-90, 1974.

Grey, G., and others: Effects of ascorbic acid on endurance performance and athletic injury. *JAMA, 211*:105, 1970.

Guggenheim, J.: Nutrition and physical fitness. *Harefuah, 85*:37-9, 1973.

Guild, W.: Pre-event nutrition, with some implications for endurance athletes. In *Exercise and Fitness*. Chicago, The Athletic Institute, 1960.

Guyton, A. C.: *Textbook of Medical Physiology*. Philadelphia, Saunders, 1971.

Haggard, H., and Greenberg, L.: *Diet and Physical Efficiency*. New Haven, Yale University Press, 1935.

Haldi, J., and Wynn, W.: Observations on efficiency of swimmers as related to some changes in pre-exercise nutriment. *J Nutr, 31*:525-32, 1946.

Haldi, J., and Wynn, W.: The effect of low and high carbohydrate meals on the blood sugar level and on work performance in strenuous exercise of short duration. *Am J Physiol, 145*:402-10, 1945.

Haldi, J., and others: Muscular efficiency in relation to the taking of food and to the height of the respiratory quotient immediately before exercise. *Am J Physiol, 121*:123-29, 1938.

Hallberg, L., and others: Menstrual blood loss and iron deficiency. *Acta Med Scand, 180*:639-50, 1966.

Hanley, D.: The catastrophic triviality. *Nutr Today, 3*:17-20, 1968.

Harger, B., and others: The caloric loss of running. *JAMA, 228*:482-83, 1974.

Harper, A.: Those pesky RDAs. *Nutr Today, 9*:15-28, March/April, 1974.

Harris, H.: *Nutrition and Physical Performance: The diet of Greek athletes.* Proceedings of the Nutrition Society, *25*:87-90, 1966.

Haymes, E.: *Iron deficiency and women athletes.* Paper presented at National ACSM meeting, New Orleans, May, 1975.

Haymes, E.: Iron deficiency and the active woman. *DGWS Research Reports, 2*:91-7, 1973.

Haymes, E.: *The effect of the physical activity level on selected hematological variables in adult women.* Paper presented at the national AAHPER convention, Houston, March, 1972.

Haymes, E., and others: *Heat tolerance of exercising lean and obese prepubertal boys.* Paper presented at national ACSM meeting, New Orleans, May, 1975.

Heald, F.: Treatment of obesity in adolescence. *Postgrad Med J, 51*:109-12, 1972.

Hebbelinck, M.: The effects of a small dose of ethyl alcohol on certain basic components of human physical performance. *Arch Int Pharmacodyn Ther, 143*:247-57, 1963.

Hebbelinck, M.: *Spierarbeid en Ethylalcohol.* Brussel, Arsica Uitgaven, 1961.

Hebbelinck, M.: The effects of a moderate dose of alcohol on a series of functions of physical performance in man. *Arch Int Pharmacodyn Ther, 120*:402-05, 1959.

Hegsted, D.: Energy needs and energy utilization. *Nutr Rev, 32*:33-8, 1974.

Hein, F.: Improvement of food selection through physical education and athletic programs. *J Sch Health, 37*:340-45, 1967.

Hein, F., and Ryan, A.: The contributions of physical activity to physical health. *Res Q Am Assoc Health Phys Ed, 31*:263-85, 1960.

Hellebrandt, F., and Dimmitt, L.: Studies in the influence of exercise on the digestive work of the stomach. III. Its effect on the relation between secretory and motor function. *Am J Physiol, 107*:364-69, 1934.

Hellebrandt, F., and Hoopes, S.: Studies in the influence of exercise on the digestive work of the stomach. I. Its effect on the secretory cycle. *Am J Physiol, 107*:348-54, 1934.

Hellebrandt, F., and Tepper, R.: Studies on the influence of exercise on the digestive work of the stomach. II. Its effect on emptying time. *Am J Physiol, 107*:355-63, 1934.

Hellebrandt, F., and others: Effect of gelatin on power of women to perform maximal anaerobic work. *Proc Soc Exp Biol Med, 43*:629-34, 1940.

Hellebrandt, F., and others: Studies on the influence of exercise on the digestive work of the stomach. IV. Its relation to the physiochemical changes in the blood. *Am J Physiol, 107*:370-77, 1934.

Henderson, Y., and Haggard, H.: The maximum power and its fuel. *Am J Physiol, 72*:264-82, 1925.

Henschel, A.: The environment and performance. In Simonson, E. (Ed.): *Physiology of Work Capacity and Fatigue*. Springfield, Thomas, 1971.

Henschel, A.: Diet and muscular fatigue. *Res Q Am Assoc Health Phys Ed, 13*:280-85, 1942.

Henschel, A., and others: Performance capacity in acute starvation with hard work. *J Appl Physiol, 6*:624-33, 1954.

Henschel. A., and others: Vitamin C and ability to work in hot environments. *Am J Trop Med Hyg, 24*:259-65, 1944.

Herbert, V., and Jacob, E.: Destruction of vitamin B_{12} by ascorbic acid. *JAMA, 230*:241, 1974.

Herbert, W.: *The effect of dehydration and subsequent rehydration on the physical working capacity of college wrestlers*. Unpublished master's thesis, Kent State University, 1969.

Herbert, W., and Ribisl, P.: Effects of dehydration upon physical working capacity of wrestlers under competitive conditions. *Res Q Am Assoc Health Phys Ed, 43*:416-22, 1972(a).

Herbert, W., and Ribisl, P.: *The effect of various degrees of rapid weight reduction and rehydration upon metabolic responses to steady state exercise*. Paper presented at national AAHPER convention, Houston, March, 1972(b).

Hermansen, L.: Oxygen transport during exercise in human subjects. *Acta Physiol Scand Suppl, 399*:9-104, 1973.

Hermansen, L.: Anaerobic energy release. *Med Sci Sports, 1*:32-8, 1969.

Hermansen, L., and others: Muscle glycogen during prolonged severe exercise. *Acta Physiol Scand, 71*:129-39, 1967.

Hettinger, T.: *Physiology of Strength*. Springfield, Thomas, 1961.

Hewitt, J., and Callaway, E.: Alkali reserve of the blood in relation to swimming performance. *Res Q Am Assoc Health Phys Ed, 7*:83-93, March, 1936.

High fat diet for weight reduction. *Nutr Rev, 20*:294-97, 1962.

Hilsendager, D., and Karpovich, P.: Ergogenic effect of glycine and niacin separately and in combination. *Res Q Am Assoc Health Phys Ed, 35*:389-92, 1964.

Hirata, I.: Pre-game meals: a discussion. *Swimming Technique, 10*:22-24, April, 1973.

Hirsch, J.: Can we modify the number of adipose cells. *Postgrad Med, 51*:83-6, 1972.

Hoitink, A.: Vitamin C and work. Leiden, *Nederl Inst V Prevent Geneesk*, 1946(a).

Hoitink, A.: Researches on the influence of vitamin C administration on the human organism, in particular in connection with the working capacity. *Acta Brev Neerl Physiol, 14*:62, 1946(b).

Holloszy, J.: Long term metabolic adaptations in muscle to endurance exercise. In Naughton, J. and Hellerstein, H. (Eds.): *Exercise Testing and Exercise Training in Coronary Heart Disease*. New York, Academic, 1973.

Holloszy, J., and others: Effects of a 6-month program of endurance exercise on the serum lipids of middle aged men. *Am J Cardiol, 14*:753-60, 1964.

Hoogerwerf, A., and Hoitink, A.: The influence of vitamin C administration on the mechanical efficiency of the human organism. *Int Z Angew Physiol, 20*:164-72, 1963.

Horstman, D.: Nutrition. In Morgan, W. (Ed.): *Ergogenic Aids and Muscular Performance*. New York, Academic Press, 1972.

Horvath, S., and others: The influence of glycine on muscular strength. *Am J Physiol, 134*:469-72, 1941.

Howley, E., and Glover, M.: The caloric costs of running and walking one mile for men and women. *Med Sci Sports, 6*:235-37, 1974.

Huenemann. R.: Food habits of obese and non-obese adolescents. *Postgrad Med, 51*:99-105, 1972.

Huenemann, R., and others: Teen-agers activities and attitudes towards activity. *J Am Diet Assoc, 51*:433-40, 1967.

Hultman, E.: Muscle glycogen stores and prolonged exercise. In Shephard, R. (Ed.): *Frontiers of Fitness*, Springfield, Thomas, 1971.

Hultman, E.: Physiological role of muscle glycogen in man, with special reference to exercise. *Cir Res*, Suppl. 1, *20*:99-114, 1967(a).

Hultman, E.: Studies on muscle metabolism of glycogen and active phosphate in man with special reference to exercise and diet. *Scand J Clin Lab Invest*, Suppl. 94, *19*:11-63, 1967(b).

Hultman, E., and Nilsson, L.: Liver glycogen as a glucose-supplying source during exercise. In Keul, J. (Ed.): *Limiting factors of physical performance*. Stuttgart, Georg Thieme, 1973.

Hultman, E., and Nilsson, L.: Liver glycogen in man. Effect of different diets and muscular exercise. In Pernow, B., and Saltin, B. (Eds.): *Muscle metabolism during exercise*. New York, Plenum, 1971.

Hursh, L.: "Coronary heart disease: risk factors and the diet debate." Chicago, National Dairy Council, 1974.

Hutcheson, R. and Hutcheson, J.: Iron and vitamin C deficiencies in a large population of children. *Health Serv Rep, 87*:232-35, 1972.

Hutchinson, R.: Meal habits and their effects on performance. *Nutr Abstr Rev, 22*:283-97, 1952.

Hutchinson, R., and Krehl, W.: The effect of food intake on performance. *Bordens Rev Nutr Res, 15*:33-52, 1959.

Huttunen, J.: Diet, energy sources and maximal performance — A review.

Duodecim, 90:455-63, 1974.

Ikai, M., and Steinhaus, A.: Some factors modifying the expression of human strength. *J Appl Physiol, 16*:157, 1961.

Issekutz, B., and others: Effect of diet on work metabolism. *J Nutr, 79*:109-16, 1963.

Jalso, S., and others: Nutritional beliefs and practices. *J Am Diet Assoc, 47*:263-68, 1965.

Jankowski, L., and Foss, M.: The energy intake of sedentary men after moderate exercise. *Med Sci Sports, 4*:11-13, 1972.

Jannot, E.: *Dietetique et Sport.* Paris, Librairie Maloine, 1968.

Jarvis, D.: *Folk medicine.* New York, Holt, 1958.

Jenkins, D.: Effects of nicotinic acid on carbohydrate and fat metabolism during exercise. *Lancet, 1*:1307-08, 1965.

Jensen, C.: Health no-no's: alcohol, nicotine, caffeine. *Scholastic Coach, 41*:76-8, Jan, 1972.

Jetzler, A., and Haffter, C.: Vitamin C — Bedarf bei einmaligar sportlicher Dauerleistung. *Wien Med Wochenshr, 89*:332, 1939.

Johnson, M., and others: Relative importance of inactivity and overeating in the energy balance of obese high school girls. *Am J Clin Nutr, 4*:37-44, 1956.

Johnson, R., and others: Exercise, dietary intake and body composition. *J Am Diet Assoc, 61*:399-403, 1972.

Johnson, W., and Black, D.: Comparison of effects of certain blood alkalinizers and glucose upon competitive endurance performance. *J Appl Physiol, 5*:577-78, 1953.

Johnson, W., and Buskirk, E.: *Science and Medicine of Exercise and Sport.* New York, Harper and Row, 1974.

Jokl, E.: Notes on doping. In Jokl, E., and Jokl, P. (Eds.): *Exercise and altitude.* Basel, S. Karger, 1968.

Jokl, E.: Nutrition and athletics: special book review. *J Assoc Phys Ment Rehabil, 19*:61-2, 1965.

Jokl, E.: *Nutrition, Exercise and Body Composition.* Springfield, Thomas, 1964.

Jokl. E., and Suzman, H.: A study of the effects of vitamin C upon physical efficiency. *Transvaal Mine Medical Officers Association Proceedings, 19*:292-300, March, 1940.

Jolliffe, N.: The preventive and therapeutic use of vitamins. *JAMA, 129*:613-17, 1945.

Jung, K.: Energy supplying processes in continuous stress described in the example of a six day cycle race. *Med Welt, 23*:1105-10, 1972.

Kaczmarek, R.: Effect of gelatin on the work output of male athletes and non-athletes and on girl subjects. *Res Q Am Assoc Health Phys Ed, 11*:109-19, 1940.

Kallen, D.: Nutrition and Society. *JAMA, 215*:94-100, 1971.

Karlsson, J., and Saltin, B.: Diet, muscle glycogen and endurance performance. *J Appl Physiol, 31*:203-06, 1971.

Karlsson, J., and Saltin, B.: Lactate, ATP and CP in working muscles during exhaustive exercise in man. *J Appl Physiol, 29*:598-602, 1970.

Karlsson, J., and others: Muscle glycogen utilization during exercise after physical training. *Acta Physiol Scand, 90*:210-17, 1974.

Karlsson, J., and others: Muscle lactate, ATP and CP levels during exercise after physical training in man. *J Appl Physiol, 33*:199-203, 1972.

Karpovich, P.: Ergogenic aids in work and sport. *Res Q Suppl, 12*:432-50, 1941.

Karpovich, P., and Millman, N.: Vitamin B and endurance. *N Engl J Med, 226*:881-82, 1942.

Karpovich, P., and Pestrecov, K.: Effect of gelatin upon muscular work in man. *Am J Physiol, 134*:300-09, 1941.

Karpovich, P., and Sinning, W.: *Physiology of Muscular Activity.* Philadelphia, Saunders, 1971.

Keller, W., and Kraut, H.: Work and nutrition. *World Rev Nutr Diet, 3*:65-81, 1959.

Kennedy, D.: *The effects of wheat germ oil on the precordial T-wave of cross-country runners.* Unpublished master's thesis, Appalachian State University, Boone, North Carolina, 1973.

Keul, J.: *Limiting factors of physical performance.* Stuttgart, Georg Thieme, 1973.

Keul, J., and Haralambie, G.: Die Wirking von Kohlenhydraten auf die Leistungsfahigkeit und die energieliefernden Substrate in Blut bei langwahrender Korperarbeit. *Dtsch Med Wochenschr, 98*:1806-17, 1973.

Keys, A.: Blood lipids in man — a brief review. *J Am Diet Assoc, 51*:508-16, 1967.

Keys, A.: Diet and incidence of heart disease. *Modern Med, 21*:90-1, July 15, 1953.

Keys, A.: Physical performance in relation to diet. *Fed Proc, 2*:164-87, 1943.

Keys, A., and Henschel, A.: Vitamin supplementation of U. S. Army rations in relation to fatigue and the ability to do muscular work. *J Nutr, 23*:259-69, 1942.

Keys, A., and Henschel, A.: High vitamin supplementation (B_1, nicotinic acid and C) and the response to intensive exercise in U. S. Army infantrymen. *Am J Physiol, 133*:350-51, 1941.

Keys, A., and others: *Human Starvation.* Minneapolis, University of Minnesota Press, 1950.

Keys, A., and others: Experimental studies on men with a restricted intake of the B vitamins. *Am J Physiol, 144*:5-42, 1945.

Keys, A., and others: The performance of normal young men on controlled thiamine intakes. *J Nutr, 26*:399-415, 1943.

King, E., and others: Failure of amino acetic acid to increase the work capacity of human subjects. *JAMA, 118*:594-97, 1942.

Klafs, C., and Arnheim, D.: *Modern Principles of Athletic Training.* St. Louis, Mosby, 1973.

Klafs, C., and Lyon, M.: *The Female Athlete.* St. Louis, Mosby, 1973.

Kline, A., and others: Comprehensive self-improvement program for inner city obese teenage girls. *J Sch Health, 39*:21-8, 1969.

Knochel, J., and Vertel, R.: Salt loading as a possible factor in the production of potassium depletion, rhabdomyolysis, and heat injury. *Lancet, 1*:659-61, 1967.

Knuttgen, H.: Potentials for development. In Larson, L. (Ed.): *Fitness, Health and Work Capacity.* New York, MacMillan, 1974.

Konishi, F.: *Exercise equivalents of Foods.* Carbondale, Southern Illinois University Press, 1973.

Konishi, F.: Food energy equivalents of various activities. *J Am Diet Assoc, 46*:186-88, 1965.

Kornhauser, S.: *The use of a 50 gram glucose solution as an ergogenic aid, pertaining to an anaerobic work task.* Unpublished master's thesis, Southern Illinois University, Carbondale, 1972.

Kourounakis, P.: Pharmacological conditioning for sporting events. *Am J Pharm, 144*:151-58, 1972.

Kozlowski, S.: Physical performance and maximal oxygen uptakes in man in exercise dehydration. *Bull Acad Pol Sci [Biol], 14*:513-19, 1966.

Kozlowski, S., and Saltin, B.: Effect of sweat loss on body fluids. *J Appl Physiol, 19*:1119-24, 1964.

Kral, J., and Hais, I.: Sweat and exercise. *J Sports Med Phys Fitness, 3*:105-12, 1963.

Krause, M., and Hunscher, M.: *Food Nutrition and Diet Therapy.* Philadelphia, Saunders, 1972.

Kraut, H., and Muller, E.: Muskelkrafte and Eiweissration. *Biochem Z, 320*:302-15, 1950.

Kraut, H., and others: Der Einfluss du Zusammensetzung des Nahrungseiweisses auf Stickstoffbilanz und Muskeltraining. *Int Z Angew Physiol, 17*:378-90, 1958.

Kraut, H., and others: Die Abhangigkeit des Muskeltrainings und des Eiweissansatzes von der Eiweissaufnahme und vom Eiweissbestand des Korpers. *Biochem Z, 324*:280-94, 1953.

Krehl, W.: The potassium depletion syndrome. *Nutr Today, 1*:20-23, June 1966(a).

Krehl, W.: Sodium-a most extraordinary dietary essential. *Nutr Today, 1*:16-18, December, 1966(b).

Krogh, A., and Lindhard, J.: The relative value of fats and carbohydrates as sources of muscular energy. *Biochem J, 14*:290-363, 1920.

LaCava, G.: *L'Alimentazione Dell' Atleta.* Milano, Societa Editrice Stampa Sportiva, 1963.

Ladell, W.: The effects of water and salt intake upon the performance of men working in hot and humid environments. *J Physiol, 127*:11-46, 1955.

Lamb, L.: Vitamin C (Ascorbic acid). *The Health Letter, 3*:1-4, 1974.

Lampman, R.: *Comparative effects of training and diet on serum lipids in man with type IV hyperlipidemia.* Paper presented at national ACSM meeting, New Orleans, May, 1975.

Larson, L. (Ed): *Fitness Health and Work Capacity.* New York, MacMillan, 1974(a).

Larson, L.: The organism at work. In Larson, L. (Ed.): *Fitness, Health and Work Capacity*. New York, MacMillan, 1974(b).

Lasagna, L., and others: Effect of potassium and magnesium aspartates on athletic performance. *JAMA, 185*:129, 1963.

Leake, C.: *The amphetamines: their actions and uses*. Springfield, Thomas, 1958.

Leveille, G., and Romsos, D.: Meal eating and obesity. *Nutr Today, 9*:4-9, November/December, 1974.

Leverton, R.: *A girl and her figure*. Chicago, National Dairy Council, 1970.

Levine, S., and others: Some changes in the chemical constituents of the blood following a marathon race. *JAMA, 82*:1778-79, 1924.

Lewis, S., and Gutin, B.: Nutrition and Endurance. *Am J Clin Nutr, 26*:1011-14, 1973.

Leyton, R.: Some practical aspects of the nutrition of athletes. *Br J Nutr, 2*:269-71, 1948.

Lincoln, J.: Calorie intake, obesity and physical activity. *Am J Clin Nutr, 25*:390-94, 1972.

Little, D., and others: Effect of water ingestion on capacity for exercise. *Res Q Am Assoc Health Phys Ed, 20*:398-401, 1949.

Lodispoto, N.: *Dietetica dello Sport*. Rome, Federazione Italiana Atletica Pesante, 1968.

Londeree, B.: *An investigation of the effect of four water replacement schedules upon exercise in the heat*. Unpublished doctoral dissertation, University of Toledo, 1966.

Londeree, B., and others: Water replacement schedules in heat stress. *Res Q Am Assoc Health Phys Ed, 40*:725-32, 1969.

Lovingood, B., and others: Effects of amphetamine (dexedrine) and caffeine on subjects exposed to heat and exercise stress. *Res Q Am Assoc Health Phys Ed, 31*:553-59, 1960.

Macaraeg, P.: High carbohydrate, low fat liquid meal for athletes. *J Sports Med Phys Fitness, 14*:259-62, 1974(a).

Macaraeg, P.: The importance of fluid and electrolytes in athletes. *J Sports Med Phys Fitness, 14*:213-17, 1974(b).

Maddox, D.: Jim Ryun: Stability and discipline. *Physician and Sportsmedicine, 2*:71-2, September, 1974.

Magazanik, A., and others: Enzyme blood levels and water balance during a marathon race. *J Appl Physiol, 36*:214-17, 1974.

Mahadeva, K., and others: Individual variations in metabolic cost of standardized exercise: food, age, sex and race. *J Physiol, (London) 121*:225-31, 1953.

Maison, G.: Failure of gelatin or amino aceticacid to increase the work ability of individual normal human muscles. *JAMA, 115*:1439-41, 1940.

Malinow, M., and Perley, A.: The effect of physical exercise on cholesterol degradation in man. *J Atherosclerosis Res, 10*:107-11, 1969.

Man, Sweat and Performance. Rutherford, New Jersey, Becton, Dickinson and Company, 1969(a).

Mann, G., and others: Exercise in the disposition of dietary calories. *N Engl J Med, 253*:349-55, 1955.

Margaria, R.: Current concepts of walking and running. In Shephard, R. (Ed.): *Frontiers of Fitness.* Springfield, Thomas, 1971.

Margaria, R.: Capacity and power of the energy processes in muscle activity: their practical relevance in athletics. *Int Z Angew Physiol, 25*:352-60, 1968.

Margaria, R., and others: Effect of alkalosis on performance and lactate formation in supramaximal exercise. *Int Z Angew Physiol, 29*:215-23, 1971.

Margaria, R., and others: The effect of some drugs on the maximal capacity of athletic performance in man. *Int Z Angew Physiol Einschl Arbeitsphysiol, 20*:281-87, 1964(a).

Margaria, R., and others: Balance and kinetics of anaerobic energy release during strenuous exercise in man. *J Appl Physiol, 19*:623-28, 1964(b).

Margaria, R., and others: Energy cost of running. *J Appl Physiol, 18*:367-70, 1963.

Margolius, S.: *Health foods: facts and fakes.* New York, Walker, 1973.

Margolius, S.: *The Great American Food Hoax.* New York, Walker, 1971.

Maron, M., and others: *Blood biochemical alterations and oxygen uptakes in response to marathon running.* Paper presented at national ACSM meeting, New Orleans, May, 1975.

Marrack, J.: The nutrition of athletes: proceedings of the nutrition society. *Br J Nutr, 2*:249-73, 1948.

Marsh, M., and Murlin, J.: Muscular efficiency on high carbohydrate and high fat diets. *J Nutr, 1*:104-37, 1928.

Marshall, T.: For soccer players, beer, tea, hot baths. *Physician and Sportsmedicine, 2*:16, August, 1974.

Mathews, D., and Fox, E.: *The Physiological Basis of Physical Education and Athletics.* Philadelphia, Saunders, 1971.

Mathews, D., and others: *A comparison of three liquids on absorption and exhaustive exercise among college men.* Paper presented at the AAHPER National Convention, Boston, April, 1969.

Mayer, J.: *Nutrition and exercise.* The Wolffe memorial lecture, National ACSM meeting, New Orleans, May, 1975.

Mayer, J.: Protein, the master builder. *Family Health, 6*:38-9, August, 1974.

Mayer, J.: *Exercise Helps You Lose Weight.* Pittsburgh Post-Gazette, Monday, May 29, 1972(a).

Mayer, J.: *Human Nutrition: Its Physiological, Medical and Social Aspects.* Springfield, Thomas, 1972(b).

Mayer, J.: *Overweight: Causes, Cost and Control.* Englewood Cliffs, Prentice-Hall, 1968.

Mayer, J.: Nutrition, exercise and cardiovascular disease. *Fed Proc, 26*:1768-71, 1967.

Mayer, J.: Obesity: Physiological considerations. *Am J Clin Nutr, 9*:530-38,

1961.

Mayer, J.: Nutrition and heart disease. *Am J Pub Health, 50*:5-10, 1960(a).

Mayer, J.: Exercise and weight control. In *Exercise and Fitness.* Chicago, The Athletic Institute, 1960(b).

Mayer, J., and Bullen, B.: Nutrition, weight control and exercise. In Johnson, W., and Buskiek, E. (Eds.): *Science and Medicine of Exercise and Sport.* New York, Harper and Row, 1974.

Mayer, J., and Bullen, B.: Nutrition and athletic performance. In *Exercise and Fitness.* Chicago, The Athletic Institute, 1960(a).

Mayer, J., and Bullen, B.: Nutrition and athletic performance. *Physiol Rev, 40*:369-97, 1960(b).

Mayer, J., and Bullen, B.: Nutrition and athletic performance. *Postgrad Med, 26*:848-56, 1959.

Mayer, J., and Stare, F.: Exercise and weight control: frequent misconceptions. *J Am Diet Assoc, 29*:340-43, 1953.

Mayo Clinic Committee on Dietetics: *Mayo Clinic Diet Manual.* Philadelphia, Saunders, 1971.

Mays, R., and Scoular, F.: Food eaten by athletes. *J Am Diet Assoc, 39*:225-27, 1961.

McCollum, E.: *A History of Nutrition.* Boston, Houghton Mifflin, 1957.

McCormick, W.: Vitamin B and physical endurance. *Med Rec, 152*:439, 1940.

Medical Commission, International Olympic Committee: *Doping.* Lausanne, Medical Commission, IOC, 1972.

Metropolitan Life Insurance Company: *How to Control Your Weight.* New York, Metropolitan Life Insurance Company, 1958.

Mickelsen, O.: Nutrition and athletics. *Food and Nutrition News, 41*:1-4, April, 1970.

Miettinen, M., and others: Effect of cholesterol in lowering diet on mortality from coronary heart disease and other causes. *Lancet, 2*:835-38, 1972.

Minard, D.: Prevention of heat casualties in Marine Corps recruits. *Milit Med, 126*:261-72, 1961.

Minnesota, University of: Laboratory of Physiological Hygiene, *Nutrition and Performance Capacity,* 1958.

Mitchell, J., and others: Respiratory weight losses during exercise. *J Appl Physiol, 32*:474-76, 1972.

Mohr, D.: Changes in waistline and abdominal girth and subcutaneous fat following isometric exercises. *Res Q Am Assoc Health Phys Ed, 36*:168-73, 1965.

Mole, P., and Johnson, R.: Disclosure by dietary modification of an exercise — induced protein catabolism in man. *J Appl Physiol, 31*:185-90, 1971.

Monagle, J., and others: Body temperature during work in man on restricted water intake and low carbohydrate diet. *Fed Proc, 15*:132, 1956.

Montague, A.: Obesity and evolution of man. *JAMA, 195*:105-07, 1966.

Montoye, H.: Vitamin B_{12} : A review. *Res Q Am Assoc Health Phys Ed, 26*:308-13, 1955.

338   *Nutritional Aspects of Athletic Performance*

Montoye, H., and others: Effects of vitamin B_{12} supplementation on physical fitness and growth of young boys. *J Appl Physiol,* 7:589-92, 1955.

Moody, D.: Fat — fact and fancy. *DGWS Research Reports: Women in Sports.* Washington, AAHPER, 1971.

Moore, H.: The meaning of food. *Am J Clin Nutr,* 5:77-82, 1957.

Morehouse, L., and Miller, A.: *Physiology of Exercise.* St. Louis, Mosby, 1971.

Morgan, W. (Ed.): *Ergogenic aids and muscular performance.* New York, Academic, 1972.

Moroff, S., and Bass, D.: Effects of overhydration on mans physiological responses to work in the heat. *J Appl Physiol,* 20:267-70, 1965.

Mueller, J.: Plain talk about a confusing matter. *Nutr Today,* 9:19-25, May/June, 1974.

Murphy, R., and Ashe, W.: Prevention of heat illness in football players. *JAMA, 194:*650-54, 1965.

Mustala, O.: Improvement of athletic performance by drugs. *Suom Laak,* 22:690-95, 1967.

Nagle, F., and others: The mitigation of physical fatigue with Spartase. *Fed Aviat Agency Rep, 63:*12, July 10, 1963.

Namyslowski, L.: Observations concerning the influence of Vitamin C on the physical fitness of sportsmen. *Sportartzliche Praxis, 3:*118-19, 1960.

Namyslowski, L.: Investigation of the Vitamin C requirement of athletes during physical exertion. *Rocz Panstw Zakl Hig,* 7:97-122, 1956.

National Dairy Council: The role of fiber in the diet. *Dairy Council Digest, 46:*1-4, 1975.

National Dairy Council: *Nutrition Source Book.* Chicago, National Dairy Council, 1970.

National Research Council: Committee on Dietary Allowances: *Recommended Dietary Allowances.* Washington, National Academy of Sciences, 1974.

Naughton, J., and Hellerstein, H.: *Exercise Testing and Exercise Training in Coronary Heart Disease.* New York, Academic, 1973.

Nelson, D.: Idiosyncrasies in training and diet. *Scholastic Coach, 30:*33-4, January, 1961.

Nelson, D.: Effects of food supplement on the performance of selected gross motor tasks. *Res Q Am Assoc Health Phys Ed, 31:*627-30, 1960.

Nelson, D.: Effects of ethyl alcohol on the performance of selected gross motor tests. *Res Q Am Assoc Health Phys Ed, 30:*312-20, 1959.

Newsholme, E., and Start, C.: *Regulation in Metabolism.* London, Wiley, 1973.

Nijakowski, F.: Assays of some vitamins of the B complex group in human blood in relation to muscular effort. *Acta Physiol Pol[Suppl], 17:*397-404, 1966.

Nocker, J.: Nutrition and performance. *Internist, 11:*269-73, 1970.

Nocker, J., and Glatzel, H.: *Die Ernahrung des Sportlers.* Nationales Olympisches Komitee fur Deutschland, 1963.

Novich, M.: Drug abuse and drugs in sports. *N Y State J Med,* 73:2597-600, 1973.

Nutrition: Magnesium reported essential for athletes. *Coach and Trainer*

Athletic Newsletter, 1:6, March, 1972(c).

Nutrition of athletes. *Nutr Rev, 7*:315-17, 1949.

O'Conner, F.: *The effect of Gatorade® upon endurance in the one mile run.* Unpublished master's thesis, University of Florida, 1967.

Olson, A., and Edelstein, E.: Spot reduction of subcutaneous adipose tissue. *Res Q Am Assoc Health Phys Ed, 39*:647, 1968.

Olson, R.: Food faddism ... why. *Nutr Rev, 16*:97-9, 1958.

Olsson, K., and Saltin, B.: Diet and fluids in training and competition. *Scand J Rehabil Med, 3*:31-8, 1971.

Orava, S., and others: Blood glucose, serum FFA and serum insulin levels after the intake of the carbohydrate rich solution before exercise in man. *J Sports Med Phys Fitness, 14*:93-102, 1974.

Organic myths. *Newsweek, 52*:March 11, 1974(a).

Oscai, L.: The role of exercise in weight control. In Wilmore, J. (Ed.): *Exercise and sport sciences reviews,* Vol. I., New York, Academic, 1973.

Oscai, L., and Holloszy, J.: *Exercise and serum triglycerides.* Paper presented at the AAHPER National Convention, Boston, April, 1969.

Oscai, L., and others: Effects of exercise on adipose tissue cellularity. *Fed Proc, 33*:1956-58, 1974(a).

Oscai, L., and others: *Effects of exercise and of food restriction in early life on adipose tissue cellularity in adult rats.* Paper presented at National American College of Sports Medicine annual meeting, Knoxville, May 10, 1974(b).

Palmer, W.: Selected physiological responses of normal young men following dehydration and rehydration. *Res Q Am Assoc Health Phys Ed, 39*:1054-59, 1968.

Pampe, W.: Hyperglykamie und korperliche Arbeit. *Arbeitsphysiologie, 5*:342-50, 1932.

Pargman, D.: Body build and dietary habits of college athletes. *Med Sci Sports, 3*:140-42, 1971.

Parizkova, J.: Body composition and exercise during growth and development. In Rarick, G. (Ed.): *Physical Activity: Human Growth and Development.* New York, Academic, 1973.

Parizkova, J.: Impact of age, diet and exercise on man's body composition. *Annals N Y Acad Sci, 110*:661-74, 1963.

Pascale, L., and others: Correlations between thickness of skinfolds and body density in 88 soldiers. *Human Biol, 28*:165-76, 1956.

Passmore, R., and Durnin, J.: *Energy, work and leisure.* London, Heinemann, 1967.

Passmore, R., and Durnin, J.: Human Energy Expenditure. *Physiol Rev, 35*:801-40, 1955.

Patton, R., and Randolph, J.: *A comparison of dextrose, Gatorade®, and Take-Five® as ergogenic aids for endurance performance.* Paper presented at National AAHPER Convention, Houston, March, 1972.

Paul, P.: FFA metabolism of normal dogs during steady-state exercise at different work loads. *J Appl Physiol, 28*:127-32, 1970.

Paul, W.: Crash diets and wrestling. *J Iowa Med Soc, 56*:835-40, 1966.

Pendergast, D., and others: *Energy cost of swimming.* Paper presented at national American College of Sports Medicine meeting, Knoxville, May 11, 1974.

Percival, L.: Experience with honey in athletic nutrition. In Jarvis, D., *Folk Medicine.* New York, Holt, 1958.

Percival, L.: Experience with honey in athletic nutrition. *Amer Bee J, 95*:390-93, 1955.

Percival, L.: *Vitamin E in athletic efficiency.* Shute Foundation for Medical Research, 3: No. 2, December, 1951.

Perkins, R., and Williams, M.: *Effect of caffeine upon maximal muscular endurance of females.* Paper presented at national AAHPER Convention, Atlantic City, March, 1975.

Pernow, B., and Saltin, B.: *Muscle Metabolism During Exercise.* New York, Plenum Press, 1971(a).

Pernow, B., and Saltin, B.: Availability of substrates and capacity for prolonged heavy exercise in man. *J Appl Physiol, 31*:416-22, 1971(b).

Physical training and cardiovascular status. *Nutr Rev, 27*:103, 1969(b).

Piehl, K.: Time course for refilling of glycogen stores in human muscle fibers following exercise-induced glycogen depletion. *Acta Physiol Scand, 90*:297-302, 1974(a).

Piehl, K.: Glycogen storage and depletion in human skeletal muscle fibers. *Acta Physiol Scand [Suppl], 402*:1-32, 1974(b).

Pitts, G., and others: Work in the heat as affected by intake of water, salt and glucose. *Am J Physiol, 142*:253-59, 1944.

Poiletman, R., and Miller, H.: The influence of wheat germ oil on the electrocardiographic T waves of the highly trained athlete. *J Sports Med Phys Fitness, 8*:26-33, 1968.

Pollock, M., and others: Effects of walking on body composition and cardiovascular function of middle aged men. *J Appl Physiol, 30*:126-30, 1971.

Pre-exercise nutriment and physical efficiency. *Nutr Rev, 4*:313-14, 1946.

Prokop, L.: Vitamins and athletic performance. *Z Ernahrungswiss, Suppl. 4*:83-91, 1965.

Prokop, L.: Vitamine und Sportsleistung. *Med u Ernahrung, 2*:174-76, 199-201, 1961.

Prokop, L.: Sport und ernahrung. In *Leberismuttel und Ernahrung.* Vienna, 1958.

Pruett, E.: Glucose and insulin during prolonged work stress in men living on different diets. *J Appl Physiol, 28*:199-208, 1970.

Ranson, R.: Nutritional guidelines for athletes. *Swimming Techniques, 10*:44, July, 1973.

Rarick, G.: *Physical Activity: Human Growth and Development.* New York, Academic, 1973.

Rasch, P., and Pierson, W.: The effect of a protein dietary supplement on muscular strength and hypertrophy. *Am J Clin Nutr, 11*:530-32, 1962.

Rasch, P., and others: Protein dietary supplementation and physical performance. *Med Sci Sports, 1*:195-99, 1969(a).

Rasch, P., and others: Effect of protein dietary supplementation on the physical performance of Marine Corps officer candidates. *Research Laboratory Report XIX: 6*:21, March, 1969(b).

Rasch, P., and others: Effects of vitamin C supplementation on cross country runners. *Sportzarztliche Praxis, 5*:10-13, Heft 1, 1962.

Ray, G., and others: Effect of gelatine on muscular fatigue. *Proc Soc Exp Biol Med, 40*:157-61, 1939.

Rechcigl, M.: Reviews relating to food, nutrition and health: a selected bibliography. *World Rev Nutr Diet, 16*:398-445, 1973.

Reeves, W.: The physiology of water in health. *Am J Orthod and Oral Surg, 32*:449-53, 1946.

Reichard, G., and others: Blood glucose metabolism in man during muscular work. *J Appl Physiol, 16*:1001-05, 1961.

Restriction of food or water and work output. *Nutr Rev, 19*:23, 1961.

Riabuschinsky, N.: The effect of phosphate on work and respiratory exchange. *Z fur Deutsch ges Exper Med, 72*:20-31, 1930.

Ribisl, P., and Herbert, W.: Effects of rapid weight reduction and subsequent rehydration upon the physical working capacity of wrestlers. *Res Q Am Assoc Health Phys Ed, 41*:536-41, 1970.

Ribisl, P., and Zuti, W.: *Energy cost of work at 10°, 25° and 40°C.* Paper presented at National American College of Sports Medicine Meeting, Philadelphia, May, 1972.

Ricci, B.: *Physiological Basis of Human Performance.* Philadelphia, Lea and Febiger, 1967.

Riendeau, R., and others: Relationship of body fat to motor fitness test scores. *Res Q Am Assoc Health Phys Ed, 29*:200-03, 1958.

Robinson, S., and Harmon, P.: The effects of training and of gelatin upon certain factors which limit muscular work. *Am J Physiol, 133*:161-69, 1941.

Roby, F.: Effect of exercise on regional subcutaneous fat accumulations. *Res Q Am Assoc Health Phys Ed, 33*:273-78, 1962.

Rochelle, R.: Blood plasma cholesterol changes during a physical training program. *J Sports Med Phys Fitness, 1*:63-70, 1961.

Rodahl, K., and others: Plasma free fatty acid in exercise. *J Appl Physiol, 19*:489-92, 1964.

Rodahl, K., and others: Effects of dietary protein on physical work capacity during severe cold stress. *J Appl Physiol, 17*:763-67, 1962.

Rose, K.: Warning for millions: intense exercise can deplete potassium. *Physician and Sportsmed, 3*:67, May, 1975.

Rose, K.: A liquid pregame meal for athletes. *JAMA, 178*:30-3, 1961.

Rose, K., and Fuenning, S.: Pre game emotional tension, gastrointestinal mobility and the feeding of athletes. *Nebr Med J, 45*:575-79, 1960.

Rose, L., and others: Serum electrolyte changes after marathon running. *J Appl Physiol, 29*:449-51, 1970.

Rowell, L.: The liver as an energy source. In Pernow, B., and Saltin, B. (Eds.): *Muscle Metabolism During Exercise.* New York, Plenum, 1971.

Rusch, H.: The taste of ambrosia. *Nutr Today, 3*:21-23, 1968.

Russians research food requirements of athletes. *Swimming Technique, 8*:59, July 1971(a).

Ryan, A.: The measurement of functions. In Larson, L. (Ed.): *Fitness, Health and Work Capacity.* New York, MacMillan, 1974.

Ryder, H.: *The effects of ingesting a liquid nutrient one hour prior to the performance of the one-mile run.* Unpublished doctoral dissertation, University of Arkansas, 1971.

Sage, J.: Effects of differing breakfast conditions and habit patterns on performance in an endurance activity. *Res Q Am Assoc Health Phys Ed, 40*:799-802, 1969.

Sakaeva, E., and Efremov, V.: Experience with additional allowance of vitamin E to sportsmen-race cyclists and skiers. *Vestn Akad Med Nauk SSSR, 27*:52-5, 1972.

Saltin, B.: Circulatory response to submaximal and maximal exercise after thermal dehydration. *J Appl Physiol, 19*:1125-32, 1964(a).

Saltin, B.: Aerobic and anaerobic work capacity after dehydration. *J Appl Physiol, 19*:1114-18, 1964(b).

Saltin, B., and Hermansen, L.: Glycogen stores and prolonged severe exercise. In Blix, G. (Ed.): *Nutrition and Physical Activity.* Uppsala, Sweden, Almqvist and Weksells, 1967.

Salt pills and leg cramps. *Physician and Sportsmed, 3*:14, May 1975(a).

Schade, M., and others: Spot reducing in overweight college women. *Res Q Am Assoc Health Phys Ed, 33*:461-71, 1962.

Schaefer, O.: The relative roles of diet and physical activity on blood lipids and obesity. *Am Heart J, 88*:673-74, 1974.

Schamadam, J., and Snively, W.: The role of potassium in diseases due to heat stress. *Ind Med Surg, 36*:785-88, 1967.

Schamadam, J., and others: Evaluation of potassium-rich electrolyte solutions as oral prophylaxis for heat stress. *Ind Med Surg, 37*:677-84, 1968.

Schenk, P.: Die Verpflegung von 4700 Wettkampfern aux 42 Nationen in Olympischen Dorf wahrend der XI Olympischen Spiele 1936 zu Berlin. *Munch med Wochenschr, 83*:1535, 1936.

Scherrer, D.: *The effect of ingesting dextrose on human performance.* Unpublished doctoral dissertation, Texas A & M University, 1971.

Scheunert, A.: *Ernahrung und Sport.* Berlin, Veb Verlag Volk und Gesundheit, 1954.

Scheunert, A., and Grafe, H.: Ernahrung und Sport. *Kleine Gesundheitsbucherei, Heft 15*:1961.

Schwartz, F.: Ascorbic acid in wound healing — a review. *J Am Diet Assoc,*

56:497-503, 1970.

Scott, D., and Pritchard, J.: Iron deficiency in healthy young college women. *JAMA, 199*:897-900, 1967.

Seelig, M.: Are American children still getting an excess of vitamin D. *Clin Pediatr (Phila), 9*:380-83, 1970.

Segurson, J., and Roby, F.: *Effect of rapid weight loss on blood and urine measurements of college wrestlers.* Paper presented at American College of Sports Medicine Annual meeting, Knoxville, May 9, 1974.

Seidl, E., and Hettinger, T.: Der Einfluss von Vitamin D_3 auf Kraft und Leistungsfahigkeit des gesunden Erwachsenen. *Int Z Angew Physiol, 16*:365-72, 1957.

Seltzer, C., and Mayer, J.: An effective weight control program in a public school system. *Am J Public Health, 60*:679-89, 1970.

Shaffer, C.: Ascorbic acid and atherosclerosis. *Am J Clin Nutr, 23*:27-30, 1970.

Sharman, I.: The effects of vitamin E and training on physiological function and athletic performance in adolescent swimmers. *Br J Nutr, 26*:265-76, 1971.

Sheehan, G.: What made Bob Kiphuth's Yale swimmers so good. *Med Times, 100*:217-22, 1972.

Shephard, R.: *Alive Man: The physiology of physical activity.* Springfield, Thomas, 1972.

Shephard, R.: *Frontiers of fitness.* Springfield, Thomas, 1971.

Shephard, R., and others: Do athletes need Vitamin E. *Physician and Sportsmedicine, 2*:57-60, September, 1974.

Sherman, H., and Smith, S.: *The Vitamins.* New York, The Chemical Catalog Co., 1922.

Sidorowicz, W., and Zawistowska, Z.: *Zywienie Sportowca i Turysty,* Warszawa, Panstwowy Zaklad, 1962.

Simka, V., and others: Mild exercise: effect on body composition and metabolism. *N Y State J Med, 74*:1563-67, 1974.

Simmons, R., and Hardt, A.: The effect of alkali ingestion on the performance of trained swimmers. *J Sports Med Phys Fitness, 13*:159-63, 1973.

Simonson, E.: Depletion of energy yielding substances. In Simonson, E. (Ed.): *Physiology of Work Capacity and Fatigue,* Springfield, Thomas, 1971(a).

Simonson, E.: Nutrition and work performance. In Simonson, E. (Ed.): *Physiology of Work Capacity and Fatigue.* Springfield, Thomas, 1971(b).

Simonson, E. (Ed.): *Physiology of work capacity and fatigue.* Springfield, Thomas, 1971(c).

Simonson, E.: Influence of nutrition on work performance. In *Nutrition Fronts in Public Health.* Nutrition Symposium Series No. 3, New York, National Vitamin Foundation, 1951.

Simonson, E., and others: The influence of vitamin B (complex) surplus on the capacity for muscular and mental work. *J Indust Hyg, 24*:83-90, 1942.

Sims, D.: An evaluation of liquid food supplements. *Scholastic Coach, 40*:28-29, December, 1970.

Singer, R., and Neeves, R.: Effect of food consumption on 200-yard freestyle swim performance. Res Q Am Assoc Health Phys Ed, 39:355-60, 1968.

Singer, R., and Weiss, S.: Effects of weight reduction on selected anthropometric, physical, and performance measures of wrestlers. Res Q Am Assoc Health Phys Ed, 39:361-69, 1968.

Skubic, V., and Hodgkins, J.: Energy expenditure of women participants in selected individual sports. J Appl Physiol, 21:133-37, 1966.

Slocum, D., and others: Wrestling and weight control. JAMA, 201:541, 1967.

Smith, R.: A new concept in controlled athletic nutrition. Evansville, E. Dalton Company, n.d.

Snellen, J.: Body temperature during exercise. Med Sci Sports, 1:39-42, 1969.

Sollman, T.: Manual of pharmacology. Philadelphia, Saunders, 1956.

Soule, R.: Dehydration and exercise performance in the heat. Paper presented at National American College of Sports Medicine meeting. Knoxville, May 9, 1974.

Southgate, D.: Assessing the energy value of the human diet. Nutr Rev, 29:131-34, 1971.

Speckmann, E.: Coronary heart disease: a scientific imbalance. Nutr Today, 10:30-3, January/February, 1975.

Spickard, A.: Heat stroke in college football and suggestions for prevention. Soc Med J, 61:791-96, 1968.

Spioch, F., and others: Influence of vitamin C upon certain functional changes and the coefficient of mechanical efficiency in humans during physical effort. Acta Physiol Pol, 17:204-15, 1966.

Sproule, B., and others: Cardiopulmonary physiological responses to heavy exercise in patients with anemia. J Clin Invest, 39:378-88, 1960.

Sprynarova, S., and Parizkova, J.: Changes in the aerobic capacity and body composition in obese boys after reduction. J Appl Physiol, 20:934-37, 1965.

Staton, W.: The influence of ascorbic acid in minimizing post-exercise muscle soreness in young men. Res Q Am Assoc Health Phys Ed, 23:356-60, 1952.

Staton, W.: The influence of soya lecithin on muscular strength. Res Q Am Assoc Health Phys Ed, 22:201-07, 1951.

Steel, J.: A nutritional study of Australian Olympic athletes. Med J Aust, 2:119-23, 1970.

Steiner, G., and Cahill, G.: Adipose tissue physiology. Ann N Y Acad Sci, 110:749-53, 1963.

Steinhaus, A.: Evidence and opinions related to swimming after meals. JOHPER, 32:59, April, 1961.

Steitz, E.: Administration of athletics in colleges and universities. Washington, NEA Publications, 1971.

Stewart, G., and others: Observations on the haemotology and the iron and protein intake of Australian Olympic athletes. Med J Aust, 2:1339-43, 1972.

Stone, I.: The genetic disease, hypoascorbemia. Acta Geneticae Medicae et

Gemellologiae, 16:52-60, 1967.

Stunkard, A., and others: The management of obesity. *Arch Intern Med, 125*:1067-72, 1970.

Talbot, D.: Vitamin supplements are essential. *Sport and Fitness Instructor,* June, 1974.

Tasler, J., and others: Gastrointestinal secretory function during physical exercise. *Acta Physiol Pol, 25*:215-26, 1974.

Tatkon, M.: *The Great Vitamin Hoax.* New York, MacMillan, 1968.

Taylor, A., and others: Skeletal muscle glycogen stores after submaximal and maximal work. *Med Sci Sports, 3*:75-8, 1971.

Taylor, H., and others: Performance capacity and effects of caloric restriction with hard physical work on young men. *J Appl Physiol, 10*:421-29, 1957.

Taylor, H., and others: Some effects of acute starvation with hard work on body weight, body fluids and metabolism. *J Appl Physiol, 6*:613-23, 1954.

Taylor, H., and others: The effect of successive fasts on the ability of men to withstand fasting during hard work. *Am J Physiol, 143*:148-55, 1945.

Taylor, H., and others: The effect of sodium chloride on the work performance of man during exposure to dry heat and experimental heat exhaustion. *Am J Physiol, 140*:439-51, 1943.

Tcheng, T., and Tipton, C.: Iowa wrestling study: anthropometric measurements and the prediction of a "minimal" body weight for high school wrestlers. *Med Sci Sports, 5*:1-10, 1973.

Tcheng, T., and others: Iowa wrestling study: lesson for physicians. ℞ *Sports and Travel, 10*:19-22, January, 1975.

Terjung, R., and others: Glycogen repletion in different types of muscle and in liver after exhausting exercise. *Am J Physiol, 226*:1387-91, 1974.

The effect of exercise on serum lipids. *Nutr Rev, 25*:197, 1967(b).

The metabolism role of vitamin E. *Nutr Rev, 23*:90-92, 1965(b).

The Nutrition Foundation: *Present Knowledge in Nutrition.* New York, The Nutrition Foundation, 1967.

The vitamin war. *Newsweek,* September 2, 1974(b).

Thompson, J.: *Sport, athletics and gymnastics in Ancient Greece.* Unpublished doctoral dissertation, Penn State University, 1971.

Thorn, G., and others: Comparison of metabolic effects of isocaloric meals of varying composition with special reference to prevention of post prandial hypoglycemic symptoms. *Ann Intern Med, 18*:913-19, 1943.

Tooshi, A., and Cureton, T.: *The effects of three different durations of endurance exercise on serum cholesterol, body composition and certain motor fitness measures in middle aged men.* Paper presented at National AAHPER Convention, Detroit, April, 1971.

Travers, P., and Campbell, W.: The organism and speed and power. In Larson, L. (Ed.): *Fitness, Health and Work Capacity.* New York, MacMillan, 1974.

Tuttle, W.: The effect of weight loss by dehydration and the withholding of food on the physiologic response of wrestlers. *Res Q Am Assoc Health Phys*

Ed, 14:158-66, 1943.

Tuttle, W., and others: Effects of breakfasts of different size and content on physiologic response of men. *J Am Diet Assoc, 27*:190-96, 1951.

Tuttle, W., and others: Effect of omitting breakfast on physiologic response of men. *J Am Diet Assoc, 26*:332-35, 1950.

Tuttle, W., and others: Influence of various levels of thiamine intake on physiologic response. III. Reaction Time. *J Am Diet Assoc, 25*:21-7, 1949(a).

Tuttle, W., and others: Effect of altered breakfast habits on physiologic response. *J Appl Physiol, 1*:545-59, 1949(b).

Ulmark, R.: The dangers of doping. *J Sports Med Phys Fitness, 3*:248-49, 1963.

United States Department of Health Education and Welfare: *Obesity and Health,* Public Health Service Publication No. 1485. Washington, U. S. Govt Printing Office, 1966.

United States Senate. *Proper and improper use of drugs by athletes.* Hearings before the subcommittee to investigate juvenile delinquency. June 18 and July 12-13, 1973. Washington, U. S. Government Printing Office, 1973.

Updyke, W., and others: *An evaluation of schedules of fluid replacement during a simulated football practice session under high temperature and humidity.* Paper presented at National American College of Sports Medicine Meeting, Madison, Wisconsin, March 25, 1966.

Upjohn, H., and others: Nutrition of athletes. *JAMA, 151*:818-19, 1953.

Vaccaro, P., and others: *Changes in body weight, hematocrit, and plasma protein concentration due to dehydration and rehydration in wrestlers.* Paper presented at National American College of Sports Medicine Meeting, New Orleans, May, 1975.

Van Handel, P., and others: *Utilization of exogenous glucose during endurance exercise.* Paper presented at National American College of Sports Medicine Meeting, New Orleans, May, 1975.

Van Huss, W.: *Vitamins and performance with emphasis on Vitamin C.* National American College of Sports Medicine meeting, Knoxville, Tennessee, May 9, 1974.

Van Huss, W.: What made the Russians run? *Nutr Today, 1*:20-3, 1966.

Van Huss, W., and others: Effect of milk consumption on endurance performance. *Res Q Am Assoc Health Phys Ed, 33*:120-28, 1962.

Van Itallie, T.: If only we knew. *Nutr Today, 3*:3-8, June, 1968.

Van Itallie, T., and Hashim, S.: Obesity in an age of caloric anxiety. *Modern Med, 38*:89-96, November 30, 1970.

Van Itallie, T., and others: Nutrition and athletic performance. In Johnson, W. (Ed.): *Science and Medicine of Exercise and Sports.* New York, Harper, 1960.

Van Itallie, T., and others: Nutrition and athletic performance. *JAMA, 162*:1120, 1956.

Venerando, A., and Torre, L.: Cocarboxylase in athletes with particular reference to non-production syndrome of muscular exercise. *Progr Med,* *8*:134-38, 1952.

Vegetarian Diets. *Am J Clin Nutr, 32*:1095, 1974(c).

Vilter, R.: Vitamins, minerals, and anemia. *JAMA, 175*:1000-01, 1961.

"Viobin Wheat Germ Oil.," Viobin Corporation, Monticello, Illinois, n.d.

Vitamin E in athletics. *Br Med J, 4*:251, 1971(b).

Vitamin supplements and performance capacity. *Nutr Rev, 8*:312-17, 1950.

Vogeler, R., and Ferguson, V.: The effect of sugar ingestion upon athletic performance. *Res Q Am Assoc Health Phys Ed, 3*:54-7, 1932.

Vytchikova, M.: Increasing the Vitamin B_1 content in the rations of athletes. *Chem Abstr, 52*:147-87, 1958.

Wachholder, K.: Steigerung des Umsatzes und des Verbrauches an Ascorbinsaure (Vitamin C) bei der Muskelarbeit. *Arbeitsphysiologie, 14*:342-62, 1951.

Wahren, J., and others: Glucose metabolism during exercise in man. In Pernow, B., and Saltin, B. (Eds.): *Muscle Metabolism During Exercise.* New York, Plenum, 1971.

Wald, G., and others: Experimental human vitamin A deficiency and ability to perform muscular exercise. *Am J Physiol, 137*:551-56, 1942.

Water depriviation and performance of athletes. *Am J Clin Nutr, 27*:1096-97, 1974(d).

Watson, G.: *Nutrition and Your Mind: The Psychochemical Sense.* New York, Harper and Row, 1972.

Watt, T., and others: Letter: Vitamin E and oxygen consumption. *Lancet, 2*:354-55, August 10, 1974.

Weinhaus, R.: The management of obesity: some recent concepts. *Missouri Medicine, 66*:719-30, 1969.

Weinstein, A.: Vitamin D poisoning. *J Tenn Med Assoc, 46*:140-42, 1953.

Weiss, B., and Laties, V.: Enhancement of human performance by caffeine and the amphetamines. *Pharmacol Rev, 14*:1-36, 1962.

Weiss, S., and Singer, R.: Weight reduction and wrestling. *Scholastic Coach, 36*:24, February, 1967.

Welch, H.: Substrate utilization in muscle — adaptations to physical effort. In Naughton, J., and Hellerstein, H. (Eds.): *Exercise testing and exercise training in Coronary heart disease,* New York, Academic, 1973.

Welch, M., and others: *Levels of RNA in response to exercise.* Paper presented at national American College of Sports Medicine meeting, New Orleans, May, 1975.

Wenzel, D., and Rutledge, C.: Effects of centrally acting drugs on human motor and psychomoter performance. *J Pharm Sci, 51*:631-44, 1962.

Westerman, R.: Fluid and electrolyte replacement in sweating athletes. *JAMA, 212*:1713, 1970.

Weswig, P., and Winkler, W.: Iron supplementation and hematological data of competition swimmers. *J Sports Med Phys Fitness, 14*:112-19, 1974.

Whipp, B., and Wasserman, K.: Efficiency of muscular work. *J Appl Physiol,* 26:644-48, 1969.

White, A., Handler, P., and Smith, E.: *Principles of Biochemistry.* New York, McGraw-Hill, 1973.

White, J.: Effect of eating a liquid meal at specific times upon subsequent performances in the one mile run. *Res Q Am Assoc Health Phys Ed,* 39:206-10, 1968.

White, P.: *Let's talk about food.* Acton, Massachusetts, Publishing Sciences Group, 1974.

Williams, J.: *Sports Medicine.* Baltimore, Williams and Wilkins, 1962.

Williams, M.: *Drugs and athletic performance.* Springfield, Thomas, 1974.

Williams, M.: *The effect of a moderate dose of alcohol on maximal heart rate and maximal endurance capacity.* Unpublished data, Old Dominion University, Norfolk, 1972.

Williams, M.: Effect of selected doses of alcohol on fatigue parameters of the forearm flexor muscles. *Res Q Am Assoc Health Phys Ed, 40:*832-40, 1969.

Wilson, E., and others: *Principles of Nutrition.* New York, Wiley, 1967.

Winick, M.: Childhood obesity. *Nutr Today, 9:*6-12, May/June, 1974.

Wirth, J., and others: *Effect of physical training on serum iron levels of college age women.* Paper presented at national American College of Sports Medicine meeting, New Orleans, May, 1975.

Wishart, G.: The efficiency and performance of a vegetarian racing cyclist under different dietary conditions. *J Physiol, 82:*189-99, 1934.

Witten, C.: The effects of three liquids on exhaustive exercise and absorption following a 2% body weight loss as a result of acute dehydration. *J Sports Med Phys Fitness, 12:*87-96, 1972.

Wolf, A.: *Thirst.* Springfield, Thomas, 1958.

Wooding, R.: *The effects of intensive physical training, weight maintenance, and nutritional intake control on the reactions of intercollegiate wrestlers to selected cardiorespiratory components.* Unpublished master's thesis, University of Washington, Seattle, 1968.

Wrightington, M.: The effect of glucose and sucrose on the respiratory quotient and muscular efficiency of exercise. *J Nutr, 24:*307-15, 1942.

Wyndham, C.: The validity of physiological determination. In Larson, L. (Ed.): *Fitness, Health and Work Capacity.* New York, MacMillan, 1974.

Wyndham, C., and others: Heat reactions of Caucasians in temperate, in hot, dry and in hot, humid climates. *J Appl Physiol, 19:*607-12, 1964.

Yakovlev, N.: *Pitanie Sportsmena.* Moscow, Fizkultura i Sport, 1967.

Yakovlev, N.: *Die Ernahrung des Sportlers am Wettkampftage.* Berlin, Sportverlag, 1956.

Yakovlev, N., and Rogozkin, V.: *Sports biochemistry in the Soviet Union.* Paper presented at the national American College of Sports Medicine meeting, New Orleans, May, 1975.

Yamaji, R.: Studies on protein metabolism in muscular exercise. I. Nitrogen metabolism in training of hard muscular exercise. *J Physiol Soc Japan,*

13:476-82, 1951(a).

Yamaji, R.: Studies on protein metabolism in muscular exercise. II. Changes of blood properties in training of hard muscular exercise. *J Physiol Soc Japan, 13*:483-89, 1951(b).

Yoshimura, H.: Anemia during physical training (sports anemia). *Nutr Rev, 28*:251-53, 1970.

Youmons, E., and others: Effects of eating at various times upon sprinting performance. *Scholastic Coach, 30*:24-26, November, 1960.

Young, D., and others: Model for evaluation of fatty acid metabolism for man during prolonged exercise. *J Appl Physiol, 23*:716-25, 1967(a).

Young, D., and others: Glucose oxidation and replacement during prolonged exercise in man. *J Appl Physiol, 23*:734-41, 1967(b).

Young, D., and others: Serum glucose and free fatty acids in man during prolonged exercise. *J Appl Physiol, 21*:1047-52, 1966.

Zaburkin, E.: Provision and requirements of sportsmen for pyridoxine and nicotinic acid. *Gig Sanit, 37*:103-04, 1972.

Zambraski, E., and others: *Iowa wrestling study. Changes in the urinary profiles of wrestlers prior to and after competition.* Paper presented at national American College of Sports Medicine meeting, New Orleans, May, 1975.

Zambraski, E., and others: Iowa wrestling study: urinary profiles of state finalists prior to competition. *Med Sci Sports, 6*:129-32, 1974.

Zauner, C., and Reese, E.: Specific training, taper and fatigue. *Swimming Technique, 10*:27-9, April, 1973.

Zauner, C., and Updyke, W.: Nutritional and physiological factors limiting performance in humans. *Swimming Technique, 10*:61-4, July, 1973.

Zuntz, N.: Ueber die Bedeutung der verschiedenen Nahrstoffe als Erzeuger der Muskelkraft. *Pfleugers Arch, 83*:557, 1901.

Zuti, W.: *A comparison of weight reduction methods that use diet and exercise.* Paper presented at National AAHPER Convention, Minneapolis, April, 1973.

Zuti, W., and Golding, L.: Equations for estimating percent fat and body density of active adult males. *Med Sci Sports, 5*:262-66, 1973.

APPENDIX A

FOOD COMPOSITION TABLE*

EXPLANATION OF APPENDIX A

Appendix A shows the food values in 615 foods commonly used in this country.

Foods listed. Foods are grouped under the following main headings: Milk; eggs; meat, poultry, fish; dry beans and peas, nuts; vegetables; fruits; grain products; fats; sugars and miscellaneous other items.

Most of the foods listed are in ready-to-eat form. Some are basic products widely used in food preparation, such as flour, fat and cornmeal.

Weight in grams — rounded to the nearest whole gram — is shown for an approximate measure of each food as it is described; if inedible parts are included in the description, both measure and weight include these parts.

The approximate measure shown for each food is in cups, ounces, pounds, some other well-known unit, or a piece of certain size. Usually, the measure shown can be calculated to larger or smaller amounts by multiplying or dividing. Because the measures are approximate (some are rounded for convenient use), calculated nutritive values for larger quantities of some food items may be less representative than those calculated for smaller quantities.

The cup measure refers to the standard measuring cup of 8 fluid ounces or 1/2 liquid pint. The ounce refers to 1/16 of a pound avoirdupois, unless fluid ounce is indicated. The weight of a fluid ounce varies according to the food measured.

Factors in general use for converting from one measure to its equivalent in another measure include those shown below.

*Courtesy of the United States Department of Agriculture

EQUIVALENTS BY VOLUME

(All measurements level)

1 quart	= 4 cups
1 cup	= 8 fluid ounces
	= 1/2 pint
	= 16 tablespoons
2 tablespoons	= 1 fluid ounce
1 tablespoon	= 3 teaspoons
1 pound regular butter	= 4 sticks
or margarine	= 2 cups
1 pound whipped butter	= 6 sticks
or margarine	= 2 8-ounce containers
	= 3 cups

EQUIVALENTS BY WEIGHT

1 pound (16 ounces)	= 453.6 grams
1 ounce	= 28.35 grams
3 1/2 ounces	= 100 grams

Food values. Values are shown for protein; fat; fatty acids; total carbohydrates; two minerals: calcium and iron; and five vitamins: vitamin A, thiamin, riboflavin, niacin, and ascorbic acid (vitamin C). Calories are shown in the column headed "Food energy." The calorie is the unit of measure for the energy furnished the body by protein, fat, and carbohydrate.

These values can be used as the basis for comparing kinds and amounts of nutrients in different foods. For some foods, the values can be used in comparing different forms of the same food.

Water content is also shown in the table because the percentage of moisture present is needed for identification and comparison of many food items.

The values for food energy (calories) and nutrients shown in Appendix A are the amounts present in the edible part of the item, that is, in only that portion of the weight of the item customarily eaten — corn without cob, meat without bone, potatoes without skin, European-type grapes without seeds. If additional parts are eaten, the skin of the potato, for example, amounts of some nutrients obtained will be somewhat greater than those shown.

For toast and for vegetables, values are without fat added, either during preparation or at the table. Values for the thiamin content of toast are about 20 percent lower than for fresh bread; it was impossible to show this loss adequately because of the small amount of thiamin present in a slice of bread. Some destruction of vitamins in vegetables, especially of ascorbic acid, may occur when foods are cut or shredded. Such losses are variable, and no deduction for these losses has been made.

Values for meat are measured as cooked, drained and without drippings. For many cuts, two sets of values are shown: meat including the fat, and meat from which the fat has been trimmed off in the kitchen or on the plate.

A variety of manufactured items, such as some of the milk products, ready-to-eat breakfast cereals, imitation cream products, fruit drinks and various mixes are included in Appendix A. Frequently these foods are fortified with one or more nutrients. If nutrients are added, this information is on the label. Values shown in this bulletin for these foods are usually based on products from several manufacturers and many differ somewhat from the values provided by any one source.

MORE INFORMATION FROM USDA

A number of other publications of the Agricultural Research Service, U. S. Department of Agriculture, give helpful information about nutrients and where they are found in foods.

Single copies of the following bulletins are free from the Office of Information, U. S. Department of Agriculture, Washington, D. C. 20250. Send your request on a post card and include your zip code.

Family Fare: A Guide to Good Nutrition .... G   1
Food and Your Weight... G 74
Conserving the Nutritive Values of Foods .... G 90
Calories and Weight: The USDA Pocket Guide..................... G 153

For a more highly technical publication with data on a much more extensive list of foods, see Agriculture Handbook No. 8,

"Composition of Foods ... raw, processed, prepared." In this handbook, data are presented for the nutrients in 100 grams of edible portion and one pound of food as purchased. The handbook is for sale by the Superintendent of Documents, U. S. Government Printing Office, Washington, D. C. 20402. The price is $1.50 per copy.

NUTRITIVE VALUES OF THE EDIBLE PART OF FOODS

[Dashes in the columns for nutrients show that no suitable value could be found although there is reason to believe that a measurable amount of the nutrient may be present]

Food, approximate measure, and weight (in grams)	Water	Food energy	Protein	Fat	Fatty acids Saturated (total)	Unsaturated Oleic	Linoleic	Carbohydrate	Calcium	Iron	Vitamin A value	Thiamin	Riboflavin	Niacin	Ascorbic acid
	Grams / Percent	Calories	Grams	Grams	Grams	Grams	Grams	Grams	Milligrams	Milligrams	International units	Milligrams	Milligrams	Milligrams	Milligrams
MILK, CHEESE, CREAM, IMITATION CREAM; RELATED PRODUCTS															
Milk:															
Fluid:															
1 Whole, 3.5% fat ---- 1 cup ------ 244	87	160	9	9	5	3	Trace	12	288	0.1	350	0.07	0.41	0.2	2
2 Nonfat (skim) ------ 1 cup ------ 245	90	90	9	Trace				12	296	.1	10	.09	.44	.2	2
3 Partly skimmed, 2% nonfat milk solids added. 1 cup ------ 246	87	145	10	5	3	2	Trace	15	352	.1	200	.10	.52	.2	2
Canned, concentrated, undiluted:															
4 Evaporated, unsweetened ---- 1 cup ------ 252	74	345	18	20	11	7	1	24	635	.3	810	.10	.86	.5	3
5 Condensed, sweetened ---- 1 cup ------ 306	27	980	25	27	15	9	1	166	802	.3	1,100	.24	1.16	.6	3
Dry, nonfat instant:															
6 Low-density (1⅓ cups needed for reconstitution to 1 qt.). 1 cup ------ 68	4	245	24	Trace				35	879	.4	[1]20	.24	1.21	.6	5
7 High-density (⅞ cup needed for reconstitution to 1 qt.). 1 cup ------ 104	4	375	37	1				54	1,345	.6	[1]30	.36	1.85	.9	7
Buttermilk:															
8 Fluid, cultured, made from skim milk. 1 cup ------ 245	90	90	9	Trace				12	296	.1	10	.10	.44	.2	2
9 Dried, packaged ------ 1 cup ------ 120	3	465	41	6	3	2	Trace	60	1,498	.7	260	.31	2.06	1.1	----
Cheese:															
Natural:															
Blue or Roquefort type:															
10 Ounce ------ 1 oz ------ 28	40	105	6	9	5	3	Trace	1	89	.1	350	.01	.17	.3	0
11 Cubic inch ------ 1 cu. in. ------ 17	40	65	4	5	3	2	Trace	Trace	54	.1	210	.01	.11	.2	0

[1] Value applies to unfortified product; value for fortified low-density product would be 1500 I.U., and the fortified high-density product would be 2290 I.U.

NUTRITIVE VALUES OF THE EDIBLE PART OF FOODS

[Dashes in the columns for nutrients show that no suitable value could be found although there is reason to believe that a measurable amount of the nutrient may be present]

	Food, approximate measure, and weight (in grams)		Water	Food energy	Protein	Fat	Fatty acids			Carbohydrate	Calcium	Iron	Vitamin A value	Thiamin	Riboflavin	Niacin	Ascorbic acid
							Saturated (total)	Unsaturated Oleic	Unsaturated Linoleic								
		Grams	Percent	Calories	Grams	Grams	Grams	Grams	Grams	Grams	Milligrams	Milligrams	International units	Milligrams	Milligrams	Milligrams	Milligrams
	MILK, CHEESE, CREAM, IMITATION CREAM; RELATED PRODUCTS—Con.																
	Cheese—Continued																
	Natural—Continued																
12	Camembert, packaged in 4-oz. pkg. with 3 wedges per pkg. 1 wedge	38	52	115	7	9	5	3	Trace	1	40	0.2	380	0.02	0.29	0.3	0
	Cheddar:																
13	Ounce 1 oz	28	37	115	7	9	5	3	Trace	1	213	.3	370	.01	.13	Trace	0
14	Cubic inch 1 cu. in.	17	37	70	4	6	3	2	Trace	Trace	129	.2	230	.01	.08	Trace	0
	Cottage, large or small curd:																
	Creamed:																
15	Package of 12-oz., net wt. 1 pkg	340	78	360	46	14	8	5	Trace	10	320	1.0	580	.10	.85	.3	0
16	Cup, curd pressed down. 1 cup	245	78	260	33	10	6	3	Trace	7	230	.7	420	.07	.61	.2	0
	Uncreamed:																
17	Package of 12-oz., net wt. 1 pkg	340	79	290	58	1	1	Trace	Trace	9	306	1.4	30	.10	.95	.3	0
18	Cup, curd pressed down. 1 cup	200	79	170	34	1	Trace	Trace	Trace	5	180	.8	20	.06	.56	.2	0
	Cream:																
19	Package of 8-oz., net wt. 1 pkg	227	51	850	18	86	48	28	3	5	141	.5	3,500	.05	.54	.2	0
20	Package of 3-oz., net wt. 1 pkg	85	51	320	7	32	18	11	1	2	53	.2	1,310	.02	.20	.1	0
21	Cubic inch 1 cu. in.	16	51	60	1	6	3	2	Trace	Trace	10	Trace	250	Trace	.04	Trace	0
	Parmesan, grated:																
22	Cup, pressed down. 1 cup	140	17	655	60	43	24	14	1	5	1,893	.7	1,760	.03	1.22	.3	0
23	Tablespoon 1 tbsp	5	17	25	2	2	1	Trace	Trace	Trace	68	Trace	60	Trace	.04	Trace	0
24	Ounce 1 oz	28	17	130	12	9	5	3	Trace	1	383	.1	360	.01	.25	.1	0
	Swiss:																
25	Ounce 1 oz	28	39	105	8	8	4	3	Trace	1	262	.3	320	Trace	.11	Trace	0
26	Cubic inch 1 cu. in.	15	39	55	4	4	2	1	Trace	Trace	139	.1	170	Trace	.06	Trace	0

No.	Food, approximate measure, and weight (in grams)	Measure	Grams	Water (%)	Food energy (cal.)	Protein (g)	Fat (g)	Saturated (total) (g)	Unsaturated Oleic (g)	Unsaturated Linoleic (g)	Carbohydrate (g)	Calcium (mg)	Iron (mg)	Vitamin A (I.U.)	Thiamin (mg)	Riboflavin (mg)	Niacin (mg)	Ascorbic acid (mg)
	Pasteurized processed cheese:																	
	American:																	
27	Ounce	1 oz.	28	40	105	7	9	5	3	Trace	1	198	.3	350	.01	.12	Trace	0
28	Cubic inch	1 cu. in.	18	40	65	4	5	3	2	Trace	Trace	122	.2	210	Trace	.07	Trace	0
	Swiss:																	
29	Ounce	1 oz.	28	40	100	8	8	4	3	Trace	1	251	.3	310	Trace	.11	Trace	0
30	Cubic inch	1 cu. in.	18	40	65	5	5	3	2	Trace	Trace	159	.2	200	Trace	.07	Trace	0
	Pasteurized process cheese food, American:																	
31	Tablespoon	1 tbsp.	14	43	45	3	3	2	1	Trace	1	80	.1	140	Trace	.08	Trace	0
32	Cubic inch	1 cu. in.	18	43	60	4	4	2	1	Trace	1	100	.1	170	Trace	.10	Trace	0
33	Pasteurized process cheese spread, American.	1 oz.	28	49	80	5	6	3	2	Trace	2	160	.2	250	Trace	.15	Trace	0
	Cream:																	
34	Half-and-half (cream and milk).	1 cup	242	80	325	8	28	15	9	1	11	261	.1	1,160	.07	.39	.1	2
35		1 tbsp.	15	80	20	1	2	1	1	Trace	1	16	Trace	70	Trace	.02	Trace	Trace
36	Light, coffee or table	1 cup	240	72	505	7	49	27	16	1	10	245	.1	2,020	.07	.36	.1	2
37		1 tbsp.	15	72	30	1	3	2	1	Trace	1	15	Trace	130	Trace	.02	Trace	Trace
38	Sour	1 cup	230	72	485	7	47	26	16	1	10	235	.1	1,930	.07	.35	.1	2
39		1 tbsp.	12	72	25	Trace	2	1	1	Trace	1	12	Trace	100	Trace	.02	Trace	Trace
40	Whipped topping (pressurized).	1 cup	60	62	155	2	14	8	5	Trace	6	67	---	570	---	.04	---	Trace
41		1 tbsp.	3	62	10	Trace	1	Trace	Trace	Trace	Trace	3	---	30	---	Trace	---	---
	Whipping, unwhipped (volume about double when whipped):																	
42	Light	1 cup	239	62	715	6	75	41	25	2	9	203	.1	3,060	.05	.29	.1	2
43		1 tbsp.	15	62	45	Trace	5	3	2	Trace	1	13	Trace	190	Trace	.02	Trace	Trace
44	Heavy	1 cup	238	57	840	5	90	50	30	3	7	179	.1	3,670	.05	.26	.1	2
45		1 tbsp.	15	57	55	Trace	6	3	2	Trace	1	11	Trace	230	Trace	.02	Trace	Trace
	Imitation cream products (made with vegetable fat):																	
	Creamers:																	
46	Powdered	1 cup	94	2	505	4	33	31	1	0	52	21	.6	²200	---	Trace	---	---
47		1 tsp.	2	2	10	Trace	1	Trace	Trace	0	1	1	Trace	²Trace	---	---	---	---
48	Liquid (frozen)	1 cup	245	77	345	3	27	25	1	0	25	29	---	²100	0	0	---	---
49		1 tbsp.	15	77	20	Trace	2	1	Trace	0	2	2	---	²10	0	0	---	---
50	Sour dressing (imitation sour cream) made with nonfat dry milk.	1 cup	235	72	440	9	38	35	1	Trace	17	277	.1	10	.07	.38	.2	1
51		1 tbsp.	12	72	20	1	2	2	Trace	Trace	1	14	Trace	Trace	Trace	Trace	---	Trace
	Whipped topping:																	
52	Pressurized	1 cup	70	61	190	1	17	15	1	0	9	5	---	²340	0	0	---	---
53		1 tbsp.	4	61	10	Trace	1	1	Trace	0	Trace	Trace	---	²20	0	0	---	---

² Contributed largely from beta-carotene used for coloring.

NUTRITIVE VALUES OF THE EDIBLE PART OF FOODS

[Dashes in the columns for nutrients show that no suitable value could be found although there is reason to believe that a measurable amount of the nutrient may be present]

	Food, approximate measure, and weight (in grams)	Water	Food energy	Protein	Fat	Fatty acids Saturated (total)	Fatty acids Unsaturated Oleic	Fatty acids Unsaturated Linoleic	Carbohydrate	Calcium	Iron	Vitamin A value	Thiamin	Riboflavin	Niacin	Ascorbic acid
		Percent	Calories	Grams	Grams	Grams	Grams	Grams	Grams	Milligrams	Milligrams	International units	Milligrams	Milligrams	Milligrams	Milligrams
	MILK, CHEESE, CREAM, IMITATION CREAM; RELATED PRODUCTS—Con.															
	Whipped topping—Continued															
54	Frozen 1 cup — 75	52	230	1	20	18	Trace	0	15	5	---	[2]560	---	0	---	---
55	1 tbsp — 4	52	10	Trace	1	1	Trace	0	1	Trace	---	[2]30	---	0	---	---
56	Powdered, made with whole milk. 1 cup — 75	58	175	3	12	10	1	Trace	15	62	Trace	[2]330	.02	.08	.1	Trace
57	1 tbsp — 4	58	10	Trace	1	1	Trace	Trace	1	3	Trace	[2]20	Trace	Trace	Trace	Trace
	Milk beverages:															
58	Cocoa, homemade — 1 cup — 250	79	245	10	12	7	4	Trace	27	295	1.0	400	.10	.45	.5	3
59	Chocolate-flavored drink made with skim milk and 2% added butterfat. 1 cup — 250	83	190	8	6	3	2	Trace	27	270	.5	210	.10	.40	.3	3
	Malted milk:															
60	Dry powder, approx. 3 heaping teaspoons per ounce. 1 oz. — 28	3	115	4	2	---	---	---	20	82	.6	290	.09	.15	.1	0
61	Beverage — 1 cup — 235	78	245	11	10	---	5	1	28	317	.7	590	.14	.49	.2	2
	Milk desserts:															
62	Custard, baked. 1 cup — 265	77	305	14	15	7	5	1	29	297	1.1	930	.11	.50	.3	1
	Ice cream:															
63	Regular (approx. 10% fat). ½ gal — 1,064	63	2,055	48	113	62	37	3	221	1,553	.5	4,680	.43	2.23	1.1	11
64	1 cup — 133	63	255	6	14	8	5	Trace	28	194	.1	590	.05	.28	.1	1
65	3 fl. oz. cup — 50	63	95	2	5	3	2	Trace	10	73	Trace	220	.02	.11	.1	1
66	Rich (approx. 16% fat). ½ gal — 1,188	63	2,635	31	191	105	63	6	214	927	.2	7,840	.24	1.31	1.2	12
67	1 cup — 148	63	330	4	24	13	8	1	27	115	Trace	980	.03	.16	.1	1
	Ice milk:															
68	Hardened — ½ gal — 1,048	67	1,595	50	53	29	17	2	235	1,635	1.0	2,200	.52	2.31	1.0	10
69	1 cup — 131	67	200	6	7	4	2	Trace	29	204	.1	280	.07	.29	.1	1
70	Soft-serve. 1 cup — 175	67	265	8	9	5	3	Trace	39	273	.2	370	.09	.39	.2	2

No.	Food	Measure	Grams	Water (%)	Food energy	Protein	Fat	Saturated	Oleic	Linoleic	Carbohydrate	Calcium	Iron	Vitamin A	Thiamine	Riboflavin	Niacin	Ascorbic acid
	Yoghurt:																	
71	Made from partially skimmed milk.	1 cup	245	89	125	8	4	2	1	Trace	13	294	.1	170	.10	.44	.2	2
72	Made from whole milk.	1 cup	245	88	150	7	8	5	3	Trace	12	272	.1	340	.07	.39	.2	2
	EGGS																	
	Eggs, large, 24 ounces per dozen:																	
	Raw or cooked in shell or with nothing added:																	
73	Whole, without shell	1 egg	50	74	80	6	6	2	3	Trace	Trace	27	1.1	590	.05	.15	Trace	0
74	White of egg	1 white	33	88	15	4	Trace	—	—	—	Trace	3	Trace	0	Trace	.09	Trace	0
75	Yolk of egg	1 yolk	17	51	60	3	5	2	2	Trace	Trace	24	.9	580	.04	.07	Trace	0
76	Scrambled with milk and fat.	1 egg	64	72	110	7	8	3	3	Trace	1	51	1.1	690	.05	.18	Trace	0
	MEAT, POULTRY, FISH, SHELLFISH; RELATED PRODUCTS																	
77	Bacon, (20 slices per lb. raw), broiled or fried, crisp.	2 slices	15	8	90	5	8	3	4	1	1	2	.5	0	.08	.05	.8	—
	Beef,² cooked:																	
	Cuts braised, simmered, or pot-roasted:																	
78	Lean and fat	3 ounces	85	53	245	23	16	8	7	Trace	0	10	2.9	30	.04	.18	3.5	—
79	Lean only	2.5 ounces	72	62	140	22	5	2	2	Trace	0	10	2.7	10	.04	.16	3.3	—
	Hamburger (ground beef), broiled:																	
80	Lean	3 ounces	85	60	185	23	10	5	4	Trace	0	10	3.0	20	.08	.20	5.1	—
81	Regular	3 ounces	85	54	245	21	17	8	8	Trace	0	9	2.7	30	.07	.18	4.6	—
	Roast, oven-cooked, no liquid added:																	
	Relatively fat, such as rib:																	
82	Lean and fat	3 ounces	85	40	375	17	34	16	15	1	0	8	2.2	70	.05	.13	3.1	—
83	Lean only	1.8 ounces	51	57	125	14	7	3	3	Trace	0	6	1.8	10	.04	.11	2.6	—
	Relatively lean, such as heel of round:																	
84	Lean and fat	3 ounces	85	62	165	25	7	3	3	Trace	0	11	3.2	10	.06	.19	4.5	—
85	Lean only	2.7 ounces	78	65	125	24	3	1	1	Trace	0	10	3.0	Trace	.06	.18	4.3	—
	Steak, broiled:																	
	Relatively fat, such as sirloin:																	
86	Lean and fat	3 ounces	85	44	330	20	27	13	12	1	0	9	2.5	50	.05	.16	4.0	—
87	Lean only	2.0 ounces	56	59	115	18	4	2	2	Trace	0	7	2.2	10	.05	.14	3.6	—
	Relatively lean, such as round:																	
88	Lean and fat	3 ounces	85	55	220	24	13	6	6	Trace	0	10	3.0	20	.07	.19	4.8	—
89	Lean only	2.4 ounces	68	61	130	21	4	2	2	Trace	0	9	2.5	10	.06	.16	4.1	—
	Beef, canned:																	
90	Corned beef	3 ounces	85	59	185	22	10	5	4	Trace	0	17	3.7	20	.01	.20	2.9	—
91	Corned beef hash	3 ounces	85	67	155	7	10	5	4	Trace	9	11	1.7	—	.01	.08	1.8	—
92	Beef, dried or chipped	2 ounces	57	48	115	19	4	2	2	Trace	0	11	2.9	—	.04	.18	2.2	—
93	Beef and vegetable stew	1 cup	235	82	210	15	10	5	4	Trace	15	28	2.8	2,810	.13	.17	4.4	15

¹ Contributed largely from beta-carotene used for coloring.

² Outer layer of fat on the cut was removed to within approximately ½-inch of the lean. Deposits of fat within the cut were not removed.

NUTRITIVE VALUES OF THE EDIBLE PART OF FOODS

[Dashes in the columns for nutrients show that no suitable value could be found although there is reason to believe that a measurable amount of the nutrient may be present]

	Food, approximate measure, and weight (in grams)	Water	Food energy	Pro-tein	Fat	Fatty acids Satu-rated (total)	Fatty acids Unsaturated Oleic	Fatty acids Unsaturated Lin-oleic	Carbo-hy-drate	Cal-cium	Iron	Vita-min A value	Thia-min	Ribo-flavin	Niacin	Ascor-bic acid
		Per cent	Calo-ries	Grams	Grams	Grams	Grams	Grams	Grams	Milli-grams	Milli-grams	Inter-national units	Milli-grams	Milli-grams	Milli-grams	Milli-grams
	MEAT, POULTRY, FISH, SHELLFISH; RELATED PRODUCTS—Continued															
94	Beef potpie, baked, 4¼-inch diam., weight before baking about 8 ounces. 1 pie -- 227 grams	55	560	23	33	9	20	2	43	32	4.1	1,860	0.25	0.27	4.5	7
	Chicken, cooked:															
95	Flesh only, broiled -- 3 ounces -- 85	71	115	20	3	1	1	1	0	8	1.4	80	.05	.16	7.4	--
	Breast, fried, ½ breast:															
96	With bone -- 3.3 ounces -- 94	58	155	25	5	1	2	1	1	9	1.3	70	.04	.17	11.2	--
97	Flesh and skin only -- 2.7 ounces -- 76	58	155	25	5	1	2	1	1	9	1.3	70	.04	.17	11.2	--
	Drumstick, fried:															
98	With bone -- 2.1 ounces -- 59	55	90	12	4	1	2	1	Trace	6	.9	50	.03	.15	2.7	--
99	Flesh and skin only -- 1.3 ounces -- 38	55	90	12	4	1	2	1	Trace	6	.9	50	.03	.15	2.7	--
100	Chicken, canned, boneless 3 ounces -- 85	65	170	18	10	3	4	2	0	18	1.3	200	.03	.11	3.7	3
101	Chicken potpie, baked 4¼-inch diam., weight before baking about 8 ounces. 1 pie -- 227	57	535	23	31	10	15	3	42	68	3.0	3,020	.25	.26	4.1	5
	Chili con carne, canned:															
102	With beans -- 1 cup -- 250	72	335	19	15	7	7	Trace	30	80	4.2	150	.08	.18	3.2	--
103	Without beans -- 1 cup -- 255	67	510	26	38	18	17	1	15	97	3.6	380	.05	.31	5.6	--
104	Heart, beef, lean, braised 3 ounces -- 85	61	160	27	5				1	5	5.0	20	.21	1.04	6.5	1
	Lamb,[3] cooked:															
105	Chop, thick, with bone, 1 chop, 4.8 ounces, broiled. 137	47	400	25	33	18	12	1	0	10	1.5	--	.14	.25	5.6	--
106	Lean and fat -- 4.0 ounces -- 112	47	400	25	33	18	12	1	0	10	1.5	--	.14	.25	5.6	--
107	Lean only -- 2.6 ounces -- 74	62	140	21	6	3	2	Trace	0	9	1.5	--	.11	.20	4.5	--
	Leg, roasted:															
108	Lean and fat -- 3 ounces -- 85	54	235	22	16	9	6	Trace	0	9	1.4	--	.13	.23	4.7	--
109	Lean only -- 2.5 ounces -- 71	62	130	20	5	3	2	Trace	0	9	1.4	--	.12	.21	4.4	--
	Shoulder, roasted:															
110	Lean and fat -- 3 ounces -- 85	50	285	18	23	13	8	1	0	9	1.0	--	.11	.20	4.0	--
111	Lean only -- 2.3 ounces -- 64	61	130	17	6	3	2	Trace	0	8	1.0	--	.10	.18	3.7	--

No.	Food, approximate measure	Weight (grams)	Water (%)	Food energy (cal.)	Protein (g)	Fat (g)	Saturated (g)	Oleic (g)	Linoleic (g)	Carbohydrate (g)	Calcium (mg)	Iron (mg)	Vitamin A (I.U.)	Thiamine (mg)	Riboflavin (mg)	Niacin (mg)	Ascorbic acid (mg)
112	Liver, beef, fried	2 ounces	57	57	130	15	6	—	—	—	3	8	5.0	30,280	.15	2.37	9.4	15
113	Ham, light cure, lean and fat, roasted.	3 ounces	85	54	245	18	19	7	8	2	0	8	2.2	0	.40	.16	3.1	—
	Luncheon meat:																	
114	Boiled ham, sliced	2 ounces	57	59	135	11	10	4	4	1	0	6	1.6	0	.25	.09	1.5	—
115	Canned, spiced or unspiced.	2 ounces	57	55	165	8	14	5	6	1	1	5	1.2	0	.18	.12	1.6	—
	Pork, fresh,[3] cooked:																	
116	Chop, thick, with bone.	1 chop, 3.5 ounces.	98	42	260	16	21	8	8	2	0	8	2.2	0	.63	.18	3.8	—
117	Lean and fat	2.3 ounces	66	42	260	16	21	8	8	2	0	8	2.2	0	.63	.18	3.8	—
118	Lean only	1.7 ounces	48	53	130	15	7	2	2	1	0	7	1.9	0	.54	.16	3.3	—
	Roast, oven-cooked, no liquid added:																	
119	Lean and fat	3 ounces	85	46	310	21	24	9	10	2	0	9	2.7	0	.78	.22	4.7	—
120	Lean only	2.4 ounces	68	55	175	20	10	3	4	1	0	9	2.6	0	.73	.21	4.4	—
	Cuts, simmered:																	
121	Lean and fat	3 ounces	85	46	320	20	26	9	11	2	0	8	2.5	0	.46	.21	4.1	—
122	Lean only	2.2 ounces	63	60	135	18	6	2	3	1	0	8	2.3	0	.42	.19	3.7	—
	Sausage:																	
123	Bologna, slice, 3-in. diam. by ⅛ inch.	2 slices	26	56	80	3	7	—	—	—	Trace	2	.5	—	.04	.06	.7	—
124	Braunschweiger, slice 2-in. diam. by ¼ inch.	2 slices	20	53	65	3	5	—	—	—	Trace	2	1.2	1,310	.03	.29	1.6	—
125	Deviled ham, canned	1 tbsp.	13	51	45	2	4	2	2	Trace	0	1	.3	0	.02	.01	.2	—
126	Frankfurter, heated (8 per lb. purchased pkg.).	1 frank.	56	57	170	7	15	—	—	—	1	3	.8	—	.08	.11	1.4	—
127	Pork links, cooked (16 links per lb. raw).	2 links	26	35	125	5	11	4	5	1	Trace	2	.6	0	.21	.09	1.0	—
128	Salami, dry type	1 oz.	28	30	130	7	11	—	—	—	Trace	4	1.0	—	.10	.07	1.5	—
129	Salami, cooked	1 oz.	28	51	90	5	7	—	—	—	Trace	3	.7	—	.07	.07	1.2	—
130	Vienna, canned (7 sausages per 5-oz. can).	1 sausage	16	63	40	2	3	—	—	—	Trace	1	.3	—	.01	.02	.4	—
	Veal, medium fat, cooked, bone removed:																	
131	Cutlet	3 oz.	85	60	185	23	9	5	4	Trace	0	9	2.7	—	.06	.21	4.6	—
132	Roast	3 oz.	85	55	230	23	14	7	6	Trace	0	10	2.9	—	.11	.26	6.6	—
	Fish and shellfish:																	
133	Bluefish, baked with table fat.	3 oz.	85	68	135	22	4	—	—	—	0	25	.6	40	.09	.08	1.6	—
	Clams:																	
134	Raw, meat only	3 oz.	85	82	65	11	1	—	—	—	2	59	5.2	90	.08	.15	1.1	8
135	Canned, solids and liquid.	3 oz.	85	86	45	7	1	—	—	—	2	47	3.5	—	.01	.09	.9	—
136	Crabmeat, canned	3 oz.	85	77	85	15	2	—	—	—	1	38	.7	—	.07	.07	1.6	—

[3] Outer layer of fat on the cut was removed to within approximately ½-inch of the lean. Deposits of fat within the cut were not removed.

NUTRITIVE VALUES OF THE EDIBLE PART OF FOODS

[Dashes in the columns for nutrients show that no suitable value could be found although there is reason to believe that a measurable amount of the nutrient may be present]

	Food, approximate measure, and weight (in grams)	Water	Food energy	Protein	Fat	Fatty acids Saturated (total)	Fatty acids Unsaturated Oleic	Fatty acids Unsaturated Linoleic	Carbohydrate	Calcium	Iron	Vitamin A value	Thiamin	Riboflavin	Niacin	Ascorbic acid
		Percent	Calories	Grams	Grams	Grams	Grams	Grams	Grams	Milligrams	Milligrams	International units	Milligrams	Milligrams	Milligrams	Milligrams
	MEAT, POULTRY, FISH, SHELLFISH; RELATED PRODUCTS—Continued															
	Fish and shellfish—Continued															
137	Fish sticks, breaded, cooked, frozen; stick 3¾ by 1 by ½ inch. 10 sticks or 8 oz. pkg. 227	66	400	38	20	5	4	10	15	25	0.9	------	0.09	0.16	3.6	------
138	Haddock, breaded, fried 3 oz. 85	66	140	17	5	1	3	Trace	5	34	1.0	------	.03	.06	2.7	2
139	Ocean perch, breaded, fried 3 oz. 85	59	195	16	11	----	----	----	6	28	1.1	------	.08	.09	1.5	------
140	Oysters, raw, meat only (13-19 med. selects). 1 cup 240	85	160	20	4	----	----	----	8	226	13.2	740	.33	.43	6.0	------
141	Salmon, pink, canned 3 oz. 85	71	120	17	5	1	1	Trace	0	⁴167	.7	60	.03	.16	6.8	------
142	Sardines, Atlantic, canned in oil, drained solids. 3 oz. 85	62	175	20	9	----	----	----	0	372	2.5	190	.02	.17	4.6	------
143	Shad, baked with table fat and bacon. 3 oz. 85	64	170	20	10	----	----	----	0	20	.5	20	.11	.22	7.3	------
144	Shrimp, canned, meat. 3 oz. 85	70	100	21	1	----	----	----	1	98	2.6	50	.01	.03	1.5	------
145	Swordfish, broiled with butter or margarine. 3 oz. 85	65	150	24	5	----	----	----	0	23	1.1	1,750	.03	.04	9.3	------
146	Tuna, canned in oil, drained solids. 3 oz. 85	61	170	24	7	2	1	1	0	7	1.6	70	.04	.10	10.1	------
	MATURE DRY BEANS AND PEAS, NUTS, PEANUTS; RELATED PRODUCTS															
147	Almonds, shelled, whole 1 cup 142	5	850	26	77	6	52	15	28	332	6.7	0	.34	1.31	5.0	Trace
	Beans, dry: Common varieties as Great Northern, navy, and others: Cooked, drained:															
148	Great Northern. 1 cup 180	69	210	14	1				38	90	4.9	0	.25	.13	1.3	0

No.	Food	Measure	Grams	Water (%)	Food energy	Protein	Fat	Saturated fatty acids	Oleic	Linoleic	Carbohydrate	Calcium	Iron	Vitamin A	Thiamine	Riboflavin	Niacin	Ascorbic acid
149	Navy (pea) Canned, solids and liquid: White with—	1 cup	190	69	225	15	1	—	—	—	40	95	5.1	0	.27	.13	1.3	0
150	Frankfurters (sliced).	1 cup	255	71	365	19	18	—	—	—	32	94	4.8	330	.18	.15	3.3	Trace
151	Pork and tomato sauce.	1 cup	255	71	310	16	7	2	3	1	49	138	4.6	330	.20	.08	1.5	5
152	Pork and sweet sauce.	1 cup	255	66	385	16	12	4	5	1	54	161	5.9	—	.15	.10	1.3	—
153	Red kidney.	1 cup	255	76	230	15	1	—	—	—	42	74	4.6	10	.13	.10	1.5	—
154	Lima, cooked, drained.	1 cup	190	64	260	16	1	—	—	—	49	55	5.9	—	.25	.11	1.3	—
155	Cashew nuts, roasted.	1 cup	140	5	785	24	64	11	45	4	41	53	5.3	140	.60	.35	2.5	—
156	Coconut, fresh, meat only: Pieces, approx. 2 by 2 by ½ inch.	1 piece	45	51	155	2	16	14	1	Trace	4	6	.8	0	.02	.01	.2	1
157	Shredded or grated, firmly packed.	1 cup	130	51	450	5	46	39	3	Trace	12	17	2.2	0	.07	.03	.7	4
158	Cowpeas or blackeye peas, dry, cooked.	1 cup	248	80	190	13	1	—	—	—	34	42	3.2	20	.41	.11	1.1	Trace
159	Peanuts, roasted, salted, halves.	1 cup	144	2	840	37	72	16	31	21	27	107	3.0	—	.46	.19	24.7	0
160	Peanut butter.	1 tbsp.	16	2	95	4	8	2	4	2	3	9	.3	—	.02	.02	2.4	0
161	Peas, split, dry, cooked.	1 cup	250	70	290	20	1	—	—	—	52	28	4.2	100	.37	.22	2.2	0
162	Pecans, halves.	1 cup	108	3	740	10	77	5	48	15	16	79	2.6	140	.93	.14	1.0	2
163	Walnuts, black or native, chopped.	1 cup	126	3	790	26	75	4	26	36	19	Trace	7.6	380	.28	.14	.9	—

VEGETABLES AND VEGETABLE PRODUCTS

No.	Food	Measure	Grams	Water (%)	Food energy	Protein	Fat	Saturated fatty acids	Oleic	Linoleic	Carbohydrate	Calcium	Iron	Vitamin A	Thiamine	Riboflavin	Niacin	Ascorbic acid
164	Asparagus, green: Cooked, drained: Spears, ½-in. diam. at base.	4 spears	60	94	10	1	Trace				2	13	.4	540	.10	.11	.8	16
165	Pieces, 1½ to 2-in. lengths.	1 cup	145	94	30	3	Trace				5	30	.9	1,310	.23	.26	2.0	38
166	Canned, solids and liquid.	1 cup	244	94	45	5	1				7	44	4.1	1,240	.15	.22	2.0	37
167	Beans: Lima, immature seeds, cooked, drained.	1 cup	170	71	190	13	1				34	80	4.3	480	.31	.17	2.2	29
168	Snap: Green: Cooked, drained.	1 cup	125	92	30	2	Trace				7	63	.8	680	.09	.11	.6	15
169	Canned, solids and liquid.	1 cup	239	94	45	2	Trace				10	81	2.9	690	.07	.10	.7	10

⁴ If bones are discarded, value will be greatly reduced.

NUTRITIVE VALUES OF THE EDIBLE PART OF FOODS

[Dashes in the columns for nutrients show that no suitable value could be found although there is reason to believe that a measurable amount of the nutrient may be present]

	Food, approximate measure, and weight (in grams)	Water	Food energy	Protein	Fat	Fatty acids Saturated (total)	Fatty acids Unsaturated Oleic	Fatty acids Unsaturated Linoleic	Carbohydrate	Calcium	Iron	Vitamin A value	Thiamin	Riboflavin	Niacin	Ascorbic acid
		Grams	Per cent	Calories	Grams	Grams	Grams	Grams	Grams	Grams	Milligrams	Milligrams	International units	Milligrams	Milligrams	Milligrams	Milligrams
	VEGETABLES AND VEGETABLE PRODUCTS—Continued																
	Beans—Continued																
	Snap—Continued																
	Yellow or wax:																
170	Cooked, drained___ 1 cup_____	125	93	30	2	Trace			6	63	0.8	290	0.09	0.11	0.6	16
171	Canned, solids and liquid. 1 cup_____	239	94	45	2	1			10	81	2.9	140	.07	.10	.7	12
172	Sprouted mung beans, cooked, drained. 1 cup_____	125	91	35	4	Trace			7	21	1.1	30	.11	.13	.9	8
	Beets:																
173	Cooked, drained, peeled: Whole beets, 2-in. diam. 2 beets_____	100	91	30	1	Trace			7	14	.5	20	.03	.04	.3	6
174	Diced or sliced_____ 1 cup_____	170	91	55	2	Trace			12	24	.9	30	.05	.07	.5	10
175	Canned, solids and liquid. 1 cup_____	246	90	85	2	Trace			19	34	1.5	20	.02	.05	.2	7
176	Beet greens, leaves and stems, cooked, drained. 1 cup_____	145	94	25	3	Trace			5	144	2.8	7,400	.10	.22	.4	22
	Blackeye peas. See Cowpeas.																
	Broccoli, cooked, drained:																
177	Whole stalks, medium size. 1 stalk_____	180	91	45	6	1			8	158	1.4	4,500	.16	.36	1.4	162
178	Stalks cut into ½-in. pieces. 1 cup_____	155	91	40	5	1			7	136	1.2	3,880	.14	.31	1.2	140
179	Chopped, yield from 10-oz. frozen pkg. 1¾ cups____	250	92	65	7	1			12	185	1.8	6,500	.15	.30	1.3	143
180	Brussels sprouts, 7–8 sprouts (1¼ to 1½ in. diam.) per cup, cooked. 1 cup_____	155	88	55	7	1			10	50	1.7	810	.12	.22	1.2	135
	Cabbage:																
	Common varieties:																

No.		Measure	Water	Food energy	Protein	Fat				Carbohydrate	Calcium	Iron	Vitamin A	Thiamine	Riboflavin	Niacin	Ascorbic acid
	Raw:																
181	Coarsely shredded or sliced.	1 cup	70	92	15	1	Trace	---	---	---	4	34	.3	90	.04	.04	.2	33
182	Finely shredded or chopped.	1 cup	90	92	20	1	Trace	---	---	---	5	44	.4	120	.05	.05	.3	42
183	Cooked.	1 cup	145	94	30	2	Trace	---	---	---	6	64	.4	190	.06	.06	.4	48
184	Red, raw, coarsely shredded.	1 cup	70	90	20	1	Trace	---	---	---	5	29	.6	30	.06	.04	.3	43
185	Savoy, raw, coarsely shredded.	1 cup	70	92	15	2	Trace	---	---	---	3	47	.6	140	.04	.06	.2	39
186	Cabbage, celery or Chinese, raw, cut in 1-in. pieces.	1 cup	75	95	10	1	Trace	---	---	---	2	32	.5	110	.03	.03	.5	19
187	Cabbage, spoon (or pakchoy), cooked.	1 cup	170	95	25	2	Trace	---	---	---	4	252	1.0	5,270	.07	.14	1.2	26
	Carrots:																
	Raw:																
188	Whole, 5½ by 1 inch, (25 thin strips).	1 carrot	50	88	20	1	Trace	---	---	---	5	18	.4	5,500	.03	.03	.3	4
189	Grated.	1 cup	110	88	45	1	Trace	---	---	---	11	41	.8	12,100	.06	.06	.7	9
190	Cooked, diced.	1 cup	145	91	45	1	Trace	---	---	---	10	48	.9	15,220	.08	.07	.7	9
191	Canned, strained or chopped (baby food).	1 ounce	28	92	10	Trace	Trace	---	---	---	2	7	.1	3,690	.01	.01	.1	1
192	Cauliflower, cooked, flowerbuds.	1 cup	120	93	25	3	Trace	---	---	---	5	25	.8	70	.11	.10	.7	66
	Celery, raw:																
193	Stalk, large outer, 8 by about 1½ inches, at root end.	1 stalk	40	94	5	Trace	Trace	---	---	---	2	16	.1	100	.01	.01	.1	4
194	Pieces, diced.	1 cup	100	94	15	1	Trace	---	---	---	4	39	.3	240	.03	.03	.3	9
195	Collards, cooked.	1 cup	190	91	55	5	1	---	---	---	9	289	1.1	10,260	.27	.37	2.4	87
	Corn, sweet:																
196	Cooked, ear 5 by 1¾ inches.[5]	1 ear	140	74	70	3	1	---	---	---	16	2	.5	[6]310	.09	.08	1.0	7
197	Canned, solids and liquid.	1 cup	256	81	170	5	2	---	---	---	40	10	1.0	[6]690	.07	.12	2.3	13
198	Cowpeas, cooked, immature seeds.	1 cup	160	72	175	13	1	---	---	---	29	38	3.4	560	.49	.18	2.3	28
	Cucumbers, 10-ounce; 7½ by about 2 inches:																
199	Raw, pared.	1 cucumber	207	96	30	1	Trace	---	---	---	7	35	.6	Trace	.07	.09	.4	23
200	Raw, pared, center slice ⅛-inch thick.	6 slices	50	96	5	Trace	Trace	---	---	---	2	8	.2	Trace	.02	.02	.1	6
201	Dandelion greens, cooked.	1 cup	180	90	60	4	1	---	---	---	12	252	3.2	21,060	.24	.29		32

[5] Measure and weight apply to entire vegetable or fruit including parts not usually eaten.

[6] Based on yellow varieties: white varieties contain only a trace of cryptoxanthin and carotenes, the pigments in corn that have biological activity.

NUTRITIVE VALUES OF THE EDIBLE PART OF FOODS

[Dashes in the columns for nutrients show that no suitable value could be found although there is reason to believe that a measurable amount of the nutrient may be present]

	Food, approximate measure, and weight (in grams)	Water	Food energy	Protein	Fat	Fatty acids Saturated (total)	Unsaturated Oleic	Linoleic	Carbohydrate	Calcium	Iron	Vitamin A value	Thiamin	Riboflavin	Niacin	Ascorbic acid
		Per cent	Calories	Grams	Grams	Grams	Grams	Grams	Grams	Milligrams	Milligrams	International units	Milligrams	Milligrams	Milligrams	Milligrams
	VEGETABLES AND VEGETABLE PRODUCTS—Continued															
202	Endive, curly (including escarole). 2 ounces___ 57 Grams	93	10	1	Trace	---			2	46	1.0	1,870	0.04	0.08	0.3	6
203	Kale, leaves including stems, cooked. 1 cup___ 110	91	30	4	1	---			4	147	1.3	8,140	---	---	---	68
	Lettuce, raw:															
204	Butterhead, as Boston types; head, 4-inch diameter. 1 head___ 220	95	30	3	Trace	---			6	77	4.4	2,130	.14	.13	.6	18
205	Crisphead, as Iceberg; head, 4¾-inch diameter. 1 head___ 454	96	60	4	Trace	---			13	91	2.3	1,500	.29	.27	1.3	29
206	Looseleaf, or bunching varieties, leaves. 2 large___ 50	94	10	1	Trace	---			2	34	.7	950	.03	.04	.2	9
207	Mushrooms, canned, solids and liquid. 1 cup___ 244	93	40	5	Trace	---			6	15	1.2	Trace	.04	.60	4.8	4
208	Mustard greens, cooked. 1 cup___ 140	93	35	3	1	---			6	193	2.5	8,120	.11	.19	.9	68
209	Okra, cooked, pod 3 by ⅝ inch. 8 pods___ 85	91	25	2	Trace	---			5	78	.4	420	.11	.15	.8	17
	Onions:															
	Mature:															
210	Raw, onion 2½-inch diameter. 1 onion___ 110	89	40	2	Trace	---			10	30	.6	40	.04	.04	.2	11
211	Cooked. 1 cup___ 210	92	60	3	Trace	---			14	50	.8	80	.06	.06	.4	14
212	Young green, small, without tops. 6 onions___ 50	88	20	1	Trace	---			5	20	.3	Trace	.02	.02	.2	12
213	Parsley, raw, chopped. 1 tablespoon___ 4	85	Trace	Trace	Trace	---			Trace	8	.2	340	Trace	.01	Trace	7
214	Parsnips, cooked. 1 cup___ 155	82	100	2	1	---			23	70	.9	50	.11	.12	.2	16
	Peas, green:															
215	Cooked. 1 cup___ 160	82	115	9	1	---			19	37	2.9	860	.44	.17	3.7	33
216	Canned, solids and liquid. 1 cup___ 249	83	165	9	1	---			31	50	4.2	1,120	.23	.13	2.2	22

No.	Food, approximate measure	Measure	Weight (g)	Water (%)	Food energy (cal.)	Protein (g)	Fat (g)	Sat. fatty acids (g)	Oleic (g)	Linoleic (g)	Carbohydrate (g)	Calcium (mg)	Iron (mg)	Vit. A (I.U.)	Thiamine (mg)	Riboflavin (mg)	Niacin (mg)	Ascorbic acid (mg)
217	Canned, strained (baby food).	1 ounce	28	86	15	1	Trace	—	—	—	3	3	.4	140	.02	.02	.4	3
218	Peppers, hot, red, without seeds, dried (ground chili powder, added seasonings).	1 tablespoon	15	8	50	2	2	—	—	—	8	40	2.3	9,750	.03	.17	1.3	2
	Peppers, sweet: Raw, about 5 per pound:																	
219	Green pod without stem and seeds.	1 pod	74	93	15	1	Trace	—	—	—	4	7	.5	310	.06	.06	.4	94
220	Cooked, boiled, drained	1 pod	73	95	15	1	Trace	—	—	—	3	7	.4	310	.05	.05	.4	70
	Potatoes, medium (about 3 per pound raw):																	
221	Baked, peeled after baking.	1 potato	99	75	90	3	Trace	—	—	—	21	9	.7	Trace	.10	.04	1.7	20
	Boiled:																	
222	Peeled after boiling	1 potato	136	80	105	3	Trace	—	—	—	23	10	.8	Trace	.13	.05	2.0	22
223	Peeled before boiling	1 potato	122	83	80	2	Trace	—	—	—	18	7	.6	Trace	.11	.04	1.4	20
224	French-fried, piece 2 by ½ by ½ inch: Cooked in deep fat	10 pieces	57	45	155	2	7	2	2	4	20	9	.7	Trace	.07	.04	1.8	12
225	Frozen, heated	10 pieces	57	53	125	2	5	1	1	2	19	5	1.0	Trace	.08	.01	1.5	12
	Mashed:																	
226	Milk added	1 cup	195	83	125	4	1	—	—	—	25	47	.8	50	.16	.10	2.0	19
227	Milk and butter added.	1 cup	195	80	185	4	8	4	3	Trace	24	47	.8	330	.16	.10	1.9	18
228	Potato chips, medium, 2-inch diameter.	10 chips	20	2	115	1	8	2	2	4	10	8	.4	Trace	.04	.01	1.0	3
229	Pumpkin, canned	1 cup	228	90	75	2	1	—	—	—	18	57	.9	14,590	.07	.12	1.3	12
230	Radishes, raw, small, without tops.	4 radishes	40	94	5	Trace	Trace	—	—	—	1	12	.4	Trace	.01	.01	.1	10
231	Sauerkraut, canned, solids and liquid.	1 cup	235	93	45	2	Trace	—	—	—	9	85	1.2	120	.07	.09	.4	33
	Spinach:																	
232	Cooked	1 cup	180	92	40	5	1	—	—	—	6	167	4.0	14,580	.13	.25	4.0	50
233	Canned, drained solids.	1 cup	180	91	45	5	1	—	—	—	6	212	4.7	14,400	.03	.21	4.7	24
	Squash: Cooked:																	
234	Summer, diced	1 cup	210	96	30	2	Trace	—	—	—	7	52	.8	820	.10	.16	.8	21
235	Winter, baked, mashed.	1 cup	205	81	130	4	1	—	—	—	32	57	1.6	8,610	.10	.27	1.6	27
	Sweetpotatoes: Cooked, medium, 5 by 2 inches, weight raw about 6 ounces:																	
236	Baked, peeled after baking.	1 sweetpotato	110	64	155	2	1	—	—	—	36	44	1.0	8,910	.10	.07	.7	24
237	Boiled, peeled after boiling.	1 sweetpotato	147	71	170	2	1	—	—	—	39	47	1.0	11,610	.13	.09	.9	25

NUTRITIVE VALUES OF THE EDIBLE PART OF FOODS

[Dashes in the columns for nutrients show that no suitable value could be found although there is reason to believe that a measurable amount of the nutrient may be present]

	Food, approximate measure, and weight (in grams)	Water	Food energy	Protein	Fat	Fatty acids Saturated (total)	Fatty acids Unsaturated Oleic	Fatty acids Unsaturated Linoleic	Carbohydrate	Calcium	Iron	Vitamin A value	Thiamin	Riboflavin	Niacin	Ascorbic acid
		Per cent	Calories	Grams	Grams	Grams	Grams	Grams	Grams	Milligrams	Milligrams	International units	Milligrams	Milligrams	Milligrams	Milligrams
	VEGETABLES AND VEGETABLE PRODUCTS—Continued															
	Sweetpotatoes—Continued															
238	Candied, 3½ by 2¼ inches. — 1 sweet-potato. — Grams 175	60	295	2	6	2	3	1	60	65	1.6	11,030	0.10	0.08	0.8	17
239	Canned, vacuum or solid pack. — 1 cup — 218	72	235	4	Trace				54	54	1.7	17,000	.10	.10	1.4	30
	Tomatoes:															
240	Raw, approx. 3-in. diam. 2⅛ in. high; wt., 7 oz. — 1 tomato — 200	94	40	2	Trace				9	24	.9	1,640	.11	.07	1.3	[7] 42
241	Canned, solids and liquid. — 1 cup — 241	94	50	2	1				10	14	1.2	2,170	.12	.07	1.7	41
	Tomato catsup:															
242	Cup — 1 cup — 273	69	290	6	1				69	60	2.2	3,820	.25	.19	4.4	41
243	Tablespoon — 1 tbsp. — 15	69	15	Trace	Trace				4	3	.1	210	.01	.01	.2	2
	Tomato juice, canned:															
244	Cup — 1 cup — 243	94	45	2	Trace				10	17	2.2	1,940	.12	.07	1.9	39
245	Glass (6 fl. oz.) — 1 glass — 182	94	35	2	Trace				8	13	1.6	1,460	.09	.05	1.5	29
246	Turnips, cooked, diced — 1 cup — 155	94	35	1	Trace				8	54	.6	Trace	.06	.08	.5	34
247	Turnip greens, cooked — 1 cup — 145	94	30	3	Trace				5	252	1.5	8,270	.15	.33	.7	68
	FRUITS AND FRUIT PRODUCTS															
248	Apples, raw (about 3 per lb.).[5] — 1 apple — 150	85	70	Trace	Trace				18	8	.4	50	.04	.02	.1	3
249	Apple juice, bottled or canned. — 1 cup — 248	88	120	Trace	Trace				30	15	1.5	---	.02	.05	.2	2
	Applesauce, canned:															
250	Sweetened — 1 cup — 255	76	230	1	Trace				61	10	1.3	100	.05	.03	.1	[8] 3
251	Unsweetened or artificially sweetened. — 1 cup — 244	88	100	1	Trace				26	10	1.2	100	.05	.02	.1	[8] 2

No.	Food, approximate measure, and weight (grams)	Water (percent)	Food energy (calories)	Protein (grams)	Fat (grams)	Saturated fatty acids (grams)	Unsaturated Oleic (grams)	Unsaturated Linoleic (grams)	Carbohydrate (grams)	Calcium (mg)	Iron (mg)	Vitamin A value (I.U.)	Thiamine (mg)	Riboflavin (mg)	Niacin (mg)	Ascorbic acid (mg)
	Apricots:															
252	Raw (about 12 per lb.)⁵ 3 apricots ... 114	85	55	1	Trace				14	18	.5	2,890	.03	.04	.7	10
253	Canned in heavy sirup 1 cup ... 259	77	220	2	Trace				57	28	.8	4,510	.05	.06	.9	10
254	Dried, uncooked (40 halves per cup) 1 cup ... 150	25	390	8	1				100	100	8.2	16,350	.02	.23	4.9	19
255	Cooked, unsweetened, fruit and liquid. 1 cup ... 285	76	240	5	1				62	63	5.1	8,550	.01	.13	2.8	8
256	Apricot nectar, canned... 1 cup ... 251	85	140	1	Trace				37	23	.5	2,380	.03	.03	.5	⁸8
	Avocados, whole fruit, raw:⁵															
257	California (mid- and late-winter; diam. 3⅛ in.). 1 avocado ... 284	74	370	5	37	7	17	5	13	22	1.3	630	.24	.43	3.5	30
258	Florida (late summer, fall; diam. 3⅝ in.). 1 avocado ... 454	78	390	4	33	7	15	4	27	30	1.8	880	.33	.61	4.9	43
259	Bananas, raw, medium size.⁵ 1 banana ... 175	76	100	1	Trace				26	10	.8	230	.06	.07	.8	12
260	Banana flakes. 1 cup ... 100	3	340	4	1				89	32	2.8	760	.18	.24	2.8	7
261	Blackberries, raw. 1 cup ... 144	84	85	2	1				19	46	1.3	290	.05	.06	.5	30
262	Blueberries, raw. 1 cup ... 140	83	85	1	1				21	21	1.4	140	.04	.08	.6	20
263	Cantaloups, raw; medium, 5-inch diameter about 1⅔ pounds.⁵ ½ melon ... 385	91	60	1	Trace				14	27	.8	⁹6,540	.08	.06	1.2	63
264	Cherries, canned, red, sour, pitted, water pack. 1 cup ... 244	88	105	2	Trace				26	37	.7	1,660	.07	.05	.5	12
265	Cranberry juice cocktail, canned. 1 cup ... 250	83	165	Trace	Trace				42	13	.8	Trace	.03	.03	.1	¹⁰40
266	Cranberry sauce, sweetened, canned, strained. 1 cup ... 277	62	405	Trace	1				104	17	.6	60	.03	.03	.1	6
267	Dates, pitted, cut. 1 cup ... 178	22	490	4	1				130	105	5.3	90	.16	.17	3.9	0
268	Figs, dried, large, 2 by 1 in. 1 fig ... 21	23	60	1	Trace				15	26	.6	20	.02	.02	.1	0
269	Fruit cocktail, canned, in heavy sirup. 1 cup ... 256	80	195	1	Trace				50	23	1.0	360	.05	.03	1.3	5

⁵ Measure and weight apply to entire vegetable or fruit including parts not usually eaten.

⁷ Year-round average. Samples marketed from November through May, average 20 milligrams per 200-gram tomato; from June through October, around 52 milligrams.

⁸ This is the amount from the fruit. Additional ascorbic acid may be added by the manufacturer. Refer to the label for this information.

⁹ Value for varieties with orange-colored flesh; value for varieties with green flesh would be about 540 I.U.

¹⁰ Value listed is based on products with label stating 30 milligrams per 6 fl. oz. serving.

NUTRITIVE VALUES OF THE EDIBLE PART OF FOODS

[Dashes in the columns for nutrients show that no suitable value could be found although there is reason to believe that a measurable amount of the nutrient may be present]

Food, approximate measure, and weight (in grams)		Water	Food energy	Protein	Fat	Fatty acids			Carbohydrate	Calcium	Iron	Vitamin A value	Thiamin	Riboflavin	Niacin	Ascorbic acid
						Saturated (total)	Unsaturated									
							Oleic	Linoleic								
	Grams	Percent	Calories	Grams	Grams	Grams	Grams	Grams	Grams	Milligrams	Milligrams	International units	Milligrams	Milligrams	Milligrams	Milligrams
FRUITS AND FRUIT PRODUCTS—Con.																
Grapefruit:																
Raw, medium, 3¾-in. diam.:[3]																
270 White ½ grapefruit.	241	89	45	1	Trace				12	19	0.5	10	0.05	0.02	0.2	44
271 Pink or red ½ grapefruit.	241	89	50	1	Trace				13	20	0.5	540	0.05	0.02	0.2	44
272 Canned, sirup pack 1 cup	254	81	180	2	Trace				45	33	.8	30	.08	.05	.5	76
Grapefruit juice:																
273 Fresh 1 cup	246	90	95	1	Trace				23	22	.5	(14)	.09	.04	.4	92
Canned, white:																
274 Unsweetened 1 cup	247	89	100	1	Trace				24	20	1.0	20	.07	.04	.4	84
275 Sweetened 1 cup	250	86	130	1	Trace				32	20	1.0	20	.07	.04	.4	78
Frozen, concentrate, unsweetened:																
276 Undiluted, can, 6 fluid ounces. 1 can	207	62	300	4	1				72	70	.8	60	.29	.12	1.4	286
277 Diluted with 3 parts water, by volume. 1 cup	247	89	100	1	Trace				24	25	.2	20	.10	.04	.5	96
278 Dehydrated crystals 4 oz.	113	1	410	6	1				102	100	1.2	80	.40	.20	2.0	396
279 Prepared with water 1 cup (1 pound yields about 1 gallon).	247	90	100	1	Trace				24	22	.2	20	.10	.05	.5	91
Grapes, raw:[5]																
280 American type (slip skin). 1 cup	153	82	65	1	1				15	15	.4	100	.05	.03	.2	3
281 European type (adherent skin). 1 cup	160	81	95	1	Trace				25	17	.6	140	.07	.04	.4	6
Grapejuice:																
282 Canned or bottled 1 cup	253	83	165	1	Trace				42	28	.8		.10	.05	.5	Trace
Frozen concentrate, sweetened:																
283 Undiluted, can, 6 fluid ounces. 1 can	216	53	395	1	Trace				100	22	.9	40	.13	.22	1.5	(14)

No.	Food	Measure	Weight (g)	Water (%)	Food energy	Protein	Fat		Carbohydrate	Calcium	Iron	Vitamin A	Thiamine	Riboflavin	Niacin	Ascorbic acid
284	Diluted with 3 parts water, by volume.	1 cup	250	86	135	1	Trace	-----	33	8	.3	10	.05	.08	.5	(12)
285	Grapejuice drink, canned.	1 cup	250	86	135	Trace	Trace	-----	35	8	.3	--	.03	.03	.3	(12)
286	Lemons, raw, 2⅛-in. diam., size 165.[5] Used for juice.	1 lemon	110	90	20	1	Trace	-----	6	19	.4	10	.03	.01	.1	39
287	Lemon juice, raw.	1 cup	244	91	60	1	Trace	-----	20	17	.5	50	.07	.02	.2	112
	Lemonade concentrate:															
288	Frozen, 6 fl. oz. per can.	1 can	219	48	430	Trace	Trace	-----	112	9	.4	40	.04	.07	.7	66
289	Diluted with 4⅓ parts water, by volume.	1 cup	248	88	110	Trace	Trace	-----	28	2	Trace	Trace	Trace	.02	.2	17
	Lime juice:															
290	Fresh.	1 cup	246	90	65	1	Trace	-----	22	22	.5	20	.05	.02	.2	79
291	Canned, unsweetened.	1 cup	246	90	65	1	Trace	-----	22	22	.5	20	.05	.02	.2	52
	Limeade concentrate, frozen:															
292	Undiluted, can, 6 fluid ounces.	1 can	218	50	410	Trace	Trace	-----	108	11	.2	Trace	.02	.02	.2	26
293	Diluted with 4⅓ parts water, by volume.	1 cup	247	90	100	Trace	Trace	-----	27	2	Trace	Trace	Trace	Trace	Trace	5
294	Oranges, raw, 2⅝-in. diam., all commercial varieties.[5]	1 orange	180	86	65	1	Trace	-----	16	54	.5	260	.13	.05	.5	66
295	Orange juice, fresh, all varieties.	1 cup	248	88	110	2	1	-----	26	27	.5	500	.22	.07	1.0	124
296	Canned, unsweetened.	1 cup	249	87	120	2	Trace	-----	28	25	1.0	500	.17	.05	.7	100
	Frozen concentrate:															
297	Undiluted, can, 6 fluid ounces.	1 can	213	55	360	5	Trace	-----	87	75	.9	1,620	.68	.11	2.8	360
298	Diluted with 3 parts water, by volume.	1 cup	249	87	120	2	Trace	-----	29	25	.2	550	.22	.02	1.0	120
299	Dehydrated crystals.	4 oz	113	1	430	6	2	-----	100	95	1.9	1,900	.76	.24	3.3	408
300	Prepared with water (1 pound yields about 1 gallon).	1 cup	248	88	115	2	1	-----	27	25	.5	500	.20	.07	1.0	109
301	Orange-apricot juice drink.	1 cup	249	87	125	1	Trace	-----	32	12	.2	1,440	.05	.02	.5	[10] 40

[5] Measure and weight apply to entire vegetable or fruit including parts not usually eaten.

[10] Value listed is based on product with label stating 30 milligrams per 6 fl. oz. serving.

[11] For white-fleshed varieties value is about 20 I.U. per cup; for red-fleshed varieties, 1,080 I.U. per cup.

[12] Present only if added by the manufacturer. Refer to the label for this information.

NUTRITIVE VALUES OF THE EDIBLE PART OF FOODS

[Dashes in the columns for nutrients show that no suitable value could be found although there is reason to believe that a measurable amount of the nutrient may be present]

Food, approximate measure, and weight (in grams)	Water	Food energy	Protein	Fat	Fatty acids Saturated (total)	Unsaturated Oleic	Unsaturated Linoleic	Carbohydrate	Calcium	Iron	Vitamin A value	Thiamin	Riboflavin	Niacin	Ascorbic acid
	Per cent	Calories	Grams	Grams	Grams	Grams	Grams	Grams	Milligrams	Milligrams	International units	Milligrams	Milligrams	Milligrams	Milligrams
FRUITS AND FRUIT PRODUCTS—Con.															
Orange and grapefruit juice:															
Frozen concentrate:															
302 Undiluted, can, 6 fluid ounces. 1 can 210	59	330	4	1				78	61	0.8	800	0.48	0.06	2.3	302
303 Diluted with 3 parts water, by volume. 1 cup 248	88	110	1	Trace				26	20	.2	270	.16	.02	.8	102
304 Papayas, raw, ½-inch cubes. 1 cup 182	89	70	1	Trace				18	36	.5	3,190	.07	.08	.5	102
Peaches:															
Raw:															
305 Whole, medium, 2-inch diameter, about 4 per pound.[5] 1 peach 114	89	35	1	Trace				10	9	.5	[13]1,320	.02	.05	1.0	7
306 Sliced. 1 cup 168	89	65	1	Trace				16	15	.8	[12]2,230	.03	.08	1.6	12
Canned, yellow-fleshed, solids and liquid: Sirup pack, heavy:															
307 Halves or slices. 1 cup 257	79	200	1	Trace				52	10	.8	1,100	.02	.06	1.4	7
308 Water pack. 1 cup 245	91	75	1	Trace				20	10	.7	1,100	.02	.06	1.4	7
309 Dried, uncooked. 1 cup 160	25	420	5	1				109	77	9.6	6,240	.02	.31	8.5	28
310 Cooked, unsweetened, 10-12 halves and juice. 1 cup 270	77	220	3	1				58	41	5.1	3,290	.01	.15	4.2	6
Frozen:															
311 Carton, 12 ounces, not thawed. 1 carton 340	76	300	1	Trace				77	14	1.7	2,210	.03	.14	2.4	[14]135
Pears:															
312 Raw, 3 by 2½-inch diameter.[5] 1 pear 182	83	100	1	1				25	13	.5	30	.04	.07	.2	7
Canned, solids and liquid: Sirup pack, heavy:															
313 Halves or slices. 1 cup 255	80	195	1	1				50	13	.5	Trace	.03	.05	.3	4

Item	Food	Measure	Grams	Water (%)	Cal.	Prot.	Fat		Carb.	Ca	Fe	Vit. A	Thiamine	Riboflavin	Niacin	Asc. acid
	Pineapple:															
314	Raw, diced	1 cup	140	85	75	1	Trace	----	19	24	.7	100	.12	.04	.3	24
	Canned, heavy sirup pack, solids and liquid:															
315	Crushed	1 cup	260	80	195	1	Trace	----	50	29	.8	120	.20	.06	.5	17
316	Sliced, slices and juice	2 small or 1 large.	122	80	90	Trace	Trace	----	24	13	.4	50	.09	.03	.2	8
317	Pineapple juice, canned	1 cup	249	86	135	1	Trace	----	34	37	.7	120	.12	.04	.5	[8]22
	Plums, all except prunes:															
318	Raw, 2-inch diameter, about 2 ounces.[5]	1 plum	60	87	25	Trace	Trace	----	7	7	.3	140	.02	.02	.3	3
	Canned, sirup pack (Italian prunes):															
319	Plums (with pits) and juice.[5]	1 cup	256	77	205	1	Trace	----	53	22	2.2	2,970	.05	.05	.9	4
	Prunes, dried, "softenized", medium:															
320	Uncooked.[5]	4 prunes	32	28	70	1	Trace	----	18	14	1.1	440	.02	.04	.4	1
321	Cooked, unsweetened, 17–18 prunes and ⅓ cup liquid.[5]	1 cup	270	66	295	2	1	----	78	60	4.5	1,860	.08	.18	1.7	2
322	Prune juice, canned or bottled.	1 cup	256	80	200	1	Trace	----	49	36	10.5	------	.03	.03	1.0	[8]5
	Raisins, seedless:															
323	Packaged, ½ oz. or 1½ tbsp. per pkg.	1 pkg.	14	18	40	Trace	Trace	----	11	9	.5	Trace	.02	.01	.1	Trace
324	Cup, pressed down.	1 cup	165	18	480	4	Trace	----	128	102	5.8	30	.18	.13	.8	2
	Raspberries, red:															
325	Raw	1 cup	123	84	70	1	1	----	17	27	1.1	160	.04	.11	1.1	31
326	Frozen, 10-ounce carton, not thawed.	1 carton	284	74	275	2	1	----	70	37	1.7	200	.06	.17	1.7	59
327	Rhubarb, cooked, sugar added.	1 cup	272	63	385	1	Trace	----	98	212	1.6	220	.06	.15	.7	17
	Strawberries:															
328	Raw, capped	1 cup	149	90	55	1	1	----	13	31	1.5	90	.04	.10	1.0	88
329	Frozen, 10-ounce carton, not thawed.	1 carton	284	71	310	1	1	----	79	40	2.0	90	.06	.17	1.5	150
330	Tangerines, raw, medium, 2⅜-in. diam., size 176.[5]	1 tangerine	116	87	40	1	Trace	----	10	34	.3	360	.05	.02	.1	27
331	Tangerine juice, canned, sweetened.	1 cup	249	87	125	1	1	----	30	45	.5	1,050	.15	.05	.2	55
332	Watermelon, raw, wedge, 4 by 8 inches (1/16 of 10 by 16-inch melon, about 2 pounds with rind).[5]	1 wedge	925	93	115	2	1	----	27	30	2.1	2,510	.13	.13	.7	30

[5] Measure and weight apply to entire vegetable or fruit including parts not usually eaten.

[8] This is the amount from the fruit. Additional ascorbic acid may be added by the manufacturer. Refer to the label for this information.

[13] Based on yellow-fleshed varieties; for white-fleshed varieties value is about 50 I.U. per 114-gram peach and 80 I.U. per cup of sliced peaches.

[14] This value includes ascorbic acid added by manufacturer.

NUTRITIVE VALUES OF THE EDIBLE PART OF FOODS

[Dashes in the columns for nutrients show that no suitable value could be found although there is reason to believe that a measurable amount of the nutrient may be present]

	Food, approximate measure, and weight (in grams)	Water	Food energy	Protein	Fat	Fatty acids Saturated (total)	Unsaturated Oleic	Unsaturated Linoleic	Carbohydrate	Calcium	Iron	Vitamin A value	Thiamin	Riboflavin	Niacin	Ascorbic acid
		Grams	Percent	Calories	Grams	Grams	Grams	Grams	Grams	Grams	Milligrams	Milligrams	International units	Milligrams	Milligrams	Milligrams	Milligrams
	GRAIN PRODUCTS																
	Bagel, 3-in. diam.:																
333	Egg _____ 1 bagel____	55	32	165	6	2	--	--	--	28	9	1.2	30	0.14	0.10	1.2	0
334	Water_____ 1 bagel____	55	29	165	6	2	--	--	--	30	8	1.2	0	.15	.11	1.4	0
335	Barley, pearled, light, uncooked. __ 1 cup _____	200	11	700	16	2	Trace	1	1	158	32	4.0	0	.24	.10	6.2	0
336	Biscuits, baking powder from home recipe with enriched flour, 2-in. diam. __ 1 biscuit_____	28	27	105	2	5	1	2	1	13	34	.4	Trace	.06	.06	.1	Trace
337	Biscuits, baking powder from mix, 2-in. diam. __ 1 biscuit_____	28	28	90	2	3	1	1	1	15	19	.6	Trace	.08	.07	.6	Trace
338	Bran flakes (40% bran), added thiamin and iron. __ 1 cup _____	35	3	105	4	1	--	--	--	28	25	12.3	0	.14	.06	2.2	0
339	Bran flakes with raisins, added thiamin and iron. __ 1 cup _____	50	7	145	4	1	--	--	--	40	28	13.5	Trace	.16	.07	2.7	0
	Breads:																
340	Boston brown bread, slice 3 by ¾ in. __ 1 slice_____	48	45	100	3	1	--	--	--	22	43	.9	0	.05	.03	.6	0
	Cracked-wheat bread:																
341	Loaf, 1 lb. _____ 1 loaf_____	454	35	1,190	40	10	2	5	2	236	399	5.0	Trace	.53	.41	5.9	Trace
342	Slice, 18 slices per loaf. __ 1 slice_____	25	35	65	2	1	--	--	--	13	22	.3	Trace	.03	.02	.3	Trace
	French or vienna bread:																
343	Enriched, 1 lb. loaf __ 1 loaf_____	454	31	1,315	41	14	3	8	2	251	195	10.0	Trace	1.27	1.00	11.3	Trace
344	Unenriched, 1 lb. loaf. __ 1 loaf_____	454	31	1,315	41	14	3	8	2	251	195	3.2	Trace	.36	.36	3.6	Trace
	Italian bread:																
345	Enriched, 1 lb. loaf __ 1 loaf_____	454	32	1,250	41	4	Trace	1	2	256	77	10.0	0	1.32	.91	11.8	0
346	Unenriched, 1 lb. loaf. __ 1 loaf_____	454	32	1,250	41	4	Trace	1	2	256	77	3.2	0	.41	.27	3.6	0

No.	Food	Measure																
348	Slice, 18 slices per loaf.	1 slice	25	35	65	2	1	--	--	--	13	18	.3	Trace	.01	.02	.2	Trace
	Rye bread:																	
	American, light (⅓ rye, ⅔ wheat):																	
349	Loaf, 1 lb.	1 loaf	454	36	1,100	41	5	--	--	--	236	340	7.3	0	.82	.32	6.4	0
350	Slice, 18 slices per loaf.	1 slice	25	36	60	2	Trace	--	--	--	13	19	.4	0	.05	.02	.4	0
351	Pumpernickel, loaf, 1 lb.	1 loaf	454	34	1,115	41	5	--	--	--	241	381	10.9	0	1.04	.64	5.4	0
	White bread, enriched:[15]																	
	Soft-crumb type:																	
352	Loaf, 1 lb.	1 loaf	454	36	1,225	39	15	3	8	2	229	381	11.3	Trace	1.13	.95	10.9	Trace
353	Slice, 18 slices per loaf.	1 slice	25	36	70	2	1	--	--	--	13	21	.6	Trace	.06	.05	.6	Trace
354	Slice, toasted.	1 slice	22	25	70	2	1	--	--	--	13	21	.6	Trace	.06	.05	.6	Trace
355	Slice, 22 slices per loaf.	1 slice	20	36	55	2	1	--	--	--	10	17	.5	Trace	.05	.04	.5	Trace
356	Slice, toasted.	1 slice	17	25	55	2	1	--	--	--	10	17	.5	Trace	.05	.04	.5	Trace
357	Loaf, 1½ lbs.	1 loaf	680	36	1,835	59	22	5	12	3	343	571	17.0	Trace	1.70	1.43	16.3	Trace
358	Slice, 24 slices per loaf.	1 slice	28	36	75	2	1	--	--	--	14	24	.7	Trace	.07	.06	.7	Trace
359	Slice, toasted.	1 slice	24	25	75	2	1	--	--	--	14	24	.7	Trace	.07	.06	.7	Trace
360	Slice, 28 slices per loaf.	1 slice	24	36	65	2	1	--	--	--	12	20	.6	Trace	.06	.05	.6	Trace
361	Slice, toasted.	1 slice	21	25	65	2	1	--	--	--	12	20	.6	Trace	.06	.05	.6	Trace
	Firm-crumb type:																	
362	Loaf, 1 lb.	1 loaf	454	35	1,245	41	17	4	10	2	228	435	11.3	Trace	1.22	.91	10.9	Trace
363	Slice, 20 slices per loaf.	1 slice	23	35	65	2	1	--	--	--	12	22	.6	Trace	.06	.05	.6	Trace
364	Slice, toasted.	1 slice	20	24	65	2	1	--	--	--	12	22	.6	Trace	.06	.05	.6	Trace
365	Loaf, 2 lbs.	1 loaf	907	35	2,495	82	34	8	20	4	455	871	22.7	Trace	2.45	1.81	21.8	Trace
366	Slice, 34 slices per loaf.	1 slice	27	35	75	2	1	--	--	--	14	26	.7	Trace	.07	.05	.6	Trace
367	Slice, toasted.	1 slice	23	35	75	2	1	--	--	--	14	26	.7	Trace	.07	.05	.6	Trace
	Whole-wheat bread, soft-crumb type:																	
368	Loaf, 1 lb.	1 loaf	454	36	1,095	41	12	2	6	2	224	381	13.6	Trace	1.36	.45	12.7	Trace
369	Slice, 16 slices per loaf.	1 slice	28	36	65	3	1	--	--	--	14	24	.8	Trace	.09	.03	.8	Trace
370	Slice, toasted.	1 slice	24	24	65	3	1	--	--	--	14	24	.8	Trace	.09	.03	.8	Trace

[15] Values for iron, thiamin, riboflavin, and niacin per pound of unenriched white bread would be as follows:

	Iron Milligrams	Thiamin Milligrams	Riboflavin Milligrams	Niacin Milligrams
Soft crumb	3.2	.31	.39	5.0
Firm crumb	3.2	.32	.59	4.1

NUTRITIVE VALUES OF THE EDIBLE PART OF FOODS

[Dashes in the columns for nutrients show that no suitable value could be found although there is reason to believe that a measurable amount of the nutrient may be present]

	Food, approximate measure, and weight (in grams)	Water	Food energy	Protein	Fat	Fatty acids			Carbohydrate	Calcium	Iron	Vitamin A value	Thiamin	Riboflavin	Niacin	Ascorbic acid
						Saturated (total)	Unsaturated									
							Oleic	Linoleic								
		Percent	Calories	Grams	Grams	Grams	Grams	Grams	Grams	Milligrams	Milligrams	International units	Milligrams	Milligrams	Milligrams	Milligrams
		Grams														
	GRAIN PRODUCTS—Continued															
	Bread—Continued															
	Whole-wheat bread, firm-crumb type:															
371	Loaf, 1 lb._____ 1 loaf_____ 454	36	1,100	48	14	3	6	3	216	449	13.6	Trace	1.18	0.54	12.7	Trace
372	Slice, 18 slices per loaf. 1 slice___ 25	36	60	3	1				12	25	.8	Trace	.06	.03	.7	Trace
373	Slice, toasted_____ 1 slice___ 21	24	60	3	1				12	25	.8	Trace	.06	.03	.7	Trace
374	Breadcrumbs, dry, grated_ 1 cup___ 100	6	390	13	5	1	2	1	73	122	3.6	Trace	.22	.30	3.5	Trace
375	Buckwheat flour, light, sifted. 1 cup___ 98	12	340	6	1				78	11	1.0	0	.08	.04	.4	0
376	Bulgur, canned, seasoned. 1 cup___ 135	56	245	8	4				44	27	1.9	0	.08	.05	4.1	0
	Cakes made from cake mixes:															
	Angelfood:															
377	Whole cake_____ 1 cake___ 635	34	1,645	36	1				377	603	1.9	0	.03	.70	.6	0
378	Piece, ½ of 10-in. diam. cake. 1 piece___ 53	34	135	3	Trace				32	50	.2	0	Trace	.06	.1	0
	Cupcakes, small, 2½ in. diam.:															
379	Without icing_____ 1 cupcake_ 25	26	90	1	3	1	1	1	14	40	.1	40	.01	.03	.1	Trace
380	With chocolate icing_ 1 cupcake._ 36	22	130	2	5	2	2	1	21	47	.3	60	.01	.04	.1	Trace
	Devil's food, 2-layer, with chocolate icing:															
381	Whole cake_____ 1 cake___1,107	24	3,755	49	136	54	58	16	645	653	8.9	1,660	.33	.89	3.3	1
382	Piece, ⅙ of 9-in. diam. cake. 1 piece___ 69	24	235	3	9	3	4	1	40	41	.6	100	.02	.06	.2	Trace
383	Cupcake, small, 2½ in. diam. 1 cupcake_ 35	24	120	2	4	1	2	Trace	20	21	.3	50	.01	.03	.1	Trace
	Gingerbread:															
384	Whole cake_____ 1 cake___ 570	37	1,575	18	39	10	19	9	291	513	9.1	Trace	.17	.51	4.6	2
385	Piece, ⅑ of 8-in. square cake. 1 piece___ 63	37	175	2	4	1	2	1	32	57	1.0	Trace	.02	.06	.5	Trace
	White, 2-layer, with chocolate icing:															
386	Whole cake_____ 1 cake___1,140	21	4,000	45	122	45	54	17	716	1,129	5.7	680	.23	.91	2.3	2

No.	Food	Measure																
387	Piece, 1/16 of 9-in. diam. cake.	1 piece	71	21	250	3	8	3	3	1	45	70	.4	40	.01	.06	.1	Trace
388	Boston cream pie; piece 1/12 of 8-in. diam.	1 piece	69	35	210	4	6	2	2	1	34	46	.3	140	.02	.08	.1	Trace
	Cakes made from home recipes:[16]																	
	Fruitcake, dark, made with enriched flour:																	
389	Loaf, 1-lb.	1 loaf	454	18	1,720	22	69	15	37	13	271	327	11.8	540	.59	.64	3.6	2
390	Slice, 1/30 of 8-in. loaf.	1 slice	15	18	55	1	2	Trace	1	Trace	9	11	.4	20	.02	.02	.1	Trace
	Plain sheet cake:																	
	Without icing:																	
391	Whole cake	1 cake	777	25	2,830	35	108	30	52	21	434	497	3.1	1,320	.16	.70	1.6	2
392	Piece, 1/9 of 9-in. square cake.	1 piece	86	25	315	4	12	3	6	2	48	55	.3	150	.02	.08	.2	Trace
393	With boiled white icing, piece, 1/9 of 9-in. square cake.	1 piece	114	23	400	4	12	3	6	2	71	56	.3	150	.02	.08	.2	Trace
	Pound:																	
394	Loaf, 8½ by 3½ by 3in.	1 loaf	514	17	2,430	29	152	34	68	17	242	108	4.1	1,440	.15	.46	1.0	0
395	Slice, ½-in. thick	1 slice	30	17	140	2	9	2	4	1	14	6	.2	80	.01	.03	.1	0
	Sponge:																	
396	Whole cake	1 cake	790	32	2,345	60	45	14	20	4	427	237	9.5	3,560	.40	1.11	1.6	Trace
397	Piece, 1/12 of 10-in. diam. cake.	1 piece	66	32	195	5	4	1	2	Trace	36	20	.8	300	.03	.09	.1	Trace
	Yellow, 2-layer, without icing:																	
398	Whole cake	1 cake	870	24	3,160	39	111	31	53	22	506	618	3.5	1,310	.17	.70	1.7	2
399	Piece, 1/16 of 9-in. diam. cake.	1 piece	54	24	200	2	7	2	3	1	32	39	.2	80	.01	.04	.1	Trace
	Yellow, 2-layer, with chocolate icing:																	
400	Whole cake	1 cake	1,203	21	4,390	51	156	55	69	23	727	818	7.2	1,920	.24	.96	2.4	Trace
401	Piece, 1/16 of 9-in. diam. cake.	1 piece	75	21	275	3	10	3	4	1	45	51	.5	120	.02	.06	.2	Trace
	Cake icings. See Sugars, Sweets.																	
	Cookies:																	
	Brownies with nuts:																	
402	Made from home recipe with enriched flour.	1 brownie	20	10	95	1	6	1	3	1	10	8	.4	40	.04	.02	.1	Trace
403	Made from mix	1 brownie	20	11	85	1	4	1	2	1	13	9	.4	20	.03	.02	.1	Trace

[16] Unenriched cake flour used unless otherwise specified.

NUTRITIVE VALUES OF THE EDIBLE PART OF FOODS

[Dashes in the columns for nutrients show that no suitable value could be found although there is reason to believe that a measurable amount of the nutrient may be present]

	Food, approximate measure, and weight (in grams)	Water	Food energy	Pro-tein	Fat	Fatty acids Satu-rated (total)	Unsaturated Oleic	Lin-oleic	Carbo-hy-drate	Cal-cium	Iron	Vita-min A value	Thia-min	Ribo-flavin	Niacin	Ascor-bic acid
		Percent	Calories	Grams	Grams	Grams	Grams	Grams	Grams	Milli-grams	Milli-grams	Inter-national units	Milli-grams	Milli-grams	Milli-grams	Milli-grams
	GRAIN PRODUCTS—Continued															
	Cookies—Continued															
	Chocolate chip:															
404	Made from home recipe with enriched flour. 1 cookie	3	50	1	3	1	1	1	6	4	0.2	10	0.01	0.01	0.1	Trace
405	Commercial 1 cookie	3	50	1	2	1	1	Trace	7	4	.2	10	Trace	Trace	Trace	Trace
406	Fig bars, commercial 1 cookie	14	50	1	1				11	11	.2	20	Trace	.01	.1	Trace
407	Sandwich, chocolate or vanilla, commercial. 1 cookie	2	50	1	2	1	1	Trace	7	2	.1	0	Trace	Trace	.1	0
	Corn flakes, added nutrients:															
408	Plain 1 cup	4	100	2	Trace				21	4	.4	0	.11	.02	.5	0
409	Sugar-covered 1 cup	2	155	2	Trace				36	5	.4	0	.16	.02	.8	0
	Corn (hominy) grits, degermed, cooked:															
410	Enriched 1 cup	87	125	3	Trace				27	2	.7	[17] 150	.10	.07	1.0	0
411	Unenriched 1 cup	87	125	3	Trace				27	2	.2	[17] 150	.05	.02	.5	0
	Cornmeal:															
412	Whole-ground, unbolted, dry. 1 cup	12	435	11	5	1	2	2	90	24	2.9	[17] 620	.46	.13	2.4	0
413	Bolted (nearly whole-grain) dry. 1 cup	12	440	11	4	Trace	1	2	91	21	2.2	[17] 590	.37	.10	2.3	0
	Degermed, enriched:															
414	Dry form 1 cup	12	500	11	2				108	8	4.0	[17] 610	.61	.36	4.8	0
415	Cooked 1 cup	88	120	3	1				26	2	1.0	[17] 140	.14	.10	1.2	0
	Degermed, unenriched:															
416	Dry form 1 cup	12	500	11	2				108	8	1.5	[17] 610	.19	.07	1.4	0
417	Cooked 1 cup	88	120	3	1				26	2	.5	[17] 140	.05	.02	.2	0
418	Corn muffins, made with enriched degermed cornmeal and enriched flour; muffin 2⅜-in. diam. 1 muffin	33	125	3	4	2	2	Trace	19	42	.7	[17] 120	.08	.09	.6	Trace

No.	Food	Measure	Grams	Water (%)	Food energy	Protein	Fat	(Saturated)	(Oleic)	(Linoleic)	Carbohydrate	Calcium	Iron	Vitamin A	Thiamin	Riboflavin	Niacin	Ascorbic acid
	with mix, egg, and milk; muffin 2⅜-in. diam.																	
420	Corn, puffed, presweetened, added nutrients.	1 cup	30	2	115	1	Trace	--	--	--	27	3	.5	0	.13	.05	.6	0
421	Corn, shredded, added nutrients.	1 cup	25	3	100	2	Trace	--	--	--	22	1	.6	0	.11	.05	.5	0
	Crackers:																	
422	Graham, 2½-in. square.	4 crackers	28	6	110	2	3	--	--	1	21	11	.4	0	.01	.06	.4	0
423	Saltines.	4 crackers	11	4	50	1	1	--	--	--	8	2	.1	0	Trace	Trace	.1	0
	Danish pastry, plain (without fruit or nuts):																	
424	Packaged ring, 12 ounces.	1 ring	340	22	1,435	25	80	24	37	15	155	170	3.1	1,050	.24	.51	2.7	Trace
425	Round piece, approx. 4¼-in. diam. by 1 in.	1 pastry	65	22	275	5	15	5	7	3	30	33	.6	200	.05	.10	.5	Trace
426	Ounce.	1 oz	28	22	120	2	7	2	3	1	13	14	.3	90	.02	.04	.2	Trace
427	Doughnuts, cake type.	1 doughnut	32	24	125	1	6	1	4	Trace	16	13	[18].4	30	[18].05	[18].05	[18].4	Trace
428	Farina, quick-cooking, enriched, cooked.	1 cup	245	89	105	3	Trace	--	--	--	22	147	[19].7	0	[19].12	[19].07	[19]1.0	0
	Macaroni, cooked:																	
	Enriched:																	
429	Cooked, firm stage (undergoes additional cooking in a food mixture).	1 cup	130	64	190	6	1	--	--	--	39	14	[19]1.4	0	[19].23	[19].14	[19]1.8	0
430	Cooked until tender.	1 cup	140	72	155	5	1	--	--	--	32	8	[19]1.3	0	[19].20	[19].11	[19]1.5	0
	Unenriched:																	
431	Cooked, firm stage (undergoes additional cooking in a food mixture).	1 cup	130	64	190	6	1	--	--	--	39	14	.7	0	.03	.03	.5	0
432	Cooked until tender.	1 cup	140	72	155	5	1	--	--	--	32	11	.6	0	.01	.01	.4	0
433	Macaroni (enriched) and cheese, baked.	1 cup	200	58	430	17	22	10	9	2	40	362	1.8	860	.20	.40	1.8	Trace
434	Canned.	1 cup	240	80	230	9	10	4	3	1	26	199	1.0	260	.12	.24	1.0	Trace
435	Muffins, with enriched white flour; muffin, 3-inch diam.	1 muffin	40	38	120	3	4	1	2	1	17	42	.6	40	.07	.09	.6	Trace
	Noodles (egg noodles), cooked:																	
436	Enriched.	1 cup	160	70	200	7	2	--	--	--	37	16	[19]1.4	110	[19].22	[19].13	[19]1.9	0
437	Unenriched.	1 cup	160	70	200	7	2	--	--	--	37	16	1.0	110	.05	.03	.6	0

[17] This value is based on product made from yellow varieties of corn; white varieties contain only a trace.

[18] Based on product made with enriched flour. With unenriched flour, approximate values per doughnut are: Iron, 0.2 milligram; thiamin, 0.01 milligram; riboflavin, 0.03 milligram; niacin, 0.2 milligram.

[19] Iron, thiamin, riboflavin, and niacin are based on the minimum levels of enrichment specified in standards of identity promulgated under the Federal Food, Drug, and Cosmetic Act.

NUTRITIVE VALUES OF THE EDIBLE PART OF FOODS

[Dashes in the columns for nutrients show that no suitable value could be found although there is reason to believe that a measurable amount of the nutrient may be present]

	Food, approximate measure, and weight (in grams)	Water	Food energy	Protein	Fat	Fatty acids			Carbohydrate	Calcium	Iron	Vitamin A value	Thiamin	Riboflavin	Niacin	Ascorbic acid
						Saturated (total)	Unsaturated Oleic	Linoleic								
		Percent	Calories	Grams	Grams	Grams	Grams	Grams	Grams	Milligrams	Milligrams	International units	Milligrams	Milligrams	Milligrams	Milligrams
	GRAIN PRODUCTS—Continued															
438	Oats (with or without corn) puffed, added nutrients. 1 cup -- 25	3	100	3	1	--	--	--	19	44	1.2	0	0.24	0.04	0.5	0
439	Oatmeal or rolled oats, cooked. 1 cup -- 240	87	130	5	2	--	--	--	23	22	1.4	0	.19	.05	.2	0
	Pancakes, 4-inch diam.:															
440	Wheat, enriched flour (home recipe). 1 cake -- 27	50	60	2	2	Trace	1	Trace	9	27	.4	30	.05	.06	.4	Trace
441	Buckwheat (made from mix with egg and milk). 1 cake -- 27	58	55	2	2	1	1	Trace	6	59	.4	60	.03	.04	.2	Trace
442	Plain or buttermilk (made from mix with egg and milk). 1 cake -- 27	51	60	2	2	1	1	Trace	9	58	.3	70	.04	.06	.2	Trace
	Pie (piecrust made with unenriched flour): Sector, 4-in, 1/7 of 9-in. diam. pie:															
443	Apple (2-crust). 1 sector -- 135	48	350	3	15	4	7	3	51	11	.4	40	.03	.03	.5	1
444	Butterscotch (1-crust). 1 sector -- 130	45	350	6	14	5	6	2	50	98	1.2	340	.04	.13	.3	Trace
445	Cherry (2-crust). 1 sector -- 135	47	350	4	15	4	7	3	52	19	.4	590	.03	.03	.7	Trace
446	Custard (1-crust). 1 sector -- 130	58	285	8	14	5	6	2	30	125	.8	300	.07	.21	.4	0
447	Lemon meringue (1-crust). 1 sector -- 120	47	305	4	12	4	6	2	45	17	.6	200	.04	.10	.2	4
448	Mince (2-crust). 1 sector -- 135	43	365	3	16	4	8	3	56	38	1.4	Trace	.09	.05	.5	1
449	Pecan (1-crust). 1 sector -- 118	20	490	6	27	4	16	5	60	55	3.3	190	.19	.08	.4	Trace
450	Pineapple chiffon (1-crust). 1 sector -- 93	41	265	6	11	3	5	2	36	22	.8	320	.04	.08	.4	1
451	Pumpkin (1-crust). 1 sector -- 130	59	275	5	15	5	6	2	32	66	.7	3,210	.04	.13	.7	Trace
	Piecrust, baked shell for pie made with:															
452	Enriched flour. 1 shell -- 180	15	900	11	60	16	28	12	79	25	3.1	0	.36	.25	3.2	0

No.	Food	Measure	Grams	Water (%)	Food energy (cal.)	Protein (g)	Fat (g)	Saturated fatty acids, total (g)	Unsaturated, Oleic (g)	Unsaturated, Linoleic (g)	Carbohydrate (g)	Calcium (mg)	Iron (mg)	Vitamin A (I.U.)	Thiamin (mg)	Riboflavin (mg)	Niacin (mg)	Ascorbic acid (mg)
454	Package, 10-oz., for double crust.	1 pkg	284	9	1,480	20	93	23	46	21	141	131	1.4	0	.11	.11	2.0	0
455	Pizza (cheese) 5½-in. sector; ⅛ of 14-in. diam. pie.	1 sector	75	45	185	7	6	2	3	Trace	27	107	.7	290	.04	.12	.7	4
	Popcorn, popped:																	
456	Plain, large kernel	1 cup	6	4	25	1	Trace	----	Trace	----	5	1	.2	----	----	.01	.1	0
457	With oil and salt	1 cup	9	3	40	1	2	----	1	1	5	1	.2	----	----	.01	.2	0
458	Sugar coated	1 cup	35	4	135	2	1	----	Trace	----	30	2	.5	----	----	.02	.4	0
	Pretzels:																	
459	Dutch, twisted	1 pretzel	16	5	60	2	1	----	----	----	12	4	.2	0	Trace	Trace	.1	0
460	Thin, twisted	1 pretzel	6	5	25	1	Trace	----	----	----	5	1	.1	0	Trace	Trace	Trace	0
461	Stick, small, 2¼ inches	10 sticks	3	5	10	Trace	Trace	----	----	----	2	1	Trace	0	Trace	Trace	Trace	0
462	Stick, regular, 3⅛ inches	5 sticks	3	5	10	Trace	Trace	----	----	----	2	1	Trace	0	Trace	Trace	Trace	0
	Rice, white: Enriched:																	
463	Raw	1 cup	185	12	670	12	1	----	----	----	149	44	[20]5.4	0	[20].81	[20].06	[20]6.5	0
464	Cooked	1 cup	205	73	225	4	Trace	----	----	----	50	21	[20]1.8	0	[20].18	[20].02	[20]2.1	0
465	Instant, ready-to-serve	1 cup	165	73	180	4	Trace	----	----	----	40	5	[20]1.3	0	[20].21	[20]--	[20]1.7	0
466	Unenriched, cooked	1 cup	205	73	225	4	Trace	----	----	----	50	21	.4	0	.04	.02	.8	0
467	Parboiled, cooked	1 cup	175	73	185	4	Trace	----	----	----	41	33	[20]1.4	0	[20].19	[20]--	[20]2.1	0
468	Rice, puffed, added nutrients.	1 cup	15	4	60	1	Trace	----	----	----	13	3	.3	0	.07	.01	.7	0
	Rolls, enriched: Cloverleaf or pan:																	
469	Home recipe	1 roll	35	26	120	3	3	1	1	1	20	16	.7	30	.09	.09	.8	Trace
470	Commercial	1 roll	28	31	85	2	2	Trace	1	Trace	15	21	.5	Trace	.08	.05	.6	Trace
471	Frankfurter or hamburger.	1 roll	40	31	120	3	2	1	1	1	21	30	.8	Trace	.11	.07	.9	Trace
472	Hard, round or rectangular.	1 roll	50	25	155	5	2	Trace	1	Trace	30	24	1.2	Trace	.13	.12	1.4	Trace
473	Rye wafers, whole-grain, 1⅞ by 3½ inches.	2 wafers	13	6	45	2	Trace	----	----	----	10	7	.5	0	.04	.03	.2	0
474	Spaghetti, cooked, tender stage, enriched.	1 cup	140	72	155	5	1	----	1	----	32	11	[19]1.3	0	[19].20	[19].11	[19]1.5	0

[19] Iron, thiamin, riboflavin, and niacin are based on the minimum levels of enrichment specified in standards of identity promulgated under the Federal Food, Drug, and Cosmetic Act.

[20] Iron, thiamin, and niacin are based on the minimum levels of enrichment specified in standards of identity promulgated under the Federal Food, Drug, and Cosmetic Act. Riboflavin is based on unenriched rice. When the minimum level of enrichment for riboflavin specified in the standards of identity becomes effective the value will be 0.12 milligram per cup of parboiled rice and of white rice.

NUTRITIVE VALUES OF THE EDIBLE PART OF FOODS

[Dashes show that no basis could be found for imputing a value although there was some reason to believe that a measurable amount of the constituent might be present]

Food, approximate measure, and weight (in grams)	Water	Food energy	Protein	Fat	Fatty acids Saturated (total)	Unsaturated Oleic	Linoleic	Carbohydrate	Calcium	Iron	Vitamin A value	Thiamin	Riboflavin	Niacin	Ascorbic acid
	Per cent	Calories	Grams	Grams	Grams	Grams	Grams	Grams	Milligrams	Milligrams	International units	Milligrams	Milligrams	Milligrams	Milligrams
GRAIN PRODUCTS—Continued															
Spaghetti with meat balls, and tomato sauce:															
475 Home recipe --- 1 cup --- 248	70	330	19	12	4	6	1	39	124	3.7	1,590	0.25	0.30	4.0	22
476 Canned --- 1 cup --- 250	78	260	12	10	2	3	4	28	53	3.3	1,000	.15	.18	2.3	5
Spaghetti in tomato sauce with cheese:															
477 Home recipe --- 1 cup --- 250	77	260	9	9	2	5	1	37	80	2.3	1,080	.25	.18	2.3	13
478 Canned --- 1 cup --- 250	80	190	6	2	1	1	1	38	40	2.8	930	.35	.28	4.5	10
479 Waffles, with enriched flour, 7-in. diam. --- 1 waffle --- 75	41	210	7	7	2	4	1	28	85	1.3	250	.13	.19	1.0	Trace
480 Waffles, made from mix, enriched, egg and milk added, 7-in. diam. --- 1 waffle --- 75	42	205	7	8	3	3	1	27	179	1.0	170	.11	.17	.7	Trace
481 Wheat, puffed, added nutrients. --- 1 cup --- 15	3	55	2	Trace				12	4	.6	0	.08	.03	1.2	0
482 Wheat, shredded, plain --- 1 biscuit --- 25	7	90	2	1				20	11	.9	0	.06	.03	1.1	0
483 Wheat flakes, added nutrients. --- 1 cup --- 30	4	105	3	Trace				24	12	1.3	0	.19	.04	1.5	0
Wheat flours:															
484 Whole-wheat, from hard wheats, stirred. --- 1 cup --- 120	12	400	16	2	Trace	1	1	85	49	4.0	0	.66	.14	5.2	0
All-purpose or family flour, enriched:															
485 Sifted --- 1 cup --- 115	12	420	12	1				88	18	[19]3.3	0	[19].51	[19].30	[19]4.0	0
486 Unsifted --- 1 cup --- 125	12	455	13	1				95	20	[19]3.6	0	[19].55	[19].33	[19]4.4	0
487 Self-rising, enriched --- 1 cup --- 125	12	440	12	1				93	331	[19]3.6	0	[19].55	[19].33	[19]4.4	0
488 Cake or pastry flour, sifted. --- 1 cup --- 96	12	350	7	1				76	16	.5	0	.03	.03	.7	0
FATS, OILS															
Butter:															
Regular, 4 sticks per pound:															
489 Stick --- ½ cup --- 113	16	810	1	92	51	30	3	1	23	0	[21]3,750				0

Item No.	Food, approximate measure	Grams	Water (%)	Food energy (cal.)	Protein (g)	Fat (g)	Saturated (g)	Oleic (g)	Linoleic (g)	Carbohydrate (g)	Calcium (mg)	Iron (mg)	Vitamin A (I.U.)	Thiamin (mg)	Riboflavin (mg)	Niacin (mg)	Ascorbic acid (mg)
491	½ stick). Pat (1-in. sq. ⅓-in. high; 90 per lb.). 1 pat	5	16	35	Trace	4	2	1	Trace	Trace	1	0	[21]170	—	—	—	0
	Whipped, 6 sticks or 2, 8-oz. containers per pound:																
492	Stick. ½ cup	76	16	540	1	61	34	20	2	Trace	20	0	[22]2,500	—	—	—	0
493	Tablespoon (approx. ⅛ stick). 1 tbsp.	9	16	65	Trace	8	4	3	Trace	Trace	3	0	[22]310	—	—	—	0
494	Pat (1¼-in. sq. ⅓-in. high; 120 per lb.). 1 pat	4	16	25	Trace	3	2	1	Trace	Trace	1	0	[21]130	—	—	—	0
	Fats, cooking:																
495	Lard. 1 cup	205	0	1,850	0	205	78	94	20	0	0	0	0	—	—	—	0
496	1 tbsp.	13	0	115	0	13	5	6	1	0	0	0	0	—	—	—	0
497	Vegetable fats. 1 cup	200	0	1,770	0	200	50	100	44	0	0	0	—	—	—	—	0
498	1 tbsp.	13	0	110	0	13	3	6	3	0	0	0	—	—	—	—	0
	Margarine: Regular, 4 sticks per pound:																
499	Stick. ½ cup	113	16	815	1	92	17	46	25	Trace	23	0	[22]3,750	—	—	—	0
500	Tablespoon (approx. ⅛ stick). 1 tbsp.	14	16	100	Trace	12	2	6	3	Trace	3	0	[22]470	—	—	—	0
501	Pat (1-in. sq. ⅓-in. high; 90 per lb.). 1 pat	5	16	35	Trace	4	1	2	1	Trace	1	0	[21]170	—	—	—	0
	Whipped, 6 sticks per pound:																
502	Stick. ½ cup	76	16	545	1	61	11	31	17	1	15	0	[22]2,500	—	—	—	0
	Soft, 2 8-oz. tubs per pound:																
503	Tub. 1 tub	227	16	1,635	1	184	34	68	68	1	45	0	[22]7,500	—	—	—	0
504	Tablespoon. 1 tbsp.	14	16	100	Trace	11	2	4	4	Trace	3	0	[22]470	—	—	—	0
	Oils, salad or cooking:																
505	Corn. 1 cup	220	0	1,945	0	220	22	62	117	0	0	0	—	0	0	0	0
506	1 tbsp.	14	0	125	0	14	1	4	7	0	0	0	—	0	0	0	0
507	Cottonseed. 1 cup	220	0	1,945	0	220	55	46	110	0	0	0	—	0	0	0	0
508	1 tbsp.	14	0	125	0	14	4	3	7	0	0	0	—	0	0	0	0
509	Olive. 1 cup	220	0	1,945	0	220	24	167	15	0	0	0	—	0	0	0	0
510	1 tbsp.	14	0	125	0	14	2	11	1	0	0	0	—	0	0	0	0
511	Peanut. 1 cup	220	0	1,945	0	220	40	103	64	0	0	0	—	0	0	0	0
512	1 tbsp.	14	0	125	0	14	3	7	4	0	0	0	—	0	0	0	0
513	Safflower. 1 cup	220	0	1,945	0	220	18	37	165	0	0	0	—	0	0	0	0
514	1 tbsp.	14	0	125	0	14	1	2	10	0	0	0	—	0	0	0	0
515	Soybean. 1 cup	220	0	1,945	0	220	33	44	114	0	0	0	—	0	0	0	0
516	1 tbsp.	14	0	125	0	14	2	3	7	0	0	0	—	0	0	0	0

[19] Iron, thiamin, riboflavin, and niacin are based on the minimum levels of enrichment specified in standards of identity promulgated under the Federal Food, Drug, and Cosmetic Act.

[21] Year-round average.

[22] Based on the average vitamin A content of fortified margarine. Federal specifications for fortified margarine require a minimum of 15,000 I.U. of vitamin A per pound.

NUTRITIVE VALUES OF THE EDIBLE PART OF FOODS

[Dashes in the columns for nutrients show that no suitable value could be found although there is reason to believe that a measurable amount of the nutrient may be present]

Food, approximate measure, and weight (in grams)	Water	Food energy	Protein	Fat	Fatty acids Saturated (total)	Unsaturated Oleic	Linoleic	Carbohydrate	Calcium	Iron	Vitamin A value	Thiamin	Riboflavin	Niacin	Ascorbic acid
	Per cent	Calories	Grams	Grams	Grams	Grams	Grams	Grams	Milligrams	Milligrams	International units	Milligrams	Milligrams	Milligrams	Milligrams
FATS, OILS—Continued															
Salad dressings:															
517 Blue cheese ------- 1 tbsp. 15	32	75	1	8	2	2	4	1	12	Trace	30	Trace	0.02	Trace	Trace
Commercial, mayonnaise type:															
518 Regular ------- 1 tbsp. 15	41	65	Trace	6	1	1	3	2	2	Trace	30	Trace	Trace	Trace	----
519 Special dietary, low-calorie. 1 tbsp. 16	81	20	Trace	2	Trace	Trace	1	1	3	Trace	40	Trace	Trace	Trace	----
French:															
520 Regular ------- 1 tbsp. 16	39	65	Trace	6	1	1	3	3	2	.1	80	.01	.03	Trace	Trace
521 Special dietary, low-fat with artificial sweeteners. 1 tbsp. 15	95	Trace	Trace	Trace	----	----	----	Trace	2	.1	40	Trace	.01	Trace	----
522 Home cooked, boiled----- 1 tbsp. 16	68	25	1	2	1	1	Trace	2	14	.1	80	.01	.03	Trace	Trace
523 Mayonnaise --------- 1 tbsp. 14	15	100	Trace	11	2	2	6	Trace	3	.1	40	Trace	.01	Trace	----
524 Thousand island------- 1 tbsp. 16	32	80	Trace	8	1	2	4	3	2	.1	50	Trace	Trace	Trace	Trace
SUGARS, SWEETS															
Cake icings:															
525 Chocolate made with milk and table fat. 1 cup 275	14	1,035	9	38	21	14	1	185	165	3.3	580	.06	.28	.6	1
526 Coconut (with boiled icing). 1 cup 166	15	605	3	13	11	1	Trace	124	10	.8	0	.02	.07	.3	0
527 Creamy fudge from mix with water only. 1 cup 245	15	830	7	16	5	8	3	183	96	2.7	Trace	.05	.20	.7	Trace
528 White, boiled --------- 1 cup 94	18	300	1	0	----	----	----	76	2	Trace	0	Trace	.03	Trace	0
Candy:															
529 Caramels, plain or chocolate. 1 oz 28	8	115	1	3	2	1	Trace	22	42	.4	Trace	.01	.05	.1	Trace
530 Chocolate, milk, plain-- 1 oz 28	1	145	2	9	5	3	Trace	16	65	.3	80	.02	.10	.1	Trace
531 Chocolate-coated peanuts. 1 oz 28	1	160	5	12	3	6	2	11	33	.4	Trace	.10	.05	2.1	Trace

No.	Food	Measure	Grams	Water (%)	Food energy (cal.)	Protein (g)	Fat (g)	Saturated (g)	Oleic (g)	Linoleic (g)	Carbohydrate (g)	Calcium (mg)	Iron (mg)	Vitamin A (I.U.)	Thiamin (mg)	Riboflavin (mg)	Niacin (mg)	Ascorbic acid (C) (mg)
532	Fondant; mints, uncoated; candy corn.	1 oz.	28	8	105	Trace	Trace	---	---	---	25	4	.3	0	Trace	Trace	Trace	0
533	Fudge, plain.	1 oz.	28	8	115	1	3	2	1	Trace	21	22	.3	Trace	.01	.03	.1	Trace
534	Gum drops.	1 oz.	28	12	100	Trace	Trace	---	---	---	25	2	.1	0	0	Trace	Trace	0
535	Hard.	1 oz.	28	1	110	0	Trace	---	---	---	28	6	.5	0	0	0	0	0
536	Marshmallows.	1 oz.	28	17	90	1	Trace	---	---	---	23	5	.5	0	0	Trace	Trace	0
	Chocolate-flavored sirup or topping:																	
537	Thin type.	1 fl. oz.	38	32	90	1	1	Trace	Trace	Trace	24	6	.6	Trace	.01	.03	.2	0
538	Fudge type.	1 fl. oz.	38	25	125	2	5	3	2	Trace	20	48	.5	60	.02	.08	.2	Trace
	Chocolate-flavored beverage powder (approx. 4 heaping teaspoons per oz.):																	
539	With nonfat dry milk.	1 oz.	28	2	100	5	1	---	---	---	20	167	.5	10	.04	.21	.2	1
540	Without nonfat dry milk.	1 oz.	28	1	100	1	1	---	---	---	25	9	.6	---	.01	.03	.1	0
541	Honey, strained or extracted.	1 tbsp.	21	17	65	Trace	0	---	---	---	17	1	.1	0	Trace	.01	.1	Trace
542	Jams and preserves.	1 tbsp.	20	29	55	Trace	Trace	---	---	---	14	4	.2	Trace	Trace	.01	Trace	Trace
543	Jellies.	1 tbsp.	18	29	50	Trace	Trace	---	---	---	13	4	.3	Trace	Trace	.01	Trace	1
	Molasses, cane:																	
544	Light (first extraction).	1 tbsp.	20	24	50	---	---	---	---	---	13	33	.9	---	.01	.01	Trace	---
545	Blackstrap (third extraction).	1 tbsp.	20	24	45	---	---	---	---	---	11	137	3.2	---	.02	.04	.4	---
	Sirups:																	
546	Sorghum.	1 tbsp.	21	23	55	---	---	---	---	---	14	35	2.6	---	---	.02	Trace	---
547	Table blends, chiefly corn, light and dark.	1 tbsp.	21	24	60	0	0	---	---	---	15	9	.8	0	0	0	0	0
	Sugars:																	
548	Brown, firm packed.	1 cup.	220	2	820	2	0	---	---	---	212	187	7.5	0	.02	.07	.4	0
	White:																	
549	Granulated.	1 cup.	200	Trace	770	0	0	---	---	---	199	0	.2	0	0	0	0	0
550	Granulated.	1 tbsp.	11	Trace	40	0	0	---	---	---	11	0	Trace	0	0	0	0	0
551	Powdered, stirred before measuring.	1 cup.	120	Trace	460	0	0	---	---	---	119	0	.1	0	0	0	0	0
	MISCELLANEOUS ITEMS																	
552	Barbecue sauce.	1 cup.	250	81	230	4	17	2	5	9	20	53	2.0	900	.03	.03	.8	13
	Beverages, alcoholic:																	
553	Beer.	12 fl. oz.	360	92	150	1	0	---	---	---	14	18	Trace	---	.01	.11	2.2	---
	Gin, rum, vodka, whiskey:																	
554	80-proof.	1½ fl. oz. jigger.	42	67	100	---	---	---	---	---	Trace	---	---	---	---	---	---	---
555	86-proof.	1½ fl. oz. jigger.	42	64	105	---	---	---	---	---	Trace	---	---	---	---	---	---	---
556	90-proof.	1½ fl. oz. jigger.	42	62	110	---	---	---	---	---	Trace	---	---	---	---	---	---	---

NUTRITIVE VALUES OF THE EDIBLE PART OF FOODS

[Dashes in the columns for nutrients show that no suitable value could be found although there is reason to believe that a measurable amount of the nutrient may be present]

	Food, approximate measure, and weight (in grams)		Water	Food energy	Protein	Fat	Fatty acids Saturated (total)	Unsaturated Oleic	Unsaturated Linoleic	Carbohydrate	Calcium	Iron	Vitamin A value	Thiamin	Riboflavin	Niacin	Ascorbic acid
		Grams	*Percent*	*Calories*	*Grams*	*Grams*	*Grams*	*Grams*	*Grams*	*Grams*	*Milligrams*	*Milligrams*	*International units*	*Milligrams*	*Milligrams*	*Milligrams*	*Milligrams*
	MISCELLANEOUS ITEMS—Continued																
	Beverages, alcoholic—Continued																
	Gin, rum, vodka, whiskey—Con.																
557	94-proof — 1½ fl. oz. jigger.	42	60	115	---					Trace							
558	100-proof — 1½ fl. oz. jigger.	42	58	125	---					Trace							
	Wines:																
559	Dessert — 3½ fl. oz. glass.	103	77	140	Trace	0				8	8	---		.01	.02	.2	---
560	Table — 3½ fl. oz. glass.	102	86	85	Trace	0				4	9	.4		Trace	.01	.1	---
	Beverages, carbonated, sweetened, nonalcoholic:																
561	Carbonated water — 12 fl. oz.	366	92	115	0	0				29	---	---	0	0	0	0	0
562	Cola type — 12 fl. oz.	369	90	145	0	0				37	---	---	0	0	0	0	0
563	Fruit-flavored sodas and Tom Collins mixes. — 12 fl. oz.	372	88	170	0	0				45	---	---	0	0	0	0	0
564	Ginger ale — 12 fl. oz.	366	92	115	0	0				29	---	---	0	0	0	0	0
565	Root beer — 12 fl. oz.	370	90	150	0	0				39	---	---	0	0	0	0	0
566	Bouillon cubes, approx. ½ in. — 1 cube	4	4	5	1	Trace				Trace	---	---					
	Chocolate:																
567	Bitter or baking — 1 oz.	28	2	145	3	15	8	6	Trace	8	22	1.9	20	.01	.07	.4	0
568	Semi-sweet, small pieces. — 1 cup	170	1	860	7	61	34	22	1	97	51	4.4	30	.02	.14	.9	0
	Gelatin:																
569	Plain, dry powder in envelope. — 1 envelope	7	13	25	6	Trace				0							
570	Dessert powder, 3-oz. package. — 1 pkg.	85	2	315	8	0				75							
571	Gelatin dessert, prepared with water. — 1 cup	240	84	140	4	0				34							

	Olives, pickled:																	
572	Green	4 medium or 3 extra large or 2 giant.	16	78	15	Trace	2	Trace	2	Trace	Trace	8	.2	40	----	----	----	----
573	Ripe: Mission	3 small or 2 large.	10	73	15	Trace	2	Trace	2	Trace	Trace	9	.1	10	Trace	Trace	----	----
	Pickles, cucumber:																	
574	Dill, medium, whole, 3¾ in. long, 1¼ in. diam.	1 pickle	65	93	10	1	Trace	----	----	----	1	17	.7	70	Trace	.01	Trace	4
575	Fresh, sliced, 1½ in. diam., ¼ in. thick.	2 slices	15	79	10	Trace	Trace	----	----	----	3	5	.3	20	Trace	Trace	Trace	1
576	Sweet, gherkin, small, whole, approx. 2½ in. long, ¾ in. diam.	1 pickle	15	61	20	Trace	Trace	----	----	----	6	2	.2	10	Trace	Trace	Trace	1
577	Relish, finely chopped, sweet.	1 tbsp.	15	63	20	Trace	Trace	----	----	----	5	3	.1	----	----	----	----	----
	Popcorn. See Grain Products.																	
578	Popsicle, 3 fl. oz. size	1 popsicle	95	80	70	0	0	0	0	0	18	0	Trace	0	0	0	0	0
	Pudding, home recipe with starch base:																	
579	Chocolate	1 cup	260	66	385	8	12	7	4	Trace	67	250	1.3	390	.05	.36	.3	1
580	Vanilla (blanc mange)	1 cup	255	76	285	9	10	5	3	Trace	41	298	Trace	410	.08	.41	.3	2
581	Pudding mix, dry form, 4-oz. package.	1 pkg.	113	2	410	3	2	1	1	Trace	103	23	1.8	Trace	.02	.08	.5	0
582	Sherbet	1 cup	193	67	260	2	2	----	----	----	59	31	Trace	120	.02	.06	Trace	4
	Soups:																	
	Canned, condensed, ready-to-serve:																	
	Prepared with an equal volume of milk:																	
583	Cream of chicken	1 cup	245	85	180	7	10	3	3	3	15	172	.5	610	.05	.27	.7	2
584	Cream of mushroom.	1 cup	245	83	215	7	14	4	4	5	16	191	.5	250	.05	.34	.7	1
585	Tomato	1 cup	250	84	175	7	7	3	2	1	23	168	.8	1,200	.10	.25	1.3	15
	Prepared with an equal volume of water:																	
586	Bean with pork	1 cup	250	84	170	8	6	1	2	2	22	63	2.3	650	.13	.08	1.0	3
587	Beef broth, bouillon consomme.	1 cup	240	96	30	5	0	----	----	----	3	Trace	.5	Trace	Trace	.02	1.2	----
588	Beef noodle	1 cup	240	93	70	4	3	1	1	1	7	7	1.0	50	.05	.07	1.0	Trace
589	Clam chowder, Manhattan type (with tomatoes, without milk).	1 cup	245	92	80	2	3	----	----	----	12	34	1.0	880	.02	.02	1.0	----
590	Cream of chicken	1 cup	240	92	95	3	6	1	2	3	8	24	.5	410	.02	.05	.5	Trace
591	Cream of mushroom.	1 cup	240	90	135	2	10	1	3	5	10	41	.5	70	.02	.12	.7	Trace
592	Minestrone	1 cup	245	90	105	5	3	----	----	----	14	37	1.0	2,350	.07	.05	1.0	----

NUTRITIVE VALUES OF THE EDIBLE PART OF FOODS

[Dashes in the columns for nutrients show that no suitable value could be found although there is reason to believe that a measurable amount of the nutrient may be present]

Food, approximate measure, and weight (in grams)	Water	Food energy	Protein	Fat	Fatty acids			Carbohydrate	Calcium	Iron	Vitamin A value	Thiamin	Riboflavin	Niacin	Ascorbic acid
					Saturated (total)	Unsaturated Oleic	Linoleic								
	Grams	Percent	Calories	Grams	Grams	Grams	Grams	Grams	Milligrams	Milligrams	International units	Milligrams	Milligrams	Milligrams	Milligrams
MISCELLANEOUS ITEMS—Continued															
Soups—Continued															
Canned, condensed, ready-to-serve—Con.															
Prepared with an equal volume of water—Con.															
593 Split pea------- 1 cup------- 245	85	145	9	3	1	2	Trace	21	29	1.5	440	0.25	0.15	1.5	1
594 Tomato------- 1 cup------- 245	90	90	2	3	Trace	1	1	16	15	.7	1,000	.05	.05	1.2	12
595 Vegetable beef --- 1 cup------- 245	92	80	5	2	---	---	---	10	12	.7	2,700	.05	.05	1.0	---
596 Vegetarian------- 1 cup------- 245	92	80	2	2	---	---	---	13	20	1.0	2,940	.05	.05	1.0	---
Dehydrated, dry form:															
597 Chicken noodle (2-oz. package). 1 pkg------- 57	6	220	8	6	2	3	1	33	34	1.4	190	.30	.15	2.4	3
598 Onion mix (1½-oz. package). 1 pkg------- 43	3	150	6	5	1	2	1	23	42	.6	30	.05	.03	.3	6
599 Tomato vegetable with noodles (2½-oz. pkg.). 1 pkg------- 71	4	245	6	6	2	3	1	45	33	1.4	1,700	.21	.13	1.8	18
Frozen, condensed:															
Clam chowder, New England type (with milk, without tomatoes):															
600 Prepared with equal volume of milk. 1 cup------- 245	83	210	9	12	•	---	---	16	240	1.0	250	.07	.29	.5	Trace
601 Prepared with equal volume of water. 1 cup------- 240	89	130	4	8	---	---	---	11	91	1.0	50	.05	.10	.5	---
Cream of potato:															
602 Prepared with equal volume of milk. 1 cup------- 245	83	185	8	10	5	3	Trace	18	208	1.0	590	.10	.27	.5	Trace
603 Prepared with equal volume of water. 1 cup------- 240	90	105	3	5	3	2	Trace	12	58	1.0	410	.05	.05	.5	---

No.	Food	Measure	Weight (grams)	Water (%)	Food energy (Cal.)	Protein (g)	Fat (g)	Saturated (total) (g)	Unsaturated Oleic (g)	Unsaturated Linoleic (g)	Carbohydrate (g)	Calcium (mg)	Iron (mg)	Vitamin A (I.U.)	Thiamine (mg)	Riboflavin (mg)	Niacin (mg)	Ascorbic acid (mg)
604	Cream of shrimp: Prepared with equal volume of milk.	1 cup	245	82	245	9	16	---	---	---	15	189	.5	290	.07	.27	.5	Trace
605	Prepared with equal volume of water.	1 cup	240	88	160	5	12	---	---	---	8	38	.5	120	.05	.05	.5	---
606	Oyster stew: Prepared with equal volume of milk.	1 cup	240	83	200	10	12	---	---	---	14	305	1.4	410	.12	.41	.5	Trace
607	Prepared with equal volume of water.	1 cup	240	90	120	6	8	---	---	---	8	158	1.4	240	.07	.19	.5	---
608	Tapioca, dry, quick-cooking.	1 cup	152	13	535	1	Trace	---	---	---	131	15	.6	0	0	0	0	0
	Tapioca desserts:																	
609	Apple.	1 cup	250	70	295	1	Trace	---	---	---	74	8	.5	30	Trace	Trace	Trace	Trace
610	Cream pudding.	1 cup	165	72	220	8	8	3	---	---	28	173	.7	480	.07	.30	.2	2
611	Tartar sauce.	1 tbsp.	14	34	75	Trace	8	1	4	1	1	3	.1	30	Trace	Trace	Trace	Trace
612	Vinegar.	1 tbsp.	15	94	Trace	Trace	0	---	---	---	1	1	.1	---	Trace	Trace	Trace	---
613	White sauce, medium.	1 cup	250	73	405	10	31	16	10	1	22	288	.5	1,150	.10	.43	.5	2
	Yeast:																	
614	Baker's, dry, active.	1 pkg.	7	5	20	3	Trace	---	---	---	3	3	1.1	Trace	.16	.38	2.6	Trace
615	Brewer's, dry.	1 tbsp.	8	5	25	3	Trace	---	---	---	3	17	1.4	Trace	1.25	.34	3.0	Trace
	Yoghurt. See Milk, Cheese, Cream, Imitation Cream.																	

RECOMMENDED DIETARY ALLOWANCES*

*From RECOMMENDED DIETARY ALLOWANCES, Eighth Edition, Publication ISBN 0-309-32216-9, Food and Nutrition Board, National Academy of Sciences - National Research Council, Washington, D.C., 1974.

FOOD AND NUTRITION BOARD, NATIONAL ACADEMY
RECOMMENDED DAILY DIETARY

Designed for the maintenance of good nutrition

| | Age | Weight | | Height | | Energy | Protein | Fat-Soluble Vitamins | | | |
| | | | | | | | | Vita-min A Activity | | Vita-min D | Vita-min E Activity[e] |
	(years)	(kg)	(lbs)	(cm)	(in)	(kcal)[b]	(g)	(RE)[c]	(IU)	(IU)	(IU)
Infants	0.0-0.5	6	14	60	24	kg × 117	kg × 2.2	420[d]	1,400	400	4
	0.5-1.0	9	20	71	28	kg × 108	kg × 2.0	400	2,000	400	5
Children	1-3	13	28	86	34	1,300	23	400	2,000	400	7
	4-6	20	44	110	44	1,800	30	500	2,500	400	9
	7-10	30	66	135	54	2,400	36	700	3,300	400	10
Males	11-14	44	97	158	63	2,800	44	1,000	5,000	400	12
	15-18	61	134	172	69	3,000	54	1,000	5,000	400	15
	19-22	67	147	172	69	3,000	54	1,000	5,000	400	15
	23-50	70	154	172	69	2,700	56	1,000	5,000		15
	51+	70	154	172	69	2,400	56	1,000	5,000		15
Females	11-14	44	97	155	62	2,400	44	800	4,000	400	12
	15-18	54	119	162	65	2,100	48	800	4,000	400	12
	19-22	58	128	162	65	2,100	46	800	4,000	400	12
	23-50	58	128	162	65	2,000	46	800	4,000		12
	51+	58	128	162	65	1,800	46	800	4,000		12
Pregnant						+300	+30	1,000	5,000	400	15
Lactating						+500	+20	1,200	6,000	400	15

[a] The allowances are intended to provide for individual variations among most normal persons as they live in the United States under usual environmental stresses. Diets should be based on a variety of common foods in order to provide other nutrients for which human requirements have been less well defined. See text for more detailed discussion of allowances and of nutrients not tabulated. See table for weights and heights by individual year of age.

[b] Kilojoules (k j) = 4.2 kcal.

[c] Retinol equivalents.

[d] Assumed to be all as retinol in milk during the first six months of life. All subsequent intakes are assumed to be half as retinol and half as β-carotene when calculated from international units. As retinol equivalents, three fourths are as retinol and one fourth as β-carotene.

[e] Total vitamine E activity, estimated to be 80 percent as α-tocopherol and 20 percent other tocopherols. See text for variation in allowances.

OF SCIENCES-NATIONAL RESEARCH COUNCIL
ALLOWANCES,[a]   Revised 1974

of practically all healthy people in the U.S.A.

Water-Soluble Vitamins							Minerals					
Ascorbic Acid (mg)	Folacin[f] (μg)	Niacin[g] (mg)	Riboflavin (mg)	Thiamin (mg)	Vitamin B_6 (mg)	Vitamin B_{12} (μg)	Calcium (mg)	Phosphorus (mg)	Iodine (μg)	Iron (mg)	Magnesium (mg)	Zinc (mg)
35	50	5	0.4	0.3	0.3	0.3	360	240	35	10	60	3
35	50	8	0.6	0.5	0.4	0.3	540	400	45	15	70	5
40	100	9	0.8	0.7	0.6	1.0	800	800	60	15	150	10
40	200	12	1.1	0.9	0.9	1.5	800	800	80	10	200	10
40	300	16	1.2	1.2	1.2	2.0	800	800	110	10	250	10
45	400	18	1.5	1.4	1.6	3.0	1,200	1,200	130	18	350	15
45	400	20	1.8	1.5	2.0	3.0	1,200	1,200	150	18	400	15
45	400	20	1.8	1.5	2.0	3.0	800	800	140	10	350	15
45	400	18	1.6	1.4	2.0	3.0	800	800	130	10	350	15
45	400	16	1.5	1.2	1.6	3.0	800	800	110	10	350	15
45	400	16	1.3	1.2	2.0	3.0	1,200	1,200	115	18	300	15
45	400	14	1.4	1.1	2.0	3.0	1,200	1,200	115	18	300	15
45	400	14	1.4	1.1	2.0	3.0	800	800	100	18	300	15
45	400	13	1.2	1.0	2.0	3.0	800	800	100	18	300	15
45	400	12	1.1	1.0	2.0	3.0	800	800	80	10	300	15
60	800	+2	+0.3	+0.3	2.5	4.0	1,200	1,200	125	18+ [h]	450	20
80	600	+4	+0.5	+0.3	2,5	4.0	1,200	1,200	150	18	450	25

[f] The folacin allowances refer to dietary sources as determined by *Lactobacillus casei* assay. Pure forms of folacin may be effective in doses less than one fourth of the recommended dietary allowance.

[g] Although allowances are expressed as niacin, it is recognized that on the average 1 mg of niacin is derived from each 60 mg of dietary tryptophan.

[h] This increased requirement cannot be met by ordinary diets; therefore, the use of supplemental iron is recommended.

APPENDIX C

SUBSTITUTES WITHIN
BASIC FOOD GROUPS*

Foods within a group can be substituted or exchanged for each other.

Milk
(1 cup whole milk contains 12 grams carbohydrate, 8 grams protein, 10 grams fat, and 170
   calories; 1 cup of skim milk contains 80 calories; 1 cup cocoa made with milk contains
   approximately 200 calories)
1 cup whole milk
1 cup skim milk
1/2 cup evaporated milk
1/4 cup powdered milk
1 cup buttermilk
1 cup cocoa

MEAT GROUP
(1 ounce contains 7 grams protein, 5 grams fat, and 75 calories)
1 ounce lean beef, lamb, pork, liver, chicken*
1 ounce fish — cod, haddock, perch, etc.
1 hot dog
1/4 cup tuna, salmon, crab, lobster
5 small oysters, shrimp, clams
3 medium sardines
1 slice cheese
1/4 cup cottage cheese
1 egg
2 tablespoons peanut butter
*1 average serving of meat or fish (such as a pork chop or 2 meatballs) is about 3 ounces

---

DARK GREEN OR DEEP YELLOW VEGETABLES (1/2 cup is one serving)
Greens and lettuce have very little carbohydrate content. The other vegetables contain
   approximately 7 grams carbohydrate and 2 grams protein and 35 calories

Broccoli*	Greens:*
Carrots	Beet greens
Chicory*	Chard
Escarole*	Collard

---

*Reprinted from *Nutrition for Athletes* with the permission of the American Alliance for
Health, Physical Education, and Recreation, 1201 Sixteenth Street, N.W., Washington,
D.C., 20036.

Pepper	Dandelion
Pumpkin	Kale
Tomatoes*	Mustard
Watercress*	Spinach
Winter squash	Turnip greens
	Lettuce*

*Low Calorie Vegetables.

CITRUS FRUITS OR SUBSTITUTE (1/2 cup is one serving)
The carbohydrate is averaged to approximately 10 grams per 1/2 cup and 40 calories

Orange	Grapefruit juice*	Tangerine
Orange juice	Cantaloupe*	Tomato juice*
Grapefruit*	Strawberries*	

*Represents low calorie fruits and vegetables

OTHER FRUITS AND VEGETABLES
Fruits (1/2 cup is approximately 10 grams carbohydrate and 40 calories)

Apple	Dates	Peach
Applesauce	Figs	Pear
Apricots	Grapes	Pineapple
Banana (1/2 small)	Grape juice (1/4 cup)	Plums
Raspberries	Honeydew melon	Raisins (2 tablespoons)
Blueberries	Mango	Pineapple juice (1/3 cup)
Cherries	Papaya	Prunes (2 medium)
		Watermelon*

Vegetables (1/2 cup is one serving)
The vegetables without the asterisk contain approximately 7 grams carbohydrate, 2 grams
    protein, and 35 calories

Asparagus*	Cucumbers*	Radishes*
Beets	Eggplant*	Rutabagas
Brussels sprouts*	Mushrooms*	Sauerkraut*
Cabbage*	Okra*	String beans*
Cauliflower*	Onions	Summer squash*
Celery*	Peas, green	Turnips

*Represents low calorie fruits and vegetables

BREAD GROUP
(1 slice of bread or 1 substitute contains 15 grams carbohydrate, 2 grams protein, and 70
    calories)

1/2 hamburger bun	1/2 cup spaghetti, noodles,	2/3 cup parsnips
1/2 hot dog bun	macaroni, etc.	1 small potato
1 cup popcorn	2 graham crackers	1/2 cup mashed potato
2 1/2" wedge pizza	5 saltines	15 potato chips — 1 ounce bag
1 slice enriched bread	6 round, thin crackers	6 pretzels, medium, or 20
		thin sticks
1 biscuit or roll	1/2 cup beans or peas	8 French fries
1 small muffin	(dried or cooked)	1/4 cup sweet potato or yams
1 small piece cornbread	(Lima or navy beans,	1 1/2 " cube sponge or angel
1/2 cup cooked cereal	split peas, cowpeas, etc.)	cake (no icing)

3/4 cup ready-to-eat cereal   1/4 cup baked beans   1/2 cup ice cream (omit
1/2 cup rice or grits   1/3 cup corn   2 fat servings)

FAT GROUP
(1 teaspoon fat contains 5 grams fat and 45 calories)

Bacon	1 slice	Cream cheese	1 tablespoon
Butter or margarine or fat spread	1 teaspoon	French dressing	1 tablespoon
		Mayonnaise	1 teaspoon
Cream (light)	2 tablespoons	Oil or cooking fat	1 teaspoon
Cream (heavy — 40%)	1 tablespoon		

SUGARS

(1 teaspoon contains	Sugar	Syrup
5 grams carbohydrate and	Jelly	Hard candy
20 calories)	Honey	Carbonated beverage (1/4 cup)

Salt used in the home should be iodized.

BASIC LOW CALORIE DIETS
WITH ALTERNATE FOODS*

---

*Courtesy of the National Dairy Council.

1000 calorie diet

DAILY MEAL PATTERN

SAMPLE MENUS

Breakfast

Fruit
Egg } or Cereal plus
Bread } ½ cup skim milk
Butter
Coffee or Tea (without
  sugar or cream)

Orange juice . . . . . . ½ cup
Oatmeal with . . . . . ½ cup
  Milk, skim . . . . ½ cup
Coffee

Grapefruit . . . . ½ small
Poached egg 1
Toast,
  whole wheat . . . . .1 slice
Butter . . . . 1 pat
Coffee

Lunch

Protein-rich food

Vegetable

Bread
Butter
Fruit
Milk

Sandwich
  Luncheon meat . . .1 slice
  American cheese . .1 slice
Bread
  whole wheat . . . .1 slice
Butter . . . . 1 pat
Carrot and celery sticks
Peach,
  fresh or canned,
  unsweetened . .1 medium
Milk, skim . . . . 1 cup

Salad
  Cottage cheese . . .½ cup
  Tomato 1
  Lettuce leaves
  French
    dressing . . . . 1 teaspoon

Saltines 5
Apple . . . . 1 small
Milk, skim . . . . 1 cup

Dinner

Protein-rich food
Vegetables, 2 or more
  servings
  1 cooked
  1 or more raw

Fruit
Beverage

Broiled beef
  patty (large) . . .4 ounces
Asparagus . . . . .½ cup
Tossed green salad
  Vinegar dressing
Melon in season
Milk, skim . . . . .½ cup
Tea

Chilled consomme
Roast chicken,
  leg and thigh
Peas . . . . .½ cup
Lettuce wedge
  Lemon juice dressing
Pineapple, fresh
  or canned
  unsweetened . . . . .½ cup
Tea

Snacks

Bouillon, consomme, raw
vegetables, unsweetened
gelatin salad or dessert,
unsweetened beverages,
or food saved from meals.

Bouillon with mushrooms
Green pepper and cucum-
ber sticks

Unsweetened gelatin
  dessert
Milk, skim . . . . 1 cup

1200 calorie diet

DAILY MEAL PATTERN	SAMPLE MENUS	

Breakfast

Fruit	Orange juice . . . . . . ½ cup	Grapefruit . . . . . . .½ small
Egg ⎫ or Cereal plus	Oatmeal with . . . . .½ cup	Poached egg 1
Bread ⎰ ½ cup milk	Milk . . . . .½ cup	Toast,
Butter	Coffee	whole wheat . . . . .1 slice
Coffee or Tea (without		Butter . . . . 1 pat
sugar or cream)		Coffee

Lunch

Protein-rich food	Sandwich	Salad
	Luncheon meat . . .1 slice	Cottage cheese . . .½ cup
	American cheese . .1 slice	Tomato 1
Vegetable	Bread,	Lettuce leaves
	whole wheat . . . .1 slice	French
	Butter . . . . 1 pat	dressing . . . . 1 teaspoon
Bread	Carrot sticks	Saltines 5
Butter	Peach,	Apricots,
Fruit	fresh or canned,	dried . . . . 4 halves
Milk	unsweetened . .1 medium	Milk . . . . 1 cup
	Milk . . . . 1 cup	

Dinner

Protein-rich food	Broiled beef	Chilled consomme
Vegetables, 2 or more	patty (large) . . .4 ounces	Roast Chicken,
servings		leg and thigh
1 cooked	Asparagus . . . . .½ cup	
1 or more raw	Tossed green salad	Peas . . . . .½ cup
	Vinegar dressing	Lettuce wedge
	Bread,	Lemon juice dressing
Bread	whole wheat . . . . .1 slice	Pineapple,
Butter	Butter . . . . 1 pat	fresh or canned,
Fruit	Cantaloupe . . . ¼ medium	unsweetened . . . . .½ cup
Milk	Milk . . . . .½ cup	Milk . . . . 1 cup
	Tea	

Snacks

Bouillon, consomme, raw	Bouillon with mushrooms	Unsweetened gelatin
vegetables, unsweetened	Green pepper and	dessert
gelatin salad or dessert,	cucumber sticks	
unsweetened beverages,		
or food saved from meals.		

1400 calorie diet

DAILY MEAL PATTERN	SAMPLE MENUS	

Breakfast

Fruit	Orange juice ......½ cup	Grapefruit ....½ small
Egg 〉 or Cereal plus	Oatmeal with .....½ cup	Poached egg 1
Bread 〉 ½ cup milk	Milk ....½ cup	Toast,
Butter	Coffee	whole wheat .....1 slice
Coffee or Tea (without		Butter .... 1 pat .
sugar or cream)		Coffee

Lunch

Protein-rich food	Sandwich	Salad
	Luncheon meat . . .1 slice	Cottage cheese . . .½ cup
	American cheese . .1 slice	Tomato 1
Vegetables	Bread,	Lettuce leaves
	whole wheat . . . .1 slice	French
	Butter .... 1 pat	dressing . . . .1 teaspoon
Bread	Carrot and celery sticks	
Butter	Peach,	Saltines 5
Fruit	fresh or canned,	Banana ....½ small
Milk	unsweetened . .1 medium	Milk ....1 cup
	Milk.......... 1 cup	

Dinner

Protein-rich food	Broiled beef	Chilled consomme
	patty (large) . . .4 ounces	Roast chicken,
Vegetables, 2 or more	Baked potato . . . .1 small	leg and thigh
servings	Butter .... 1 pat	Grits ....½ cup
1 cooked	Asparagus ....½ cup	Butter .... 1 pat
1 or more raw	Tossed green salad	Peas.............½ cup
	French	Lettuce wedge
Bread	dressing . . . .1 teaspoon	Lemon juice dressing
Butter	Cantaloupe . . . ¼ medium	Pineapple,
Fruit	Milk ....½ cup	fresh or canned,
Milk	Tea	unsweetened .....½ cup
		Milk ....1 cup

Snacks

Bread	Bouillon	Graham crackers 2
Butter	Saltines 5	Butter .... 1 pat
Fruit	Butter .... 1 pat	Grapes ....½ cup
	Apple ....1 small	

1800 calorie diet

DAILY MEAL PATTERN		SAMPLE MENUS

Breakfast

Fruit	Orange juice ......½ cup	Grapefruit ....½ small
Egg ⎫ or Cereal plus	Oatmeal with .....½ cup	Poached egg 1
Bread ⎭ ½ cup milk	Milk ....½ cup	Toast,
Butter	Bacon :......... 1 strip	whole wheat ....2 slices
Coffee or Tea (without	Toast,	Butter ....2 pats
sugar or cream)	whole wheat .....1 slice	Milk ....1 cup
	Butter .... 1 pat	Coffee
	Coffee	

Lunch

Protein-rich food	Bouillon	Salad
	Sandwich	Cottage cheese ...½ cup
Vegetable	Luncheon meat ...1 slice	Tomato 1
	American cheese ..1 slice	Romaine leaves 2
	Bread,	Lemon juice dressing
Bread	whole wheat ...2 slices	
Butter	Butter ....2 pats	Toast,
Fruit	Carrot sticks	whole wheat 2
Milk	Peach,	Butter 2
	fresh or canned,	Cantaloupe ...¼ medium
	unsweetened ..1 medium	Milk ....1 cup
	Milk ....1 cup	

Dinner

Protein-rich food	Broiled beef	Chilled consomme
Vegetables, 2 or more	patty (large) ...4 ounces	Roast chicken,
servings	Hamburger Bun 1	leg and thigh
1 cooked	Butter ....2 pats	Baked potato ....1 small
1 or more raw	Sliced tomato	Butter ....2 pats
Bread	Tossed green salad	Peas.............½ cup
Butter	French	Lettuce wedge
Fruit	dressing ....1 teaspoon	French
Milk	Strawberries in	dressing ....1 teaspoon
	unsweetened gelatin	Bread,
	dessert	whole wheat .....1 slice
	Milk ....½ cup	Pineapple,
	Tea	fresh or canned,
		unsweetened .....½ cup
		Tea

Snacks

Fruit	Grapes ....½ cup	Dried apricots ... 4 halves
Bread	Graham crackers 2	Saltines 5
Milk	Milk ....1 cup	Butter .... 1 pat
		Yogurt, plain .....1 cup

TASTE-TEMPTING TIPS

Low-calorie diets allow a wide variety of common foods. Meals can be varied, although the cooking method should not add extra calories.

Add zest to cooked vegetables and salads with fresh parsley, chives, dill, fennel, green or red pepper, pimento strips, or a few drops of lemon, garlic, or onion juice.

For snacks and/or meals use bouillon or consomme as an appetizer; a soup, plain or with vegetables from List 2; or as the cooking liquid for rice, potatoes, or other vegetables.

Unflavored gelatin and fruit or vegetable juice plus raw vegetables from List 2 make good salads for meals or snacks.

Tasty low-calorie salad dressings can be made by using vinegar, pickle juice, lemon juice, tomato juice, or yogurt as the base. For variety, add seasoned salt and pepper, garlic, dry mustard, dill, tarragon, or paprika. Use as desired. If oil is added, use as a butter alternate.

Use tangy yogurt or buttermilk in place of sour cream with potatoes, salads, and meat.

Other flavor-enhancing ideas:

... with meat: bay leaf, dry mustard, sage, marjoram, paprika, thyme, curry, garlic, rosemary, oregano, onion, green pepper, lemon juice, parsley.

... with egg: curry, dry mustard, green pepper, mushrooms, onion, parsley, tomato.

... with vegetables: lemon juice, green pepper, tomato, onion, parsley, mushrooms, marjoram, dill, mace, basil, plain yogurt, or buttermilk.

Dishes like stews or casseroles are simply combinations of foods. The foods allowed on your diet may be combined any way you desire.

All extra food or larger servings add calories. Sweeteners such as sugar, honey, and syrup are high in calories and low in nutrients and, therefore, have been omitted. Fried foods are not included because all fats are high in calories. The butter allowance may be used for frying rather than with your bread.

Alternates for 1 Cup Skim Milk: average 88 Calories
1/2 cup cottage cheese
3/4 cup plain yogurt
1 cup buttermilk
1 glass whole milk (if you omit butter allowance)

Alternates for Meat: average 208 Calories
oo 3 ounces boiled, broiled, roasted meat with all visible fat removed—about 1/4 pound raw meat
oo 1 slice of beef about 3″ by 3″ by 1/2″
oo 1 ground beef patty, 3″ in diameter, 1″ thick
o leg and thigh of chicken
o fish fillet, 3″ by 3″ by 1/2″
o 2/3 cup canned fish, packed in water
2 tablespoons peanut butter
oo 3 eggs
2 slices American or Swiss cheese
3/4 cup cottage cheese
oo 2/3 cup dried beans or peas
oo 2/3 cup chilli con carne with beans
1 1/4 frankfurter (8 per pound)
2 slices bologna

Alternates for Vegetables:
List 1, 1/2 cup cooked: average 40 Calories

Vitamin A	Others
carrots	beets
o squash, winter	o peas
pumpkin	onions
	rutabagas
Vitamin C	turnips
o tomato juice	

List 2, 1/2 cup cooked, as much raw as desired:
average 13 Calories

Vitamin A	Others	
broccoli	asparagus	green beans
o greens	brussels sprouts	green onions
peppers, chili	cauliflower	lettuce
tomato	celery	parsley
Vitamin C	chives	radishes
broccoli	cucumber	sauerkraut
cabbage	o endive	o romaine
o greens	o escarole	squash, summer
green pepper		mushrooms
tomato		

Alternates for Fruit: fresh and unsweetened: average 55 Calories

Vitamin C		Others	
cantaloupe	1/4 medium	apple	1 small
grapefruit	1/2 small	applesauce	1/2 cup
grapefruit juice	1/2 cup	blackberries	1 cup
orange	1 small	banana	1/2 small
orange juice	1/2 cup	blueberries	2/3 cup
strawberries	1 cup	cherries	1/2 cup
tangerine	1 medium	grapes	1/2 cup
o watermelon	1 cup	honeydew	1/8 medium
		peach	1 medium
Vitamin A		pear	1 small
apricots, fresh	2	pineapple	1/2 cup
dried	4 halves	pineapple	
cantaloupe	1/4 medium	juice	1/3 cup
o watermelon	1 cup	plums	2 small
		prunes	2
		raisins	2 tablespoons
		raspberries	1 cup

Alternates for Grain Products: average 60 Calories
o (whole wheat, enriched, or fortified grain products)

bread	1 slice	grits, cooked	1/2 cup
crackers		rice, cooked	1/4 cup
graham	2	noodles, cooked	1/3 cup
oyster	10	pasta, cooked	1/2 cup
saltines	5		
pancake, 4″	1	Vegetables	
roll, frankfurter	1/2	green lima	
roll, hamburger	1/2	beans	1/2 cup
tortilla, 6″	1	corn	1/2 cup
cereal, cooked;	1/2 cup	parsnips	1/2 cup
ready-to-eat,	3/4 cup	potato	1 small
unsweetened			

Alternates for 1 Teaspoon Butter: average 36 Calories
1 teaspoon oil or cooking fat
1 teaspoon mayonnaise
1 teaspoon French dressing
1 tablespoon sour cream
1 tablespoon half and half
1 slice crisp bacon

＊Iron-rich foods:
oIndicates that one serving contributes 5 to 14 percent of the U.S. Recommended
Daily Allowance.
ooIndicates that one serving contributes 15 to 23 percent.
NOTE:
Liver and other variety meats contribute over 40 percent of the recommended
allowance of iron.

APPENDIX E

HEIGHT AND WEIGHT TABLES
FOR BOYS AND GIRLS*

*From Krause, M. and Hunscher, M.: FOOD, NUTRITION AND DIET THERAPY, Courtesy of W. B. Saunders Company, Philadelphia, Pennsylvania.

Boys

(Weight is Expressed in Pounds)

Ht. Ins.	5 Yrs.	6 Yrs.	7 Yrs.	8 Yrs.	9 Yrs.	10 Yrs.	11 Yrs.	12 Yrs.	13 Yrs.	14 Yrs.	15 Yrs.	16 Yrs.	17 Yrs.	18 Yrs.	19 Yrs.	Ht. Ins.
38	34	34														38
39	35	35														39
40	36	36														40
41	38	38	38													41
42	39	39	39	39												42
43	41	41	41	41												43
44	44	44	44	44												44
45	46	46	46	46	46											45
46	47	48	48	48	48											46
47	49	50	50	50	50	50										47
48		52	53	53	53	53										48
49		55	55	55	55	55	55									49
50		57	58	58	58	58	58	58								50
51			61	61	61	61	61	61								51
52			63	64	64	64	64	64	64							52
53			66	67	67	67	67	68	68							53
54				70	70	70	70	71	71	72						54
55				72	72	73	73	74	74	74						55
56				75	76	77	77	77	78	78	80					56
57					79	80	81	81	82	83	83					57
58					83	84	84	85	85	86	87					58
59						87	88	89	89	90	90	90				59
60						91	92	92	93	94	95	96				60
61							95	96	97	99	100	103	106			61
62							100	101	102	103	104	107	111	116		62
63							105	106	107	108	110	113	118	123	127	63
64								109	111	113	115	117	121	126	130	64
65								114	117	118	120	122	127	131	134	65
66									119	122	125	128	132	136	139	66
67									124	128	130	134	136	139	142	67
68										134	134	137	141	143	147	68
69										137	139	143	146	149	152	69
70										143	144	145	148	151	155	70
71										148	150	151	152	154	159	71
72											153	155	156	158	163	72
73											157	160	162	164	167	73
74											160	164	168	180	171	74

The following percentages of net weight have been added for clothing (shoes and sweaters not included): 35 to 64 pounds: 3.5 percent; 64 pounds and over: 2.0 per cent.

Girls

(Weight is Expressed in Pounds)

Ht. Ins.	5 Yrs.	6 Yrs.	7 Yrs.	8 Yrs.	9 Yrs.	10 Yrs.	11 Yrs.	12 Yrs.	13 Yrs.	14 Yrs.	15 Yrs.	16 Yrs.	17 Yrs.	18 Yrs.	Ht. Ins.
38	33	33													38
39	34	34													39
40	36	36	36												40
41	37	37	37												41
42	39	39	39												42
43	41	41	41	41											43
44	42	42	42	42											44
45	45	45	45	45	45										45
46	47	47	47	48	48										46
47	49	50	50	50	50	50									47
48		52	52	52	52	53									48
49		54	54	55	55	56	56								49
50		56	56	57	58	59	61	62							50
51			59	60	61	61	63	65							51
52			63	64	64	64	65	67							52
53			66	67	67	68	68	69	71						53
54				69	70	70	71	71	73						54
55				72	74	74	74	75	77	78					55
56					76	78	78	79	81	83					56
57					80	82	82	82	84	88	92				57
58						84	86	86	88	93	96	101			58
59						87	90	90	92	96	100	103	104		59
60						91	95	95	97	101	105	108	109	111	60
61							99	100	101	105	108	112	113	116	61
62							104	105	106	109	113	115	117	118	62
63								110	110	112	116	117	119	120	63
64								114	115	117	119	120	122	123	64
65								118	120	121	122	123	125	126	65
66									124	124	125	128	129	130	66
67									128	130	131	133	133	135	67
68									131	133	135	136	138	138	68
69										135	137	138	140	142	69
70										136	138	140	142	144	70
71										138	140	142	144	145	71

The following percentages of net weight have been added for clothing (shoes and sweaters not included): 35 to 65 pounds: 3.0 per cent; 66 to 82 pounds: 2.5 per cent; 83 pounds and over: 2 per cent.

PREDICTION FORMULAE FOR BODY FAT

EVALUATION OF BODY FAT FROM
SKINFOLD MEASUREMENTS

A. In order to make accurate measurements, it is important to use calipers which have the pressure built into the instrument itself. Standardized procedures should be followed when taking any skinfold measurement.
Briefly:
    1. a full fold of fat should be pinched up from the underlying tissue by the thumb and forefinger of one hand.
    2. while the fold is held firmly between the fingers, the calipers should be applied to the fold beneath the fingers.
    3. take recordings to the nearest half mm.
    4. duplicate the measurements until two consecutive measurements agree within one mm.
B. With fat calipers, take the following measurements. Females are measured at X and Z, while males are measured at X, Y and Z
    X — abdominal skinfold in mm. The measure is taken at the midaxillary line at waist level.
    Y — chest skinfold in mm, at the level of xiphold in the midaxillary line.
    Z — arm skinfold in mm. Triceps: skinfold is made at the back of the upper arm, at a level midway between the tip of the acromial process of the scapula and the tip of the elbow. Lift the skinfold parallel to the long axis of the arm while the elbow is flexed to 90°, but take the measurement with the arm hanging loosely at the side.
C. Computation of Density. Skinfold technique (women)
Young women, aged 17-25
Density = 1.0764 - .00081 (X) - .00088 (Z)
Conversion of density to body fat

$$\text{Percent body fat} = 100 \left\{ \frac{4.201}{\text{Density}} - 3.813 \right\}$$

D. Skinfold Technique (men)

Calculation of specific gravity from skinfold measurements via method of Brozek and Keys, with conversion to percent body fat by method of Rathbun and Pace.

Specific gravity = $1.1017 - 0.000282(X) - 0.000736(Y) - 0.000883(Z)$

Conversion of specific gravity to percent body fat.

$$\text{Percent fat} = 100 \left\{ \frac{5.548}{\text{sp.gr.}} - 5.044 \right\}$$

AMERICAN COLLEGE OF SPORTS MEDICINE POSITION STATEMENT ON HEAT INJURIES*

AMERICAN COLLEGE OF SPORTS MEDICINE

POSITION STATEMENT ON

Prevention of Heat Injuries During Distance Running

PURPOSE OF POSITION STATEMENT

The Purpose of this Position Statement is:

(a) To alert local, national and international sponsors of distance running events of the health hazards of heat injury during distance running and

(b) To inform said sponsors of injury preventative actions that may reduce the frequency of this type of injury.

The recommendations address only the manner in which distance running sports activities may be conducted to further reduce incidence of heat injury among normal athletes conditioned to participate in distance running. The recommendations are advisory only.

Recommendations concerning the ingested quantity and content of fluid are merely a partial preventative to heat injury. The physiology of each individual athlete varies: strict compliance with these recommendations and the current rules governing distance running may not reduce the incidence of heat injuries among those so inclined to such injury.

Based on research findings and current rules governing distance running competition, it is the position of the American College of

---

*From *Med Sci Sports*, 7:vii, 1975.

Sports Medicine that:

1. Distance races (> 16 km or 10 miles) should *not* be conducted when the wet bulb temperature — globe temperature exceeds 28° C (82.4° F).

2. During periods of the year, when the daylight dry bulb temperature often exceeds 27° C (80° F), distance races should be conducted before 9:00 A.M. or after 4:00 P.M.

3. It is the responsibility of the race sponsors to provide fluids which contain small amounts of sugar (less that 2.5 g glucose per 100 ml of water) and electrolytes (less than 10 mEq sodium and 5 mEq potassium per liter of solution.)

4. Runners should be encouraged to frequently ingest fluids during competition and to consume 400-500 ml (13-17 oz.) of fluid 10-15 minutes before competition.

5. Rules prohibiting the administration of fluids during the first 10 kilometers (6.2 miles) of a marathon race should be amended to permit fluid ingestion at frequent intervals along the race course. In light of the high sweat rates and body temperatures during distance running in the heat, race sponsors should provide "water stations" at 3-4 kilometer (2-2.5 mile) intervals for all races of 16 kilometers (10 miles) or more.

6. Runners should be instructed in how to recognize the early warning symptoms that precede heat injury. Recognition of symptoms, cessation of running, and proper treatment can prevent heat injury. Early warning symptoms include the following: piloerection on chest and upper arms, chilling, throbbing pressure in the head, unsteadiness, nausea, and dry skin.

7. Race sponsors should make prior arrangements with medical personnel for the care of cases of heat injury. Responsible and informed personnel should supervise each "feeding station." Organizational personnel should reserve the right to stop runners who exhibit clear signs of heat stroke or heat exhaustion.

It is the position of the American College of Sports Medicine that policies established by local, national, and international sponsors of distance running events should adhere to these guidelines. Failure to adhere to these guidelines may jeopardize the health of competitors through heat injury.

APPENDIX H

METRIC SYSTEM AND EQUIVALENTS*

*From Krause, M., and Hunscher, M.: FOOD, NUTRITION AND DIET THERAPY, 1972. Courtesy of W. B. Saunders Company, Philadelphia.

THE METRIC SYSTEM AND EQUIVALENTS

To measure ingredients, a standardized system has been established which is interpreted on an international basis. However, in our country we also employ another set of measure and weight. In the field of dietetics, both systems are employed. The following tables give the quantities of the measures besides stating equivalents. With this information it is possible to calculate in either system of measure and weight.

Level Measures and Weights

60 drops	=	1 teaspoon
		5 cc.
		5 grams
4 saltspoons	=	1 teaspoon
		5 grams
3 teaspoons	=	1 tablespoon
		15 cc.
		15 grams
1 dessert spoon	=	10 cc.
2 tablespoons	=	30 cc.
		30 grams
		1 ounce (fluid)
4 tablespoons	=	¼ cup
		60 cc.
		60 grams
8 tablespoons	=	½ cup
		120 cc.
		120 grams
16 tablespoons	=	1 cup
		240 grams
		250 ml. or mil. (fluid)
		8 ounces (fluid)
		½ pound
2 cups	=	1 pint
		480 grams
		500 ml. or mil. (fluid)
		16 ounces (fluid)
		1 pound
4 cups	=	2 pints
		1 quart
		1000 or 960 cc.
		1000 ml. or mil. (fluid)
		1 kilogram
		2.2 pounds
4 quarts	=	1 gallon
8 quarts	=	1 peck
2 gallons	=	1 peck
4 pecks	=	1 bushel
8 gallons	=	1 bushel

Household Measurement Equivalents in Grams

For easy computing purposes, the cubic centimeter (cc.) is considered equivalent to 1 gram:

1 cc. = 1 gram

For easy computing purposes, one ounce equals 30 grams or 30 cubic centimeters.

1 quart	= 960 grams
1 pint	= 480 grams
1 cup	= 240 grams
½ cup	= 120 grams
1 soup cup	= 120 grams
1 glass (8 ounces)	= 240 grams
½ glass (4 ounces)	= 120 grams
1 orange juice glass	= 100 to 120 grams
1 tablespoon	= 15 grams
1 teaspoon	= 5 grams

Comparison of Avoirdupois and Metric Weights

Ounces to Grams	Grams to Ounces
1 = 28.35	1 = 0.035

Pounds to Kilograms	Kilograms to Pounds
1 = 0.454	1 = 2.205

Comparison of United States and Metric Liquid Measure

Ounces (Fluid) to Milliliters	Milliliters to Ounces (Fluid)
1 = 29.573	1 = 0.034

Quarts to Liters	Liters to Quarts
1 = 0.946	1 = 1.057

Gallons to Liters	Liters to Gallons
1 = 3.785	1 = 0.264

Measures of Weight

1 gram	=	0.035	ounce
1 kilogram	=	2.21	pounds
1 ounce	=	28.35	grams
1 pound	=	453.6	grams

GLOSSARY

Acetaldehyde — an intermediate breakdown product of alcohol.

Acetic Acid — a naturally-occurring saturated fatty acid; a precursor for the Krebs cycle when converted into acetyl CoA.

Acetoacetic Acid — one of the ketone bodies, an intermediate by-product of fatty acid degradation under some circumstances.

Acetyl CoA — the major fuel for the oxidative processes in the body, the Krebs cycle; the major sources are derived from the metabolism of glucose and fatty acids.

ADH — anti-diuretic hormone.

Aerobic — relating to energy processes which occur in the presence of oxygen.

Alactacid — the portion of the oxygen debt that is not accounted for by lactate production.

Alanine — a nonessential amino acid.

Alcohol — a colorless liquid with depressant effects; ethyl alcohol or ethanol.

Aldosterone — the main electrolyte-regulating hormone secreted by the adrenal cortex; primarily controls sodium balance.

Alkaline Salts — buffering salts such as sodium bicarbonate used to counteract acidity in various parts of the body.

Alkalinizer — an agent that causes alkalinization, or making a substance alkaline.

Alpha-tocopherol — the most biologically active alcohol in vitamin E; a main constituent of wheat germ oil.

Amino Acids — the chief structure of protein, some being essential in human nutrition.

Aminoacetic Acid — a colorless powder, derivable from many proteins and ofttimes used as a dietary supplement; glycine; glycocoll.

Ammonia — a metabolic byproduct of the oxidation of glutamate; may be formed into urea for excretion from the body.

Amphetamines — synthetic stimulants of the central nervous system.

Amylase — an enzyme that catabolyzes starches into smaller compounds.

Anabolic Steroids — chemical compounds similar to testosterone that facilitate the building of muscular tissue with minimal androgenic effects.

Anaerobic — relating to energy processes which occur in the absence of oxygen.

Antidiuretic Hormone — a hormone secreted by the pituitary gland that suppresses the secretion of urine.

Arachidonic Acid — an unsaturated fatty acid which is a main constituent of lecithin.

413

Arginine — an essential amino acid.
Arteriosclerosis — hardening of the arteries.
Ascorbic Acid — vitamin C.
Asparagine — an amide of aspartic acid, a nonessential amino acid.
Aspartates — salts of aspartic acid, a nonessential amino acid.
Atherosclerosis — a specific form of arteriosclerosis, characterized by the formation of plaques on the inner layers of the arterial wall.
ATP — abbreviation for adenosine triphosphate, one of the prime energy sources in the body.

BAL — blood alcohol level; the concentration of alcohol in the blood.
Basal Metabolic Rate — BMR; measurement of energy expenditure under resting, postabsorptive conditions.
Benzedrine — trademark for a preparation of amphetamine.
Betahydroxybutryic Acid — an intermediate metabolite produced in the oxidation of fat; one of the ketone bodies.
Blood Sugar — glucose, the form by which carbohydrate is carried in the blood; normal range is 70-120 mg/100 ml.
BMR — Basal Metabolic Rate

Caffeine — a stimulant of the central nervous system
Carotene — a provitamin which may be converted into vitamin A in the body.
Cholecalciferol — the product of irradiation of 7-dehydrocholesterol found in the skin.
Cholesterol — a fatlike pearly substance, an alcohol, found in all animal fats and oils; a main constituent of some body tissues and substances.
Chylomicron — a particle of emulsified fat found in the blood during the digestion of fat.
Citric Acid — major acid of limes, lemons and other citric fruits; an intermediate product of the Krebs cycle.
Citric Acid Cycle — the Krebs cycle.
Cobalamin — the cobalt-containing complex common to all members of the vitamin B_{12} group; often used to designate cyanocobalamin.
Cocaine — a crystalline alkaloid used as a systemic stimulant or local anaesthetic.
Collective Food Faddism — the patterning of food habits after a particular individual or group of individuals.
Cyanocobalamin — vitamin B_{12}, used in treatment of pernicious anemia.
Cystine — a nonessential amino acid.
Cytochrome — any one of a class of compounds found in man that play an important role in oxidative processes.

D_1 — an impure mixture of calciferol with another sterol.
D_2 — calciferol; ergocalciferol; formed from the irradiation of ergosterol.
D_3 — prepared by the activation of 7-dehydrocholesterol; cholecalciferol.

Deamination — removal of an amino group from an amino body, such as amino acids.

Dextrose — a white crystalline powder, $C_6H_{12}O_6 \cdot H_2O$; d-glucose.

Dietetics — the science and study of dietary principles.

Disaccharide — any one of a class of sugars that yields two monosaccharides on hydrolysis; sucrose, lactose and maltose.

Doping — the use of drugs in athletics in order to achieve a physiological or psychological advantage.

Double-blind — an experimental design in which neither the investigator nor the subject has knowledge of the treatment used.

DPN — abbreviation for diphosphopyridine nucleotide, a coenzyme serving as an electron carrier in energy processes; also known as NAD.

Energade — a commercial glucose-electrolyte solution.

Energol — a commercial compound containing vitamin E; purported as being an ergogenic aid.

Ergocalciferol — calciferol; vitamin D_2; an antirachitic vitamin.

Ergogenic Aids — agents which are utilized in attempts to increase work capacity.

Ergosterol — a sterol present in animal tissues which when irradiated by ultraviolet rays forms vitamin D_2.

Ethanol — alcohol; ethyl alcohol.

Ethyl Alcohol — alcohol; the basic alcohol for human consumption.

Fast Twitch Fibers — muscle fibers characterized by high contractile speed.

Fatty Acid — any one of a number of aliphatic acids containing only carbon, hydrogen and oxygen. They may be saturated or unsaturated.

FDA — Food and Drug Administration.

Ferritin — the iron-apoferritin complex.

Ferrous Ascorbate — an iron supplement compound.

Ferrous Citrate — an iron supplement compound.

Ferrous Fumarate — an iron supplement compound.

FFA — free fatty acids.

Fibrinolysis — the splitting up of fibrin, or clots, by enzymic action.

Flavoprotein — a conjugated protein which serves as an electron carrier in the energy processes; FAD.

Folacin — folic acid.

Folic Acid — a water soluble vitamin which may be essential in preventing certain types of anemia.

Free Fatty Acids — formed by the hydrolysis of triglycerides.

Fructose — levulose, or fruit sugar, found in all sweet fruits.

FT Fibers — fast twitch fibers.

Galactose — a monosaccharide resembling glucose in most of its properties, but is less soluble and less sweet.

Gatorade — a commercial glucose electrolyte solution.

Gelatin — a product obtained by partial hydrolysis of collagen or white connective tissue; used as a food.

Gluconeogenesis — the formation of carbohydrates from molecules which are not themselves carbohydrates, such as protein or fat.

Glucoreceptors — receptors in the body that respond to glucose concentration in the blood; may be involved in regulation of hunger.

Glucose — a monosaccharide, a thick syrupy sweet liquid.

Glucose-electrolyte Solution — a solution of varient proportions of glucose, sodium, potassium, and other electrolytes designed to replace sweat losses.

Glucose-U-C^{14} — radioactive isotope of glucose in order to trace its metabolic pathways.

Glucose-6-phosphate — an intermediate product in carbohydrate metabolism.

Glutamic Acid — a non-essential amino acid.

Glutamine — an amide of glutamic acid.

Glycine — aminoacetic acid.

Glycerol — glycerin; a clear syrupy liquid; a part of triglycerides along with fatty acids.

Glycocoll — aminoacetic acid.

Glycogen — a polysaccharide which is the chief carbohydrate storage form in animals. Stored in the liver and muscle; also known as animal starch.

Glycogen Storage Techniques — dietary techniques used to increase the storage of glycogen in the liver and muscles.

Glycogen Synthetase — enzyme used in the formation of glycogen from glucose.

Glycogenic Amino Acids — amino acids that may be converted to carbohydrates.

Glycogenolysis — the splitting of glycogen in the body.

Glycolysis — the degradation of sugars into smaller compounds. Main quantitative anaerobic energy process in the muscle tissue.

Hemeprotein — a combination of heme, the iron protoporphyrin, and protein.

Hemochromotosis — a disorder of iron metabolism characterized by excess deposition of iron in the tissues. May result from excess iron salt administration.

Hemosiderin — an insoluble form of storage iron.

Histidine — an essential amino acid.

Hyperglycemia — abnormally increased content of sugar in the blood.

Hyperhydration — a state of increased water content of the body.

Hyperkalemia — abnormally high potassium content in the blood.

Hyperketonemia — abnormal increase in the ketone bodies in the blood.

Hyperlipemia — abnormal excessive levels of fat in the blood.

Hypernatremia — excess sodium concentration in the blood.

Hyperplasia — abnormal increase in the number of normal cells in a tissue.

Hyperplastic Obesity — obesity caused by an increase in the number of normal adipose tissue cells.

Hypertrophic obesity — obesity due to an increase in the size of the fat cells.

Hypervitaminosis — a condition due to an excess of vitamins, usually A or D.

Hypoglycemia — an abnormal decrease in the sugar content of the blood.

Hypohydration — dehydration; a state of decreased water content of the body.

Hypokalemia — abnormally low potassium content of the blood.

Hyponatremia — abnormally low sodium content of the blood.

Hypotonic — having an osmotic pressure lower than that of the solution to which it is compared.

IAAF — International Amateur Athletic Federation.

Instant Replay — a glucose-electrolyte solution.

Insulin — a hormone secreted by the pancreas that regulates carbohydrate metabolism

International unit — IU; an international activity standard for a given vitamin or other substance.

In Vitro — within a glass or test tube; outside the living body.

In Vivo — within the living body.

Ischemia — deficiency of blood in a body part.

Isoleucine — an essential amino acid.

Isosmotic — having the same osmotic pressure.

Isotonic — pertaining to a state of equal tension or activity, i.e. equal osmotic pressures between two solutions.

IU — International Unit.

Ketogenic Amino Acids — amino acids capable of being converted into ketone bodies.

Ketone Bodies — intermediate products of fatty acids and some amino acids under certain conditions. Acetocetic acid, betahydroxybutyric acid, and acetone are ketone bodies.

KG-M — kilogram-meter; a unit of work representing the energy needed to raise 1 kilogram to a height of one meter.

Kilocalorie — a large calorie, the unit most often used in describing the energy content of foods.

KPM — kilopondmeter; KGM or kilogram-meter.

Krebs Cycle — the main oxidative reaction sequence in the body that generates ATP.

Lactacid — term referring to the portion of the oxygen debt which is accounted for by anaerobic glycolysis resulting in lactic acid production.

Lactic Acid — the anaerobic end product of glycolysis; it has been implicated as a causative factor in the etiology of fatigue.

Lactoovovegetarian — a vegetarian who uses milk and eggs in addition to vegetables in his diet.

Lactose — a white crystalline disaccharide which yields glucose and galactose upon hydrolysis. Also called milk sugar.

Lecithin — a monoaminomonophosphatide, said to have the therapeutic properties of phosphorus.

Leucine — an essential amino acid.

Linoleic Acid — an unsaturated fatty acid.

Lipase — an enzyme that catabolyzes fats (triglycerides) into fatty acids and glycerol.

Lipid — any one of a group of organic substances which are insoluble in water, but soluble in alcohol and other fat solvents.

Lipolysis — the decomposition of fat.

Lipopolysaccharide — a compound involving the combination of lipid and carbohydrate.

Lipoprotein — a combination of lipid and protein, possessing the general properties of proteins. Practically all the lipids of the plasma are present in this form.

Lysine — an essential amino acid.

Maltose — a white crystalline disaccharide.

Maximal Oxygen Uptake — the ability of the body to utilize oxygen for energy purposes; reflects the maximal capacity of cardiac output and arterial-venous oxygen difference.

MAX VO$_2$ — maximal oxygen uptake.

MDR — minimal daily requirements.

MET — a unit of measurement of energy expenditure; 1 MET equals approximately 3.5 ml O$_2$/Kg body weight/minute.

Metabolic Obesity — obesity caused by a biochemical disturbance in the metabolism other than in the regulatory center.

Methionine -- an essential amino acid.

Minim — a unit of liquid measure, the equivalent of 0.0616 milliliter.

Minimal Daily Requirement — the amount of a given nutrient necessary to prevent a deficiency.

Monosaccharide — a simple sugar; a carbohydrate which cannot be hydrolyzed. Glucose is a hexose monosaccharide.

Monounsaturated Fat — a fat which contains one double bond and hence may add various atoms.

NAD — nicotinamide adenine dinucleotide, an electron carrier in the energy processes of the body; DPN.

Needle Biopsy Technique — a biopsy of material obtained by inserting a needle in the appropriate tissue.

Niacin — vitamin B$_3$; nicotinamide; nicotinic acid; a component of certain coenzymes of oxidative processes.

Nicotinamide — the amide of nicotinic acid; vitamin B$_3$; niacin.

Nicotinic Acid — niacin.

Nitrogen Retention — the retention of nitrogen, or protein substances, in the body necessary for tissue building.

Nutrament — a commercial liquid meal.

Octacosanol — a solid white alcohol extracted from the germ, or embryo, of the wheat kernel.

Oleic Acid — an unsaturated fatty acid.

Olympade — a commercial glucose-electrolyte solution.

Organic Foods — foods grown and packaged without the use of artificial chemicals.

Ornithine — an amino acid formed from arginine.

Oxygen Debt — elevated oxygen consumption following an exercise task; it represents the anaerobic aspects of the exercise.

Palmitic Acid — a saturated fatty acid.

Palmitoleic Acid — an unsaturated fatty acid.

Pantothenate — a salt of pantothenic acid.

Pantothenic Acid — a vitamin of the B complex.

PC — phosphocreatine.

Pepsin — enzyme in the gastric juice that initiates breakdown of some peptide linkages in protein.

Periactin — trademark for preparations of cyproheptadine hydrochloride; used as an antihistamine.

Phenylalanine — an essential amino acid.

Phosphagen — a compound such as phosphocreatine which is a source of high-energy phosphate.

Phosphates — salts of phosphoric acid, purported to possess ergogenic qualities.

Phosphocreatine — a high energy compound occurring in the muscle, composed of creatine and phosphoric acid.

Phosphoglycerides — compounds that are derivatives of glycerol phosphate.

Phospholipid — a lipid containing phosphorus, which in hydrolysis yields fatty acids, glycerin and a nitrogenous compound. Lecithin is an example.

Phosphorylation — the process of introducing the phosphate group into an organic molecule.

Phosphotidate — a phosphoglyceride.

Placebo — an inactive substance utilized in experimental studies in order to determine the efficacy of medicaments.

Polysaccharide — a carbohydrate which on hydrolysis yields more than ten monosaccharides.

Polyunsaturated Fats — a fat which contains two or more double bonds.

Potassium Citrate — the potassium salt of citric acid.

PP — pellagra-preventing vitamin, niacin.

PRE — progressive resistive exercise.

Progressive Resistive Exercise — a training technique, primarily with weights, whereby resistance is increased as the individual develops increased strength levels.

Proline — a nonessential amino acid.

Protease — a general term for a proteolytic enzyme; catabolyzes protein.

Protein Tablets — usually synthetic protein, highly complex polypeptides made in the laboratory and possessing most of the characteristics of native protein.

PWC — physical working capacity.

PWC$_{170}$ Test — a submaximal test which predicts maximal work capacity from a submaximal heart rate.

Pyridoxine — a component of the vitamin B complex.

Rating of Perceived Exertion — a subjective rating, on a numerical scale, of the difficulty of a given work task.

RDA — Recommended Dietary Allowances.

Recommended Dietary Allowances — the levels of intake of essential nutrients considered to be adequate to meet the known nutritional needs of practically all healthy persons.

Regulatory Obesity — an impairment in the central control mechanism, such as the hypothalamus, may disturb control of food intake and cause obesity.

Respiratory Quotient — during rest, a general indicator of the type of food being metabolised in the body.

Retinol — vitamin A$_1$.

Riboflavin — vitamin B$_2$.

Risk Factor — a statistical expression of probability.

RPE — rating of perceived exertion.

RQ — respiratory quotient.

Saturated Fats — fats which have all chemical affinities satisfied, and hence have no double bonds.

SDA — specific dynamic action.

Serine — a nonessential amino acid.

Slow Twitch Fibers — muscle fibers that are predominently involved in sustained contractions, as contrasted to fast twitch fibers.

Sodium Bicarbonate — an alkalizing agent; commonly known as baking soda.

Sodium Citrate — an alkalizing agent.

Spartase — trademark for a preparation of potassium and magnesium aspartates.

Specific Dynamic Action — the effect of carbohydrates, fats and proteins ingestion upon the metabolic rate; the metabolic rate is elevated, more so by protein.

Sports Anemia — anemia which may develop during early stages of training as protein is utilized for muscle formation rather than hemoglobin formation.

ST Fibers — slow twitch fibers.

Starch — a polysaccharide from various plant tissues.

Stearic Acid — a saturated fatty acid.

Submaximal Exercise Task — an exercise task below maximal capacity.

Sucrose — a disaccharide, extensively used as a sweetening agent.

Sustagen — a commercial glucose-electrolyte fluid replacement solution.

Take-Five — a commercial glucose-electrolyte fluid replacement solution.

Thiamine — vitamin B_1.

Thiamine Hydrochloride — a vitamin supplement.

Threonine — an essential amino acid.

Tocopherol — an alcohol which has the properties of vitamin E; found in wheat germ oil.

Trace Elements — those elements essential to the body but needed in no more than several milligrams/day.

Transferrin — a serum globulin that binds and transports iron.

Tricarboxylic Cycle — the Krebs cycle.

Triglyceride — one of the many fats formed by the union of glycerol and fatty acids.

Tryptophan — an essential amino acid.

Tyrosine — a nonessential amino acid.

United States Pharmacopia Units — the unit used by the United States Pharmacopia in expressing the potency of various preparations.

Unsaturated Fats — fat that contains double or triple bonds, and hence can add atoms.

Urea — the chief nitrogenous constituent of the urine, and the final product of the decomposition of proteins in the body.

USP — United States Pharmacopia.

Valine — an essential amino acid.

Vegan — an extreme vegetarian who has no animal protein in his diet.

Vegetarian — one whose food is exclusively of vegetable origin.

Vegetarianism — the practice of using only vegetables in the diet.

Vitamin — a general term for a number of substances deemed essential for the normal metabolic functioning of the body.

Vitamin A — an unsaturated aliphatic alcohol; deficiency causes visual and skin problems.

Vitamin B_1 — thiamine; the antineuritic vitamin.

Vitamin B_2 — riboflavin.

Vitamin B_3 — niacin; the antipellagra vitamin.

Vitamin B_6 — pyridoxine.

Vitamin B_{12} —cyanocobalamin.

Vitamin B Complex — a term to designate a class of water soluble vitamins that tend to occur together in nature.

Vitamin C — ascorbic acid; the antiscorbutic vitamin.

Vitamin D — any one of related sterols which have antirachitic properties.

Vitamin E — alpha-tocopherol, one of three tocopherols. The so-called "fertility" vitamin.

Watt/pulse — amount of mechanical work done per heart beat.

Watts — a unit of electrical power of work.

WBGT — wet bulb globe thermometer.

Wet Bulb Globe Thermometer — a device which takes into account the various factors determining heat stress: air temperature, air movement, radiation heat and humidity.

Wet Bulb Thermometer — a thermometer with a wet wick surrounding the bulb, thus evaluating humidity effects upon the air temperature.

Wetzel Grid — a direct reading chart for evaluating body growth and development during the school years.

Wheat Germ — the embryo of wheat which contains tocopherol, thiamine, riboflavin and other vitamins.

Wheat Germ Oil — oil derived from the germ of wheat kernels; rich in vitamin E.

AUTHOR INDEX

Abrahams, A., 11, 52
Addison, V., 312
Aftergood, L., 99, 147, 163
Ahlborg, H., 229, 230
Ahlman, K., 179, 182
Albrink, M., 85
Alfin-Slater, R., 99, 147, 163
American Alliance for Health, Physical
  Education and Recreation, 22, 189, 246,
  295-296, 306, 393-95
American Medical Association, 274
Amundson, L., 278, 279
Anderson, H., 165
Archdeacon, J., 123
Arnheim, D., 116, 159, 245
Arnold, M., 210, 211
Arterbury, T., 218
Ashe, W., 203
Asmussen, E., 83, 238
Asprey, G., 310
Astrand, P., 34, 36, 41, 48, 52, 53, 54, 65, 66,
  68, 69, 74, 96, 102, 159, 176, 181, 188, 205,
  225, 228, 284
Atzler, E., 215

Bailey, D., 143
Bair, G., 118
Bajusz, E., 84, 85, 86, 87, 88, 89, 90, 91, 156,
  157, 158
Baker, E., 136, 137, 139, 144
Baldwin, K., 63
Balke, B., 36
Ball, J., 310
Banister, E., 35, 37
Banister, R., 16
Barborka, C., 134
Barkue, H., 165
Barnes, F., 135
Bass, D., 185
Basu, N., 139
Beetham, W., 177

Bell, C., 57
Benade, A., 56
Bencsik, J., 132
Bennion, M., 269
Bensley, E., 282
Berard, L., 6
Bergstrom, J., 26, 33, 51, 54, 58, 59, 60, 65,
  70, 126, 159
Berland, T., 102, 260
Berry, W., 11
Berryman, G., 131
Berven, H., 146
Best, C., 50
Bialecki, M., 125
Bicknell, F., 121
Bideau, D., 6
Bierring, E., 72
Black, D., 227
Black, E., 70
Blanchard, D., 108, 253
Blank, L., 185
Blix, G., 14, 19, 67, 282
Bloom, W., 269
Blyth, C., 180, 184
Bobb, A., 18, 282
Bock, W., 181
Boddy, K., 138
Bogart, J., 6, 12, 68, 103, 290-291
Bohm, W., 11
Boje, O., 5, 53, 122, 141, 215, 216, 234, 238,
  240, 242
Bolliger, A., 193
Bosco, J., 178
Bourne, G., 120, 139, 148
Bradfield, R., 35
Brannon, D., 313
Bray, G., 31
British Committee on Medical Aspects of
  Food, 88
Brooke, J., 57, 60, 69
Brown, S., 35, 37

423

Brozek, J., 121, 220, 250
Brunner, H., 139
Bugyi, G., 243
Bullen, B., 17, 29, 31, 120, 150, 156, 163, 166, 233, 244, 265
Burt, J., 180, 183, 184
Burton, B., 45, 102
Buskirk, E., 48, 103, 111, 117, 127, 159, 162, 167, 177, 180, 205, 244, 250, 298, 299, 300, 301
Bynyan, J., 147

Cade, J., 187, 188, 198
Caldwell, L., 231
Callaway, E., 227
Campbell, D., 93, 94
Campbell, R., 14
Campbell, W., 103, 106
Canning, H., 270
Cantone, A., 92
Carlson, B., 121, 130, 133
Carlson, L., 82, 83, 92, 126
Carpenter, J., 236, 241
Carpenter, T., 72
Caspari, W., 303
Castle, B., 185
Celejowa, I., 103
Cerretelli, P., 32, 42
Chaikelis, A., 213
Cho, M., 22
Christakis, G., 270
Christensen, E., 44, 50, 59, 72
Christophe, J., 55
Clarke, H., 256, 268, 269
Clarke, K., 20, 281
Clausen, D., 149
Committee on Iron Deficiency, 162, 163
Committee on Nutrition, American Heart Association, 88, 89, 91
Committee on Nutrition Misinformation, 205
Conner, W., 85, 89
Consolazio, C., 105, 174, 232, 276, 277
Cooper, D., 278, 307
Coopersmith, S., 235
Corbin, C., 265
Corliss, R., 93
Costill, D., 41, 42, 54, 56, 60, 61, 62, 66, 73, 178, 179, 181, 183, 186, 191, 193, 194, 195,

196, 197
Coulson, L., 224
Council on Drugs, 229
Craig, F., 180
Creff, A., 6
Crooks, M., 109, 253
Csik, L., 132
Cummings, E., 180
Cureton, T., 10, 18, 21, 93, 116, 137, 149, 218, 219, 220, 221, 222, 223, 225

Damon, A., 250
Darden, E., 13, 52, 103, 111, 190
Darling, R., 110
Daum, K., 312
Davies, C., 165, 166, 167
Davies, G., 57
Davis, T., 113, 163
Daws, T., 277
Debigne, G., 6
DeLuca, H., 145
Dennig, H., 215, 226
Denton, D., 157
Depinto, A., 188
deVries, H., 61, 225, 232, 266
deWijn, J., 164, 166
Dill, D., 50, 53, 226
Dowdy, R., 156
Doyle, J., 85, 86
Drummond, G., 70
Dudleston, A., 269
DuPain, R., 139
Durnin, J., 5, 15, 37, 40, 42, 244, 254, 275, 314

Early, R., 121, 130, 133
Eaves, C., 198
Edelstein, E., 269
Edgerton, V., 165, 166
Efremov, V., 149
Egana, E., 131
Ekblom, B., 204
Embden, G., 216
Engel, R., 14, 22
Ericsson, P., 167
Evans, W., 231

Fallis, N., 231
Feeley, R., 90

Ferguson, V., 209
Field, E., 311
Fischbach, E., 235, 240, 242
Fischer, I., 303
Fleming, A., 19, 96, 208
Flinn, F., 216
Foley, P., 185
Foltz, E., 133
Fordtran, J., 194
Foss, M., 267
Fox, E., 41, 42, 174, 186, 189
Fox, F., 141
Fox, S., 38, 39
Frankau, I., 125, 135
Frederick, R., 273
Friedman, T., 132
Fryer, B., 22
Fuenning, S., 305
Fujioka, H., 229, 230
Fukui, T., 230
Fulton, E., 224

Ganslen, R., 242
Gardiner, E., 8
Gardner, G., 166
Gemmill, C., 72
General Health and Fitness Corporation
  Report, 96
Giese, M., 93
Glatzel, H., 6, 116, 117
Glover, M., 42, 43
Godin, G., 39
Goldman, R., 250
Gollnick, P., 63, 66, 74
Goode, R., 93
Gordon, B., 52
Gordon, E., 262
Gould, L., 234
Gounelle, H., 122
Grafe, H., 6, 116
Grande, F., 265
Gray, D., 266
Green, J., 147
Green, L., 60, 69
Greenberg, L., 312
Greenleaf, J., 178, 185, 186
Gregg, W., 261
Grenier, R., 264
Grey, G., 143, 144

Gutin, B., 75
Guyton, A., 80, 192, 202, 206

Haffter, C., 141
Haggard, H., 52, 312
Hais, I., 205
Haldi, J., 51, 310
Hallberg, L., 163
Handler, P., 20, 29, 31, 45, 46, 47, 49, 76, 80-
  82, 97-98, 100-101, 118, 125, 127-129, 145-
  47, 159, 161-62, 167, 285
Hanley, D., 17, 137
Hansen, O., 44, 50, 59, 72
Haralambie, G., 52
Hardt, A., 228
Harger, B., 41, 42
Harmon, P., 214
Harper, A., 21, 286
Harris, H., 8
Hashim, S., 258
Haymes, E., 103, 111, 117, 127, 159, 162,
  164, 167, 244, 250, 300, 301
Heald, F., 245, 256, 263
Hebbelinck, M., 236, 237, 238
Hein, F., 23
Hellebrandt, F., 214
Hellerstein, H., 85, 91, 282
Henderson, Y., 52
Henschel, A., 53, 134, 141, 202, 276
Herbert, V., 137
Herbert, W., 179, 182, 196, 274
Hermansen, L., 57, 60, 61, 65, 67, 68, 69, 74,
  166
Hettinger, T., 138, 142, 146
Hewitt, J., 227
Hilsendager, D., 125, 215
Hirata, I., 128, 304, 307
Hirsch, J., 258
Hodgkins, J., 35
Hoitink, A., 139, 140
Holloszy, J., 75, 92, 93
Homa, M., 103
Hoogerwerf, A., 140
Horstman, D., 19, 21, 54, 59, 111, 137, 138,
  306, 307
Horvath, S., 214
Howley, E., 42, 43
Huenemann, R., 264
Hultman, E., 54, 56, 57, 58, 59, 60, 61, 64, 65,

69, 159
Hunscher, M., 17, 71, 78, 79, 285, 289, 293-94, 404-06, 411-12
Hursh, L., 84, 86, 87, 90
Hutcheson, J., 163
Hutcheson, R., 163
Hutchinson, R., 304

Ikai, M., 237
Issekutz, B., 73
Ivy, A., 132

Jacob, E., 137
Jalso, S., 14
Jankowski, L., 267
Jannot, E., 6
Jarvis, D., 210, 211
Jenkins, D., 126
Jensen, C., 233
Jetzler, A., 141
Johnson, H., 105
Johnson, R., 105
Johnson, W., 227
Jokl, E., 11, 141, 234
Jung, K., 73

Kaczmarek, R., 212, 213
Karlsson, J., 33, 69, 75
Karpovich, P., 52, 53, 122, 125, 132, 209, 214, 215, 217, 227, 312
Karvonen, M., 179, 182
Keller, W., 217
Kennedy, D., 224
Keul, J., 52
Keys, A., 86, 120, 123, 131, 134, 250, 275
King, D., 74
King, E., 214
Klafs, C., 116, 159, 245
Knochel, J., 191
Knuttgen, H., 54
Konishi, F., 271
Kourounakis, P., 240
Kozlowski, S., 178, 181, 187
Kral, J., 205
Krause, M., 17, 71, 78, 79, 285, 289, 293-94, 404-06, 411-12
Kraut, H., 106, 217
Krehl, W., 157, 158
Krogh, A., 44, 59, 72

LaCava, G., 6
Ladell, W., 196
Lamb, L., 136, 137, 138, 143
Lampman, R., 92, 94
Larson, L., 37
Laties, V., 242
Leake, C., 241
Lehmann, G., 215
Leveille, G., 263
Levine, S., 50
Lewis, S., 75
Lindhard, J., 44, 59, 72
Little, D., 185
Lodispoto, N., 6
Londeree, B., 184
Loutfi, M., 139
Lovingood, B., 242

Macaraeg, P., 191, 192, 193, 308
Maddox, D., 115
Magazanik, A., 177
Mahadeva, K., 39
Maison, G., 213
Malinow, M., 94
Margaria, R., 33, 41, 42, 43, 142, 228, 242
Margolius, S., 14
Maron, M., 50
Marrack, J., 116
Marsh, M., 72
Mathews, D., 186, 189, 198
Mayer, J., 9, 16, 17, 22, 29, 31, 55, 86, 99, 120, 150, 156-57, 163, 166, 244-45, 250-51, 255-59, 261, 264, 266, 269-70, 275, 278-79, 297, 306
Mays, R., 11
McCollum, E., 7, 212, 302, 303
McCormick, W., 122
Medical Commission, International Olympic Committee, 208
Metropolitan Life Insurance Company, 249
Miettinen, M., 86
Miller, A., 37
Miller, H., 224
Millman, N., 122
Minard, D., 203
Minnesota, University of, 275
Mitchell, J., 265
Mohr, D., 269

Mole, P., 105
Montague, A., 264
Montoye, H., 128, 129
Moody, D., 269
Moore, H., 7
Morehouse, L., 37
Morgan, W., 3
Moroff, S., 185
Mossfeldt, F., 92
Mueller, J., 84, 85, 86, 87, 88, 91
Muller, E., 106
Murlin, J., 72, 123
Murphy, R., 203
Mustala, O., 240

Nagle, F., 231
Namyslowski, L., 139, 141
National Dairy Council, 286, 396-403
National Research Council: Committee on
    Dietary Allowances, 16, 76, 77, 99, 102,
    121, 122, 124, 127, 136-37, 145, 148, 153,
    155, 157, 160, 163, 205, 246, 286, 287
Naughton, J., 38, 39, 85, 91, 282
Neeves, R., 310
Nelson, D., 22, 217, 236, 237, 238, 311
Newsholme, E., 47, 50, 73, 75, 79, 80
Nijakowski, F., 121, 129
Nilsson, L., 61
Nocker, J., 6, 116, 117

O'Conner, F., 198
Olson, A., 269
Olson, R., 14, 17, 120
Orava, S., 210
Oro, L., 126
Oscai, L., 92, 267, 269, 272

Pagliuchi, D., 6
Palmer, W., 182
Pampe, W., 51, 209
Pargman, D., 299
Parizkova, J., 268
Partridge, R., 50
Pascale, L., 250
Passmore, R., 37, 40, 42, 244, 275
Patton, R., 198
Paul, W., 278
Pendergast, D., 43
Percival, L., 148, 211, 219

Perkins, R., 243
Perley, A., 94
Pernow, B., 74
Pestrecov, K., 214
Piehl, K., 62, 63, 64, 69, 75
Pierson, W., 107, 108
Pitts, G., 195
Pletcher, P., 265
Pohndorf, R., 221
Poiletman, R., 224
Prescott, F., 121
Prokop, L., 116
Pruett, E., 50, 61, 66

Randolph, J., 198
Ranson, R., 18
Rasch, P., 105, 106, 107, 108, 139, 142, 144
Ray, G., 139, 212
Rechcigl, M., 6
Reese, E., 66
Reichard, G., 56
Riabuschinsky, N., 216
Ribisl, P., 174, 179, 182, 196, 274
Riendeau, R., 256
Robinson, S., 214
Roby, F., 269
Rochelle, R., 93
Rodahl, K., 34, 36, 41, 48, 53, 54, 66, 69, 102,
    110, 159, 176, 181, 188, 205, 225, 228, 284
Rogozkin, V., 116
Romsos, D., 263
Rose, K., 190, 192, 193, 305, 307
Rose, L., 155, 187, 193
Rowell, L., 61
Rutledge, C., 241
Ryder, H., 309

Sage, J., 313
Sakaeva, E., 149
Saltin, B., 33, 57, 60, 65, 67, 68, 69, 74, 178,
    179, 180, 181, 187, 194
Schade, M., 269
Schaefer, O., 94
Schamadam, J., 191, 192
Schendel, H., 103, 111
Schenk, P., 11
Scherrer, D., 209
Scheunert, A., 116
Schwartz, F., 145

Scoular, F., 11
Seelig, M., 146
Seidl, E., 146
Seltzer, C., 270
Shaffer, C., 136
Sharman, I., 150
Sheehan, G., 16
Shephard, R., 39, 151, 152, 234, 235, 236, 239
Sherman, H., 116
Sidorowicz, W., 6
Simka, V., 269
Simmons, R., 228
Simonson, E., 16, 18, 21, 49, 50, 73, 99, 133, 307
Sims, D., 108, 253
Singer, R., 273, 310
Sinning, W., 52, 53, 132, 209, 217, 227, 312
Skubic, V., 35
Slocum, D., 273, 278, 281
Smith, E., 20, 29, 31, 45, 46, 47, 49, 76, 80-82, 97-98, 100-01, 118, 125, 127-29, 145-47, 159, 161-62, 167, 285
Smith, S., 116
Snellen, J., 176, 177
Snively, W., 191
Sollman, T., 235
Soule, R., 185
Sparks, K., 197
Speckmann, E., 87
Spickard, A., 204
Spioch, F., 140
Sproule, B., 165
Start, C., 47, 50, 73, 75, 79, 80
Staton, W., 144, 215, 216
Steel, J., 12, 123
Steinhaus, A., 237
Steitz, E., 298-99
Stewart, G., 163
Stone, I., 136
Stunkard, A., 263
Suzman, H., 141

Talbot, D., 115
Tatkon, M., 8, 114, 115, 118, 145
Taylor, A., 63, 75
Taylor, H., 188, 276, 277, 278
Tcheng, T., 278, 280
Terjung, R., 63

Thompson, J., 8
Tipton, C., 280
Tooshi, A., 93
Travers, P., 103, 106
Tuttle, W., 123, 274, 312, 313

Ulmark, R., 235
United States Senate, 5, 15, 18, 115, 137, 146
Updyke, W., 117, 159, 183, 219

Vaccaro, P., 182
Van Haaren, J., 166, 167
Van Handel, P., 58
Van Huss, W., 115, 137, 139, 142, 144, 311
Van Itallie, T., 9, 21, 137, 158, 258
Vertel, R., 191
Vogeler, R., 209
Vytchikova, M., 122

Wachholder, K., 138
Wahren, J., 56
Wald, G., 119
Watson, G., 120
Watt, T., 151
Weinhaus, R., 256
Weinstein, A., 146
Weiss, B., 242
Weiss, S., 273
Welch, H., 72
Wenzel, D., 241
Westerman, R., 205
Weswig, P., 167
White, A., 20, 29, 31, 45, 46, 47, 49, 76, 80-82, 97-98, 100-101, 118, 125, 127-29, 145-47, 159, 161-62, 167, 285
White, J., 308
White, P., 89, 116, 119, 147, 154, 155, 159, 166, 211, 284, 301, 306
Williams, J., 16, 21, 116
Williams, M., 6, 110, 168, 234, 236, 237, 238, 240, 243
Wilson, E., 32, 171, 312
Winick, M., 256, 258, 259
Winkler, W., 167
Wirth, J., 164
Wishart, G., 96, 303
Witten, C., 197
Wooding, R., 309
Wrightington, M., 209

Wyndham, C., 28, 205
Wynn, W., 51, 310

Yakovlev, N., 7, 116
Yamaji, R., 103, 104
Yoshimura, H., 104, 105, 106
Youmons, E., 310

Young, D., 56, 82

Zambraski, E., 169, 177, 182
Zauner, C., 66, 117, 159, 219
Zawistowska, Z., 6
Zuntz, N., 44, 72, 76
Zuti, W., 174, 269

SUBJECT INDEX

A

AAHPER, 295-96
  fitness test, 313
AAU, 240
Acclimitization
  to heat, 205-06
Acetyl CoA, 26, 27, 48, 71, 78-81, 121, 129
Acidosis
  pre-game meal, 306
Adenosine triphosphate (see ATP)
Adipose tissue, 245
Alactacid energy source, 32-33
Alanine, 46, 56, 98
Alcohol, 6, 208, 241-42
  as ergogenic aid, 232-39
  caloric content, 263
  effect on physical performance, 236-39
  effect on physiological responses to exer-
    cise, 236
  effect on psychomotor performance, 235-
    36
  metabolism, 233
  physiological effects, 234
Aldosterone, 188, 191-92
  effect on sodium, 157
Alkaline salts, 10, 208, 225-29
Alpha-tocopherol (see Vitamin E)
American College of Sports Medicine, 199,
  207, 409-10
American Heart Association, 83, 87, 89, 91
American Medical Association, 255, 261,
  274, 278, 281
Americans
  dietary habits, 113
Aminoacetic acid (see glycine)
Amino acids, 97-99, 101
  and vitamin C, 136
  essential, 98
  glycogenic, 46-47, 71, 101
  ketogenic, 71, 101

table of, 98
Ammonia, 101
Amphetamines, 3-5, 240-41, 262
Anabolic steroids, 3-5, 110, 152, 253
Anemia
  and copper, 156
  and physical performance, 161-65
  and vitamin C deficiency, 136
  iron deficiency, 128, 163
  pernicious, 302
  and vitamin B_{12} , 128
Anemia, sports (see sports Anemia)
Anoretics, 262
Antidiuretic hormone, 172-73
Apoferritin, 161-62
Arginine, 98, 285
Arteriosclerosis, 83
Ascorbic acid, 134-35, 218, 285
  (see also Vitamin C)
  content in foods, 351-89
  RDA, 391
Asparagine, 98
Asparaginic acid, 229
Aspartates, 208
  as ergogenic foods, 229-32
Astrand dietary regimen, 68
Atherosclerosis, 84-86
Athletes
  anemia in, 163-64
  college, diet of, 282-83
  diets of, 10-13
  endurance, 300
  energy requirement, 297-300
  feeding of, 282-314
  female, 300-01
  Greek, 302
  heat, guidelines for exercise in, 206-07
  iron deficiency in, 163-64
  Olympic, 11-12, 17, 52
  and use of vitamins, 115
  professional, 17

431

vegetarian, 301-04
ATP, 24-26, 32-33, 48, 121, 155, 229-30

B

Basal metabolic rate, 30-32, 37
  factors affecting, 31
  of females, 31
  of males, 31
Basic food groups, 287
Beer, 233, 235
Benzedrine, 5
Benzocaine, 262
Biotin, 119, 130, 285
Blood alcohol level, 234
Blood doping, 168
Blood glucose (see also glucose, blood)
  use during exercise, 52-58
Body composition, 247-51
  (see also body fat)
  and exercise, 268
  changes from exercise, 265
Body fat, 244-45
  prediction of, 407-08
Body image
  and obesity, 256
Body mass
  relation to athletics, 244
Body temperature (see Temperature, body)
Body water compartments, 170
Body weight (see weight, body)
Books, nutrition, 6-7
Breakfast
  and physical performance, 312-14
B Vitamins (see Vitamin B)

C

Caffeine, 6, 208, 218
  as ergogenic aid, 239-43
  effect on physical performance, 241-43
Calcium, 134, 145-46, 153-55, 211, 285, 303,
    306
  content in foods, 351-89
  in basic four food groups, 290-91
  RDA, 392
Caloric balance
  negative, 297

Caloric concept
  in weight control, 245-47
Caloric content
  of electrolyte solutions, 193
Caloric costs of
  running, 37-43
  swimming, 37-43
  various activities, 37-43
    table of, 38-39
  walking, 37-43
Caloric requirement
  of athletics, 297-300
Caloric values
  of carbohydrates, 28
  of fat, 28
  of protein, 28
Calorie, 27-30
  definition, 27
Calories
  content in foods, 351-89
  daily intake
    determination of, 295-96
  in alcohol, 233
  in body fat, 261
  recommendation for males, 246
  recommendation for females, 246
Carbohydrate
  absorption of, 28
  and physical performance, 51-58
    intake prior to, 51-52
    intake during, 52-58
  as energy source, 70-74
  caloric value of, 28-29, 45
  content in foods, 351-89
  dietary
    and coronary heart disease, 90
  digestion of, 45
  function of, 45
  in breakfast, 312
  in pre-game meal, 305-06
  metabolism of in humans, 46-49
  respiratory quotient, 29
  role in physical activity, 44-75
  sources of, 44-45
  specific dynamic action of, 31
  storage in human body, 46-49
  types of, 44-45
  water of oxidation, 171
Cardiac output

effect of dehydration, 180-81
Cardiovascular efficiency
  effect of glucose on, 52
Carotene, 118
Charmis of Sparta, 8
Chloride, 153, 156-58, 170, 186, 193
Chlorine, 285
Cholecalciferol, 145
Cholesterol, 13, 77-80, 84-85
  and coronary heart disease, 82-95
  serum, effect of exercise on, 92-94
Choline, 119, 220, 285
Chromium, 153, 156
Chylomicrons, 79, 82
Citric acid cycle, 25-26, 70-71, 79-81
Coaches
  nutritional information of, 22
Cobalamin, 134
  (see also cyanocobalamin and Vitamin
    B_{12})
Cobalt, 128, 153, 156
Coca-Cola, 197-98, 210
Cocaine, 5
Coffee, 239-42, 305
Composition of food
  table of, 351-89
Conduction, 175
Convection, 175
Cooper, Kenneth, 40, 272
Copper, 153, 156, 285
Coronary heart disease
  and dietary fat, 83-95
  and exercise, 40
  and obesity, 256
  risk factors in, 84
  role of exercise in prevention, 91-95
Cramps, heat, 200-01
Creatine phosphate, 230
  (see also phosphocreatine)
Cyanocobalamin, 119, 128-29
  (see also vitamin B_{12})
  and physical performance, 128-29
  effect on endurance, 129
  effect on heart rate, 129
  effect on strength, 129
Cyclamates, 13
Cystine, 98
Cytochromes, 25, 26

D

Dehydration, 182, 199
  and physical performance, 177-81
  Boston Marathon, in, 177
  by metabolic stress, 178
  by thermal stress, 178
  effect on strength, 178-79
  for athletics, 177-78
  health hazards, 278
  techniques
    in wrestling, 273-74
Delta-tocopherol (see vitamin E)
Dextrose, 218, 306
  as ergogenic food, 209-10
  tablets, 52
Diabetes, 260
  and obesity, 256
Diet
  adequate, 288-92
  and blood lipids, 88-92
  and body glycogen stores, 64-70
  and coronary heart disease, 85-91
  athletes (see also athletes, diets of)
    special considerations, 297-314
  balanced, 261
  high carbohydrate, 68
  high protein, 99
  Key's ideal, 11
  low calorie, 295-97, 396-403
  low protein, 99
Dieting principles, 260-64
Diglycerides, 77
Diphosphopyridine nucleotide (see DPN
    and NAD)
Disaccharide, 45
Distance running (see also marathon run-
    ning)
  and dehydration, 181-82
Diuretics, 279
Doping, 4-5, 208, 240
DPN, 25-27
Dromeus of Stymphalus, 8
Drugs, reducing, 262

E

Education
  against nutritional quackery, 20-23

against obesity, 265
diet and coronary heart disease, 91
nutrition and exercise, 259
of athletes, 314
physical, of obese, 269-72
Efficiency
carbohydrates versus fat, 70-74
effect of glucose, 209
effect on niacin, 126
effect of vitamin C, 140
Electrolytes, 207
(see also salt and specific elements)
and physical performance, 186-99
loss in sweat, 186-87
replacement, 300
solutions of, 57, 192-99
(see also Gatorade)
and heat cramps, 201
composition, 193
and gastric emptying, 195
recommended, 195
effect on maximal performance, 197-99
ergogenic aspects, 195-99
glucose effect on absorption, 194
in distance running, 410
Endurance
and vegetarianism, 303
effect of
alcohol, 236-37
anemia, 165
aspartates, 229-32
caffeine, 242-43
cyanocobalamin, 129
glycine, 213-15
glycogen loading, 59-70
niacin, 125-26
thiamine, 122-23
vitamin A, 119
vitamin B, 132-33
complex deficiency, 131
vitamin C, 139-44
vitamin E, 149-51
wheat germ oil, 218-25
Energade, 187
Energol, 148, 218
Energy, 24-43
balance, 244
negative, 244
positive, 244

content in foods, 351-89
cost of
running, 37-43
swimming, 38-43
various activities, 38-39
walking, 37-43
equivalent values, 28
expenditure, 30-43
and weight control, 266
calculation of, 37-40
during physical activity, 35-43
methods of measuring in humans, 35-36
in basic four food groups, 290-91
major sources of, in humans, 24
measures of, 27-30
requirements of athletics, 297-300
sources
during exercise, 32-35
carbohydrate versus fat, 70-74
effect of physical activity, 75
percentual contribution
aerobic, 33-34
anaerobic, 33-34
protein, 96
submaximal work, 54
in fat, 82-83
in non-humans, 70
protein, 70-71, 97
types of, 43
Ergocalciferol, 145
Ergogenic aids, 10
theory for use, 3
Ergogenic foods, 208-43
alcohol, 232-29
alkaline salts, 225-29
aspartates, 229-32
caffeine, 239-43
dextrose, 209-10
gelatin, 212-15
glucose, 209-10
honey, 210-12
lecithin, 215-16
multiple supplements, 217-18
phosphates, 216-17
wheat germ oil, 218-25
Ergosterol, 145
Ethyl alcohol (see alcohol)
Eurymenes of Samos, 8
Evaporation, of sweat, 176-77

Exercise
  and blood lipids, 91-95
  and coronary heart disease, 83-95
  and obesity, 91
  and serum cholesterol levels, 92-94
  and weight reduction, 264-72
  effect on carbohydrate utilization, 47-75
  effect on fat mobilization, 70-75, 82-83
  for preschool children, 272
  for weight reduction, recommended pro-
    gram, 271-72
  in heat, guidelines, for, 206-07
  mechanisms of weight loss, 265
  metabolic aftereffects, 266
  misconceptions in weight control, 266-67

F

FAD, 25-27
Faddism, 5
  nutritional, in athletes, 13-20
Fat
  absorption of, 28
  and acidosis, 83
  body
    caloric content, 245
    methods of determination, 247-51
    mobilization during exercise, 268
    prediction of, 407-08
    use during exercise, 70-74
  caloric value of, 28-29
  content in foods, 351-89
  dietary, and coronary heart disease, 83-95
  digestion of, 78
  energy source, 70-74, 76
    during exercise, 82-83
    effect of physical training, 75
  energy store, 80
  functions in humans, 76
  in pre-game meal, 305-06
  metabolism of, 78-82
    and Krebs cycle, 81-82
  respiratory quotient, 29
  role during physical activity, 76-95
  saturated, 13, 303
    and coronary heart disease, 86-91
  sources of, 76-78
  specific dynamic action, 31
  storage of, 78-82

  types of, 76-78
  water of oxidation, 171
Fatigue
  and aspartates, 230-31
  and blood glucose, 47-59
  and liver glycogen, 47-49
  and muscle glycogen, 47-49
Fatty acids
  and vitamin E, 148
  formation of, 78
  metabolic pathways, 79, 81-82
  monounsaturated, 77
  polyunsaturated, 77, 285
  saturated, 77
    content in foods, 351-89
  unsaturated, 77
    content in foods, 351-89
Females
  athlete, 300-01
    and body fat, 244
    iron requirements, 160-68
  body fat, 250
  exercise in heat, 207
  heat illness, 202
Ferritin, 161-62
Ferrous ascorbate, 160
Ferrous citrate, 160
Ferrous fumarate, 160
Ferrous sulfate, 160
FFA, 73-74, 79, 82
  plasma
    during exercise, 82-83
    effect of niacin, 126
Fiber, dietary, 286
FISM, 240
Flavin adenine dinucleotide (see FAD)
Fluid replacement (see also water, body, re-
    hydration)
  effect on blood volume, 196
  in distance running, 410
Fluorine, 153, 285
Folacin, 130
  RDA, 392
Folic acid, 119, 130, 285
Food
  composition
    table of values, 351-89
  functions of, 282-83
  groups, basic, 287-92

daily requirements, 289-94
substitutes within, 393-95
guide, daily, 289
scoreboard, 295-96
substitutes, 393-95
Food and Drug Administration, 20
Football, 169, 177
and dehydration, 181-82
and exercise in heat, 174
guidelines, 206-07
and salt tablets, 188-90
deaths, 168, 183
heat illnesses, 199-207
Frazier, Walt, 302
Free fatty acids (see FFA)
Fructose, 45, 51
in honey, 211

G

Galactose, 45
Gatorade, 22, 59, 187, 193, 196-98
(see also electrolytes, solutions)
Gelatin, 10, 22, 105, 208, 212-15
Gluconeogenesis, 46-47, 56, 312
in starvation, 275
Glucose, 5, 44-46, 72, 194, 208, 227, 410
absorption of during exercise, 55
and glucostatic theory, 257-58
as ergogenic food, 209-10
blood
and physical performance, 49-59
sources and fate of, 46
effect of pre-performance intake, 51-52
electrolyte solutions, 193
(see also electrolytes, solutions)
in pre-game meal, 306
in solution
effect on absorption time, 194
ingestion
adverse effects, 52
effect on ratings of perceived exertion, 5
practical aspects, 58-59
intake
during exercise, 52-58
solutions
composition, 58
hypertonic, effects of, 58
Glucose-U-C^{14}, 56

Glucose-6-phosphate, 46-49
Glucostatic theory
of food intake regulation, 257
Glutamic acid, 98
Glutamine, 98
Glycerol, 56, 76-80
metabolism of, 81-82
Glycerol-3-phosphate, 80
Glycine, 98, 125, 212-15
Glycocoll (see glycine)
Glycogen, 32, 45, 47, 211, 229-30
and potassium, 159, 192
depletion of, 65-68
liver, 47-49, 53, 55-56, 61-62
muscle, 47-49, 54-56, 74, 126, 306
effect of diet, 64-70
effect of physical training, 75
importance during exercise, 60-61
in fast twitch fibers, 62-63, 66
in slow twitch fibers, 62-63, 66
methods to increase, 64-70
selective depletion of, 62-63
stores, 48
time for depletion and repletion, 63-64
storage, 282, 300
disadvantages of, 69
mechanisms of, 69
techniques, 10, 12, 44, 59-70
synthetase, 69
Glycolysis, 26, 46, 48, 70-71, 74, 125, 130, 225
Greek athletes, 8, 302

H

Health hazards
of making weight in athletics, 278-81
Heart rate
effects of
cyanocobalamin, 128
dehydration, 179-83
hyperhydration, 185
rehydration, 182-83
vitamin A, 119
Heat
acclimitization to, 205-06
body
loss of, mechanisms, 175
environmental

energy costs of exercise in, 174
exercise in
  guidelines, 206-07
  loss of electrolytes, 186-87
exhaustion
  salt depletion, 200-01
  water depletion, 200-01
illnesses, 199-207
  prevention of, 202-07, 409-10
stroke, 200-02
Height and weight tables
adults, 249
boys, 405
girls, 406
Hemochromotosis, 168
Hemoglobin
and protein supplementation
(see sports anemia)
Hemosiderin, 161
liver accumulation, 167
Hillary, Sir Edward, 169
Hippocrates, 255, 264
Histidine, 98, 285
Honey, 22, 44, 52, 210-12, 305-06
effects on physical performance, 211-12
Humidity, 177, 203, 206
Hunger, 13
Hypercholesteremia, 256
(see also cholesterol)
Hyperglycemia, 210
Hyperhydration, 171, 282
(see also water, body)
Hyperkalemia, 158-59, 192
Hyperlipidemia, 91-92
Hypernatremia, 157
Hypertension
and obesity, 256
Hyperthermia, 199
Hypervitaminosis
vitamin A, 118
vitamin D, 145-46
Hypnosis, 3-4
Hypoglycemia, 47-48, 53, 58-62, 312
and physical performance, 49-59
in starvation, 275
symptoms of, 48
Hypohydration, 171
Hypokalemia, 158-59, 190
Hypokinetism

and obesity, 264
Hyponatremia, 157
Hypothalamus, 201, 257-58, 266
role in temperature regulation, 175-76

I

IAAF, (see International Amateur Athletic
  Federation)
Illnesses, heat, 199-207
Inactivity
and obesity, 264
Incaparina, 98
Inositol, 119
Instant Breakfast, 19, 308-09
Instant Replay, 187
International Amateur Athletic Federation, 4, 240
International Olympic Committee, 4-6,
  208, 235, 240
International Units, 119
IOC, (see International Olympic Committee)
Iodine, 153-54, 285
  RDA, 392
Iron, 22, 27, 115, 134, 153-54, 211, 285, 301,
  303
and females, 160
and physical performance, 159-68
content in foods, 351-89
deficiency, 116
  American women, 163
  athletes, 163-64
in basic four food groups, 290-91
metabolism of, 160-62
plasma level, 161
RDA, 160-61, 392
sources of, 160
supplementation
  to anemic subjects, 166
  to athletes, 165-68
  to elderly subjects, 167
  to females, 166
  to swimmers, 167
Isoleucine, 98, 285

K

Ketone bodies

in starvation, 275
Kilocalorie (see Calorie)
Krebs cycle (see Citric Acid cycle)

L

Lactic acid, 22, 32-33, 46, 154, 225, 228, 23?
Lactoovovegetarian, 302
Lactose, 45
Lecithin, 12, 78, 208, 215-16
Leucine, 98, 285
Linoleic acid, 77, 218, 285
Lipids, 76-77
  blood, 79-80
  and diet, 88-92
Lipogenesis, 81
Lipopolysaccharides, 77
Lipoproteins, 77, 79-80, 82, 86, 92
Liquid meal, 305
  pre-game, 307-09
Liver
  and protein metabolism, 101
  damage in dehydration, 278
  glycogen (see glycogen, liver)
Low calorie diets, 396-403
Lysine, 98, 285

M

Magnesium, 153-55, 170, 186, 193, 211, 285
  and marathon running, 155
  aspartates, 229, 231-32
  loss in sweat, 187
  RDA, 155, 392
Making weight, in athletics, 272-81
Maltose, 45
Manganese, 153, 156, 285
Marathon, 57, 410
  Boston, dehydration in, 177
  running, 50, 155, 186
  and aspartates, 230
  in environmental heat, 174
  water replacement, 183-84
Maximal oxygen uptake
  effect of
    caffeine, 242-43
    dehydration, 180-81
    gelatin, 214
    in anemic subjects, 165

starvation, 276
vitamin C, 142-43
vitamin E, 149, 151
wheat germ oil, 223
Meals, pre-game, 304-11
Megavitamins, 113
Menstrual flow
  iron loss, 161, 163
Meredith age-height-weight chart, 248
MET, 36-39
  definition, 36
Methionine, 98, 104, 285, 303
Metrecal, 263
Metric system, 412
Milk
  in pre-game meal, 311
Milo of Croton, 8
Minerals
  functions of, 153
  major, 153
  role in physical activity, 153-68
  supplements, 12, 18
  trace elements, 153, 156
Minimal daily requirement
  of vitamins, 114
Molybdenum, 153, 285
Monoglycerides, 77
Monosaccharides, 45-46
Monounsaturated fatty acids, 88-89
Multiple supplements, 217-18
Multivitamins, 22, 208
  and colds, 135
  and physical performance, 134-36
Muscle cramps
  and magnesium, 155
Muscle glycogen (see glycogen, muscle)
Muscle hypertrophy
  effect of protein supplementation, 107
Muscle soreness
  and vitamin C, 144-45
Muscle tissue
  and protein supplementation, 102-12

N

NAD, 26-27, 125
  (see also DPN)
NADP, 125
National Basketball Association, 302

National Collegiate Athletic Association, 4
(see also NCAA)
NCAA, 240
Niacin, 27, 116, 119-20, 124-27, 215, 285, 301
(see also nicotinamide and nicotinic acid)
content in foods, 351-89
effect on endurance, 125-26
effect on FFA, 126
effect on physical performance, 125-27
in basic four food groups, 290-91
metabolic role, 125
RDA, 392
Nicotinamide, 116
(see also niacin and nicotinic acid)
Nicotinamide adenine dinucleotide phosphate (see NADP)
Nicotinic acid, 116, 211
(see also niacin and nicotinamide)
and FFA release, 74
Nitrogen balance, 99
negative, 101
positive, 101, 103
Nitrogen losses, 102-03, 105
Nomogram
energy cost of running, 41
Normohydration, 171
Nurmi, Pavlo, 302
Nutrament, 108, 253, 307-09
Nutrients
essential, 285
in basic four food groups, 290-91
pharmacological effect, 21
Nutrition
basic, 284-97
science of, history, 9

O

Obesity, 254-72
(see also weight, body)
and coronary heart disease, 88
and heat illness, 202
childhood, 258
creeping, 259
disadvantages of, 255-57
effect on motor performance, 256-57
effect of physical education, 269-72
energy expenditure in exercise, 266
etiology of, 257-59
hyperplastic, 258
hypertrophic, 258
metabolic, 258
prevention, 259-72
regulatory, 257
spot reducing, 269
treatment, 259-72
versus overweight, 254
Octacosanol, 218-25
Oleic fatty acid, 77
Olympade, 187
Olympic games, 6, 8-9, 11, 18, 50, 52, 137, 218, 235, 241
Orange juice, 142-43
Ornithine, 98
Osmoreceptors
in body water regulation, 172-73
Overeaters Anonymous, 263
Overhydration (see water, body hyperhydration)
Overweight
versus obesity, 254
Oxygen
caloric equivalents, 28-29, 35
consumption
effect of dehydration, 179-80
cost, of various activities, 37-43
debt, 225
alactacid, 36
and alkaline salts, 226
and vitamin C, 137
lactacid, 36
uptake
and energy expenditure, 36
effect of vitamin A, 119

P

Pantothenic acid, 27, 119, 129-30, 134, 285
levels after exercise, 130
Para-aminobenzoic acid, 119, 130
Palmitic fatty acid, 77
Palmitoleic fatty acid, 77
Perceived exertion (see ratings of perceived exertion)
Periactin, 254
Phenylalanine, 98, 285
Phosphagens, 75
Phosphatase, hepatic, 46

Phosphates, 5, 12, 145, 153-54, 208, 216-17
Phosphocreatine, 26, 32-33, 212, 229
Phosphoglycerides, 77
Phospholipids, 79-80
Phosphorus, 134, 153-55, 193, 211, 285, 306
  RDA, 392
Phosphorylation, oxidative, 26
Phosphotidates, 77
Physical education majors
  nutritional knowledge of, 22
Polypeptides, 99
Polysaccharides, 45
Polyunsaturated fatty acids, 88-89
Potassium 153-54, 156, 158-59, 169-70, 186,
    193, 199, 207, 211, 285, 306, 410
  aspartates, 229-32
  citrate, 225-26, 228
  depletion during exercise, 190-92
  in body fat determination, 250
  losses in sweat, 187
  phosphate, 216
Power, effect of
  alcohol, 237
  protein supplements, 106-07
Pre-game meals, 304-11
  composition, 305
  liquid, 307-09
  nonrecommended foods, 311
  solid, 309-11
Progressive resistive exercise training
  and protein supplementation, 107-08, 110
  in weight gaining, 252
Proline, 98
Prometol, 218
Proteases, 99
Protein
  absorption of, 28
  anabolism, and testosterone, 110
  and the nervous system, 104
  and physical performance, 110
  and vegetarianism, 302-03
  anemia (see sports anemia)
  animal, 98-99
  as energy source, 70-71, 97
    during exercise, 96
  caloric value of, 28-29
  catabolism, exercise effects, 105
  content in foods, 351-89
  daily needs of athletes, 111-12

  dietary, metabolic fate, 100
  digestion of, 98-99
  efficiency of utilization, 99
  exercise in heat, 207
  function of, in humans, 97
  in basic four food groups, 290-91
  in breakfast, 312
  in diets of athletes, 12
  in pre-game meal, 305-07
  loss during starvation, 275
  metabolism of, 71, 100-02
  needs
    and athletic trauma, 103
    during physical training, 102-12
  RDA, 391
  respiratory quotient, 29
  role in physical activity, 96-112
  sources of, 97-100
  specific dynamic action, 31, 102, 261
  storage of, in humans, 100-02
  supplements, 5, 18-20, 102-12, 224, 252-53
    effect on
      body weight, 107-09
      muscle hypertrophy, 107
      power, 106-07
      strength, 106-07
  tablets, 208
  types of, 97-100
  vegetable, 98
  water of oxidation, 171
Psychomotor performance
  effect of
    alcohol, 235-36
    caffeine, 241-42
    vitamin B, 132
    vitamin C, 142
Pyridoxal, 127
Pyridoxamine, 127
Pyridoxine, 119, 127, 134, 285
  (see also vitamin B_6)

Q

Quackery, nutritional
  education against, 14
  in athletics, 13-20

R

Radiation, 175

Ratings of perceived exertion
effects of
caffeine, 243
glucose, 57
RDA, 114, 284-88, 390-92
(see also specific nutrients)
magnesium, 155
pantothenic acid, 129
protein, 99, 102
riboflavin, 124
vitamin A, 118
vitamin B_{12}, 128
vitamin C, 136
vitamin D, 145
vitamin E, 147
Reaction time
effect of
alcohol, 236
caffeine, 241-42
Recommended Dietary Allowances (see RDA)
Redoxon, 140
Research
needs, 20-23, 144, 152
Russian, 18, 103-04, 116, 226
and cyanocobalamin, 128
and iron, 159
and vitamin A, 119
and vitamin C, 140
Respiratory quotient, 29, 35, 56, 72, 126
Retinol (see Vitamin A)
Riboflavin, 27, 119-20, 124, 131-35, 211, 285, 301, 303
(see also vitamin B_2)
content in foods, 351-89
in basic four food groups, 290-91
RDA, 392
Royal Jelly, 129
Runners
effect of alkaline salts, 227
heat illness in, 199-207
Running
energy cost of, 37-43

S

Salt, 207
(see also sodium)
alkaline (see alkaline salts)

and coronary heart disease, 90, 157
losses in sweat, 189
replacement, 189-191
during exercise, 196
tablets, 15, 187-90
Saturated fats (see fat, saturated)
Selenium, 153, 285
Serine, 98
Skinfolds
and body fat, 250-51
triceps, 251
Sling psychrometer, 203
Slow sodium, 190
Soccer
dehydration in, 181-82
Socrates, 225
Sodium, 153-54, 156-58, 186, 193, 285, 306, 410
(see also salt and electrolytes)
and coronary heart disease, 157
deficiency, 158
losses in sweat, 157-58, 187, 189
Sodium acid phosphate, 227
Sodium bicarbonate, 225-29
Sodium chloride (see salt)
Sodium citrate, 218, 225-28
Sodium phosphate, 216, 218, 225
Sodium sulfate, 225
Soya lecithin (see lecithin)
Spartase, 231
Specific dynamic action, 174
in dieting, 261
of food, 31
of protein, 102
Specific heat
of human body, 176
Speed
effect of alcohol, 238
Sport drinks (see electrolytes, solutions)
Sports anemia, 103-06, 164, 301
Sportti-C, 210
Spot reducing, 269
Starvation, 262
effect on physical performance, 274-78
partial, 277-78
Stearic fatty acid, 77
Steroids, 77
Strength
effects of

alcohol, 236-37
aspartates, 231-32
caffeine, 243
cyanocobalamin, 129
dehydration, 178-79
glycine, 213-14
lecithin, 216
protein supplements, 106-07
thiamine, 123
vitamin B, 131-33
wheat germ oil, 218-25
Stroke, heat (see heat stroke)
Stroke volume
effect of dehydration, 180-81
Sucrose, 45, 51, 56, 228, 277, 306
Superhydration (see water, body, hyperhydration)
Supplements, multiple (see multiple supplements)
Supplements, protein
(see protein supplements)
Supplements, vitamin, 297
Sustagen, 193, 307-08
(see also electrolyte solutions)
Sweat
loss of electrolytes, 186-87
replacement, 410
role in temperature regulation, 176-77
sodium content, 158
Sweating
and body weight loss, 265
in acclimatized man, 206
in heat illness, 201
Swimming performance
effect of
alkaline salts, 227-28
vitamin E, 150-51

T

Take Five, 187, 198
(see also electrolyte solutions)
Temperature, body
and hyperhydration, 184-85
increase during exercise, 175
regulation
during exercise, 175-76
in humans, 173-77
Temperature, environmental, 203

Tennis
fluid losses, 193
Testosterone, 253
THAM, 226
Thermometer
dry bulb, 203
globe, 204
wet bulb, 203, 410
wet bulb globe, 204
Thiamine, 119-24, 131-35, 218, 285, 301
(see also vitamin B_1)
and physical performance, 121-24
content in foods, 351-89
deficiency effects, 121
effects on
endurance, 122-23
strength, 123
in basic four food groups, 290-91
RDA, 392
role in metabolism, 120-21
Thirst quenchers (see electrolyte solutions)
Threonine, 98, 285
Tocopherol, 147
(see also vitamin E)
Tocotrienol, 147
TOPS, 263
Training, physical
and protein needs, 102-12
effect on energy sources during exercise, 75
Transferrin, 161-62
Tricarboxylic acid cycle (see citric acid cycle)
Triglycerides, 47, 77
body storage, 80
muscle, 73-74
serum, effect of exercise, 91-95
Trometamol, 226
Tryptophan, 98, 285
Tyrosine, 98

U

United States Pharmacopia Units (see USP)
Urea, 101-02
USP, 114

V

Valine, 98, 285

DATE DUE

HIGHSMITH 45-102   PRINTED IN U.S.A.